Health Behavior Change and Treatment Adherence

Health Behavior Change and Treatment Adherence

Evidence-based Guidelines for Improving Healthcare

Second Edition

M. ROBIN DIMATTEO
LESLIE R. MARTIN
KELLY B. HASKARD-ZOLNIEREK

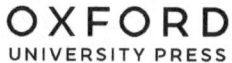

OXFORD
UNIVERSITY PRESS

Oxford University Press is a department of the University of Oxford.
It furthers the University's objective of excellence in research, scholarship,
and education by publishing worldwide. Oxford is a registered trademark of
Oxford University Press in the UK and in certain other countries.

Published in the United States of America by Oxford University Press
198 Madison Avenue, New York, NY 10016, United States of America.

© Oxford University Press 2025

First Edition published in 2010
Second Edition published in 2025

All rights reserved. No part of this publication may be reproduced, stored in a retrieval system, transmitted, used for text and data mining, or used for training artificial intelligence, in any form or by any means, without the prior permission in writing of Oxford University Press, or as expressly permitted by law, by license or under terms agreed with the appropriate reprographics rights organization. Inquiries concerning reproduction outside the scope of the above should be sent to the Rights Department, Oxford University Press, at the address above

You must not circulate this work in any other form
and you must impose this same condition on any acquirer

Library of Congress Cataloging-in-Publication Data
Names: Martin, Leslie R., author. | DiMatteo, M. Robin, author. |
Haskard-Zolnierek, Kelly B., 1978- author.
Title: Health behavior change and treatment adherence / M. Robin DiMatteo,
Leslie R. Martin, Kelly B. Haskard-Zolnierek.
Description: Second edition. | New York : Oxford University Press, 2025. |
Leslie R. Martin's name appears first in the previous edition. |
Includes bibliographical references and index. |
Identifiers: LCCN 2024042739 (print) | LCCN 2024042740 (ebook) |
ISBN 9780197778586 (hardback) | ISBN 9780197778593 |
ISBN 9780197778609 (epub) | ISBN 9780197778616
Subjects: MESH: Health Behavior | Evidence-Based Medicine |
Treatment Adherence and Compliance | Professional-Patient Relations |
Social Determinants of Health | Case Reports
Classification: LCC R727.43 (print) | LCC R727.43 (ebook) |
NLM W 85 | DDC 613—dc23/eng/20241204
LC record available at https://lccn.loc.gov/2024042739
LC ebook record available at https://lccn.loc.gov/2024042740

DOI: 10.1093/oso/9780197778586.001.0001

Printed by Sheridan Books, Inc., United States of America

To Michael Esnard and Gia DiNicola, with admiration, gratitude, and love. (MRD)

To Dickie Wrightsil, who supports my health. (LRM)

To Jamie Zolnierek, who seized a "teachable moment" as a motivation to change and inspires me daily. To Kirra, Elena, and Scott Zolnierek, for being the greatest joys of my life. (KBHZ)

Contents

List of Figures	xiv
List of Tables	xv
List of Case Studies	xvi
Preface to the Second Edition	xviii

Introduction	1
Good intentions	2
A framework for understanding health behavior change and treatment adherence	3
Goals of this book	4
References	5
1. An Overview of Health Behavior Change and Treatment Adherence	6
Levels of health behavior: primary, secondary, and tertiary prevention	7
Primary prevention	8
Healthy diet: nutrition, healthy weight, and obesity	9
Healthy eating	10
Obesity	11
Smoking, alcohol use, substance use, and sexual risk behaviors	12
Communicable respiratory disease prevention	15
Physical activity and exercise	16
Secondary prevention: disease screening	20
Tertiary prevention: adherence to medical treatments	21
Unintentional and intentional nonadherence	21
The prevalence of nonadherence	22
Costs and consequences of nonadherence	24
Financial costs	24
Human costs	25
Why health behavior change and adherence sometimes fail	25
A social-ecological perspective on health behavior and adherence	26
Summary	28
Tools for instruction and self-study	29
Learning objectives	29
Review questions	30

Prompts for discussion and further study	30
Suggested reading	30
References	31

2. Models of Health Behavior Change and Treatment Adherence — 37

Understanding irrational health-related behaviors	38
Theoretical models of health behavior and treatment adherence	39
Health Belief Model	40
Theory of Reasoned Action	43
Theory of Planned Behavior	45
Transtheoretical Model	46
Social Cognitive Models	49
Precaution Adoption Process Model	51
Information-Motivation-Strategy Model	52
Cognitive dissonance reduction and behavior change	54
A multilevel determinants approach	55
Summary	57
Tools for instruction and self-study	58
Learning objectives	58
Review questions	59
Prompts for discussion and further study	59
Suggested reading	60
References	60

3. Trust and Interpersonal Communication in the Provider-Patient Relationship — 64

The roles of provider and patient	65
Models of the practitioner-patient relationship	68
Paternalism	68
Consumerism	69
Expertise	69
Mutuality	70
Trust	71
The elements of interpersonal communication	71
Practitioner-patient communication	72
Physical environment	73
Verbal communication	74
Open-ended questions	75
Refraining from interruption	77
Providing clear information	78
Patients' verbalizations	78
Nonverbal communication	81
Indicators of distress	82

Physical pain and sensitivity cues	82
Empathy	83
Empathy and the actor-observer asymmetry	85
Summary	87
Tools for instruction and self-study	88
Learning objectives	88
Review questions	88
Prompts for discussion and further study	89
Suggested reading	89
References	89

4. Communication and Decision-Making — 97

Health Literacy	97
Information processing and recall	99
Focusing attention and encoding	100
Memory storage	101
Emotion and memory	101
Chronic stress	103
Self-enhancement bias	103
Cultural context	104
Additional factors affecting understanding and recall	105
Strategies for improving memory and recall	106
Tailoring information	106
Memory aids	107
Ordering of information	108
Mnemonics and chunking	108
Decision-making	108
Evaluating risk in making medical decisions	109
Medical decision analysis	110
A crash course in Bayesian methods	110
Understanding risks and risk reduction	113
Odds ratios	113
Risk ratios	114
Hazard ratios	116
Risk ratios and correlation	117
The landscape of study results and the value of meta-analysis	118
Cumulative and interactive effects	120
Patient involvement in decision-making	121
Tools for participatory decision-making	122
Joint decision-making and maximizing quality-adjusted life years	125
Joining the perspectives of providers and patients	126
Summary	127
Tools for instruction and self-study	128
Learning objectives	128

Review questions	128
Prompts for discussion and further study	129
Suggested reading	129
References	129

5. Persuasion and Motivation — 137

- Persuasion — 137
  - Resistance to persuasion — 139
  - Persuasive messages — 140
    - Expertise and other forms of power — 142
    - Liking — 142
    - Scarcity, reciprocity, and consistency — 143
    - Fear induction — 144
    - Teachable moments — 144
    - Message framing — 145
    - Expectations — 146
- Goal setting — 146
  - Goal pursuit — 148
  - Optimism — 149
  - Self-efficacy — 150
  - Perceptions of benefits and costs — 151
- Goal framing — 152
  - Targeting goals — 153
- Motivation — 156
  - Motivational interviewing, motivational communication — 158
- From persuasion and motivation to behavior change — 162
- Summary — 162
- Tools for instruction and self-study — 163
  - Learning objectives — 163
  - Review questions — 164
  - Prompts for discussion and further study — 164
  - Suggested reading — 165
- References — 165

6. Habits — 170

- Habits defined — 172
  - The "new" habit science — 172
- The basics of behavioral analysis and change — 173
  - Forming habits — 173
    - Classical conditioning — 174
    - Operant conditioning — 174
    - Rewards for behaviors — 175
    - Maintaining habits and reinforcement schedules — 175
  - Behavioral contracts and contingency plans — 177

Intrinsic motivation	178
Breaking bad habits	179
The habit of not doing	181
Very small behavior changes	182
Self-knowledge and personality	183
Choosing the right environments	186
Balancing habits with mindfulness	188
Managing barriers to behavior change	189
Self-monitoring and regulating	190
The Health Behavior Internalization Model	192
Managing ups and downs	194
Cognitive Behavioral Therapy and a habit of moving	196
Summary	197
Tools for instruction and self-study	198
Learning objectives	198
Review questions	198
Prompts for discussion and further study	199
Suggested reading	199
References	200

7. **Health Behavior and Adherence in a Sociocultural Context** — 204

Social cognitive models	204
Family	205
Social support	206
Culture: a deeper dive	211
Social norms and comparisons	213
Social comparison processes	214
Social media	217
Health professionals and vaccination-related decisions	220
Disparities and the death gap	223
Racism, discrimination, and disparities in medical care	225
A cultural distrust of medicine	227
Trauma, stress, and health vulnerabilities	228
What health professionals can do	233
Culturally informed medical care and communication	234
Summary	235
Tools for instruction and self-study	236
Learning objectives	236
Review questions	236
Prompts for discussion and further study	237
Suggested reading	237
References	238

CONTENTS

8. Using Teams and Technology to Deliver Better Care	248
Medical teams	249
Planning and agenda-setting for the medical visit	250
Models of care for the whole person	251
Group visits	255
Technologies in health and healthcare	256
Definitions of key terms in the digital health sphere	257
eHealth	258
Information-seeking and management using the internet and artificial intelligence	258
Automated healthcare systems and health information technology	261
Decision aids	262
Virtual support groups	263
Medication packaging technology	263
Technologies for medical communication and medical care	264
Telehealth and telemedicine	264
Telemedicine and the provider-patient relationship, health behavior, and treatment adherence	265
Limitations of telemedicine	265
Artificial intelligence in patient care	268
Can AI help with medical diagnosis?	271
How do physicians and patients feel about AI?	272
Use with caution	273
Mobile health (mHealth) technologies for healthcare and treatment adherence	273
How mHealth tools support habits and behavior change	275
Summary	278
Tools for instruction and self-study	279
Learning objectives	279
Review questions	279
Prompts for discussion and further study	280
Suggested reading	280
References	280
9. Individuals in the Context of Medical Systems and Public Policy	290
The big picture	292
Stakeholders in health: who owns the risk?	293
Costs, health insurance, and access to care	294
Integrated care systems	296
Public health and the public good	297
Health education	298

Government supported programs for health behavior change	300
Laws and public policy mandates	300
Laws and women's healthcare	302
Public health and the COVID-19 pandemic	304
Implementation science and research on health behavior change	305
Health behavior change: now and in the future	306
Summary	309
Tools for instruction and self-study	309
Learning objectives	309
Review questions	310
Prompts for discussion and further study	311
Suggested reading	311
References	311
Index	315

List of Figures

Figure 2.1 Health Belief Model	42
Figure 2.2 Theory of Reasoned Action	44
Figure 2.3 Theory of Planned Behavior	46
Figure 2.4 Transtheoretical Model	48
Figure 2.5 Social Cognitive Theory	50
Figure 2.6 Precaution Adoption Process Model	52
Figure 2.7 Information-Motivation-Strategy Model	53
Figure 4.1 Sample Decision Tree	124

List of Tables

Table 1.1	Myths and Realities About Patient Adherence and Health Behavior Change	26
Table 3.1	Repertoire of Doctor-Patient Relationships and Their Appropriate Contexts	70
Table 4.1	What Health Professionals Can Do to Help Patients Remember Medical Information	102
Table 4.2	Illustration of the Influence of Base Rates on Risk Ratios and Correlations	117
Table 5.1	Summary of Elements of Persuasive Messages in Healthcare	141
Table 5.2	Examples of Persuasive Power in Use	142
Table 5.3	Strategies for Increasing Patients' Self-Efficacy	151
Table 6.1	Brief Descriptions of the "Big Five" Personality Traits	184
Table 6.2	Sample Nudges, Prompts, and Associated Health Behaviors	188
Table 6.3	Lapses and Reactions	195
Table 7.1	Examples of Family Influences on Health Behavior	207
Table 9.1	Common Barriers to Adherence and Strategies for Addressing Them	291

List of Case Studies

Case Study 1.1	Celia	15
Case Study 1.2	Elders and Exercise	19
Case Study 2.1	Carl	38
Case Study 2.2	Martine	54
Case Study 2.3	Rosalie	55
Case Study 3.1	Damien	64
Case Study 3.2	Sylvia and Alvin	67
Case Study 3.3	Simplified Illustrations of Medical Interviews Using Closed-Ended versus Open-Ended Questions	76
Case Study 3.4	Chronological Story Development in Two Patients	80
Case Study 3.5	Asking about Adherence	86
Case Study 4.1	Sample Decision Tree and a Simplified (Hypothetical) Medical Decision Analysis	123
Case Study 5.1	What Persuaded and Motivated People to Get the COVID-19 Vaccination?	138
Case Study 5.2	The Sturgis Motorcycle Rally, July 2020	140
Case Study 5.3	Modifying but Not Discouraging Maisie's Goals	154
Case Study 5.4	A Father's Motivation to Help His Daughter	156
Case Study 5.5	The Stages of Change and Motivational Interviewing Applied to Mercedes' Exercise Regimen	159
Case Study 6.1	Gabriel	171
Case Study 6.2	Examples of Reinforcement Schedules for Health Behavior Change in Action	176
Case Study 6.3	Gabriel and His Habit of "Not Doing"	181
Case Study 6.4	Gabriel and Small Habits	182
Case Study 6.5	Daniel's Adoption of Meditation for Stress Reduction	191
Case Study 7.1	Frank and Mrs. Tomasetti	209
Case Study 7.2	Travius	218
Case Study 7.3	Racial Bias and Pain Communication	224
Case Study 7.4	Cassandra	231
Case Study 8.1	Group Health Education in Action	256

Case Study 8.2 A Different Type of Tech Issue   266
Case Study 8.3 Example of AI Compared to Human Physician
                Communication   270
Case Study 8.4 Using a Digital App to Self-Monitor Eating Behavior
                and Exercise   276
Case Study 9.1 Helen, Darlene, and the Price of Cigarettes and Soda   300

Preface to the Second Edition

Nearly a decade and a half ago, in 2010, we published the first edition of *Health Behavior Change and Treatment Adherence*. In it, we synthesized what, to that point, had become a vast literature on preventive health behavior change and adherence to medical treatment. Our goal was to examine health communication, persuasion, motivation, social influence, and habit formation, focusing on elements of primary health promotion and disease prevention. We examined ways to improve health actions such as exercise, weight loss, stress management, and smoking cessation, and improve medication-taking for such conditions as diabetes and hypertension. We offered practical guidance to health professionals and those in training as they faced the challenges of helping their patients to eat better, be more physically active, follow disease screening guidelines, and adhere to prescribed treatments.

In this second edition, we have reorganized and restructured the material of the first edition around the simple unifying principles described in the Introduction. We have updated references to the vast and continually growing scholarly literature, and presented new research developments in medicine, public health, and psychological/behavioral science that deal with issues of health behavior change and adherence to treatment. We focus more attention on adherence in clinical medical practice, elucidating the challenges of effectively following complex treatments for diabetes, cancer, cardiovascular disease, HIV, and other conditions. We examine resistance to lifestyle change and vaccination in the management of communicable disease. We assess some of the social and psychological factors that challenged U.S. health policy through the COVID-19 pandemic and that shape current plans to face future health emergencies. We consider that while the United States has arguably the most sophisticated medical technology (and the highest medical costs) in the world, its healthcare outcomes fall far below those of many other developed nations. In this book, we see that the best treatments may not necessarily be the most expensive ones, but rather the ones that truly match the social, psychological, and behavioral needs of individuals and address the many contextual factors that drive health outcomes.

In this expanded edition, we offer a considerable amount of new material: evidence-based, scientific strategies for habit formation and maintenance, as well as demotivation of unhealthy behaviors. We address in more detail the social context of individuals (including influence through social media) and the interpersonal and intrapersonal elements affecting their adherence and health behavior change. We expand on issues of trust in health professionals and in health authorities; the effects of health messages, knowledge, and information; communication effectiveness; understanding, persuasion, and personal motivation; and new and developing models of health behavior. We examine socioeconomic disparities and inequities in health, healthcare, and environmental risk as well as vulnerable populations, diversity, equity, and inclusion in culturally-informed care. We consider socioeconomic determinants of wellness, environmental determinants of health maintenance and disease management, and the increasing recognition of vulnerabilities including mental health challenges and trauma as drivers of health and health behaviors.

In this updated volume, we also expand on the role of multidisciplinary healthcare teams in providing direction and support for health behavior change and adherence, and offer a detailed analysis of the role of, and options for, technologies in medicine, psychology, and behavior change. We examine such topics as digital health and virtual medical visits that (unlike 15 years ago) are now commonplace. We consider provider-patient communication in the context of an increasing role for artificial intelligence (AI), as well as a wide array of technological aids to medical care delivery and adherence such as health behavior apps.

In this second edition, we analyze individual behavioral choices within a complex network of stakeholders in healthcare; we consider elements of patients' experiences as they navigate health insurance and service availability (or lack thereof). We also examine the prevention and management of communicable and chronic diseases at the population level, and emphasize that the implementation of health policy requires the cooperation of human beings, some of whom may be resistant to change.

In this second edition, we again offer a succinct, readable, practical, and usable format, applying theoretical concepts and empirical findings to real world problems. We offer numerous case studies (which are composites, with all potentially identifying information changed). These case studies highlight applications of theoretical and empirical issues and offer the health professional, in training or in practice, an opportunity to apply the book's theoretical concepts and empirical analyses to challenging, real-world health problems. Our goal in this second edition is to provoke thought and action in policy and practice, encouraging the reader to use a "health behavior and treatment adherence lens" to look at various health-related phenomena, whether at a societal level or at an individual level.

We are, all three, university professors with many decades of combined experience teaching undergraduate, graduate, medical, nursing, and allied health professional students. We also lecture regularly to practicing healthcare providers and healthcare administrators throughout the United States. Thus, we are particularly attuned to the potential value of this book for instruction and self-study, and we offer additional support toward this end.

At the conclusion of each chapter, we offer a unique and practical section called Tools for Instruction and Self-Study. It contains: Learning Objectives (based on Bloom's Taxonomy), Review Questions, Prompts for Discussion and Further Study, and Suggested Reading. These latter are books that one or more of us has read and, in many cases, used as supplemental reading in our own classes. We endeavor to make this material accessible to students and their instructors in a broad range of disciplines, and to assist instructors in their class preparations and students in their mastery of the material.

Our goals in this book are to untangle the complexities involved in understanding the change and maintenance of health behaviors, to summarize key ideas (braced by theory and research), and to offer engaging examples and case studies. We look forward to reaching a broad audience with this second edition, including a wide variety of healthcare professionals, in practice and training, in fields such as nursing, medicine, allied health, chiropractic, physical therapy, dentistry, clinical/health psychology, social work, healthcare administration, and public health. This book is also broadly applicable to researchers and to graduate and advanced undergraduate students in the social and behavioral sciences. It can serve as a valuable resource for faculty, students, and practitioners who are focused on health education and coaching in medical practices, private practice settings, hospitals, and healthcare systems, as well as those who are developing and implementing health policy.

We are grateful to our editors at Oxford University Press, Nadina Persaud and Sarah Ebel, for their enthusiasm and expert guidance. We each acknowledge those who supported our efforts in writing this book. Robin thanks Anne Kim, Nancy Dye Leer, and Nicole Miller; Leslie thanks Helen Regan and Giancarlo Valdez; and Kelly thanks Krista Howard.

Introduction

The past decade has seen a vast array of new and impressive medical technologies, medications, and vaccines introduced to prevent, manage, or even cure many medical conditions that once engendered fear and hopelessness. Some chronic diseases continue to require (sometimes extensive) self-management, but they now have far more options for care than ever before. More medical information is available to patients than at any time in history; significant advances have transformed medical communication and have vastly expanded healthcare access using digital mobile technologies. Options for self-management have proliferated with mobile phone applications; vaccines to prevent severe illness and death from communicable diseases have been developed and produced in an astoundingly short period of time.

During this decade, we have also become increasingly aware that medical advances are beneficial only insofar as patients have access to them, and actually use them. Vaccines only work if they become "shots in arms." Medications only work if they are taken properly. Behavioral intentions (e.g., to exercise, to eat better) only help if they are implemented. Chronic diseases stay manageable, and medical crises are avoided, only if patients actually follow the directives given to them by their healthcare teams.

Still, medication nonadherence, vaccination avoidance, and resistance to health behavior change remain frustratingly high. Since the 1948 publication of the first research study on treatment compliance (with antibiotic therapy for children with rheumatic fever)[1] and the first scholarly book on treatment compliance and health behavior change in 1982,[2] the term *compliance* has been replaced with *adherence* in the hope of shifting views of the practitioner-patient relationship. Indeed, during the latter two decades of the 20th century, the provider-patient relationship changed rather dramatically from generally one-sided and characterized by physician power and dominance to a more equal provider-patient partnership with decisions made jointly and problems solved together. The first two decades of the 21st century have brought a proliferation of decision aids, of technologies that give patients unprecedented control of their own health and healthcare, and of methods for behavioral self-management. And yet, behavior-mediated health risks including obesity, cigarette smoking, heavy use of alcohol, sedentary lifestyle, unsafe sex practices, refusal of life-saving vaccinations for communicable diseases, and failure to follow treatments for acute and chronic conditions have remained as common and problematic as they were in the previous 50 years. And, in some cases, these health risks have increased.

Nonadherence to medical treatment has recently been described as an "epidemic hidden in plain sight."[3] Indeed, in the hectic process of healthcare delivery, relatively little attention tends to be paid to what happens after the patient leaves their medical visit. Health professionals provide their patients with hard-won diagnoses and solutions to their medical problems and offer them expert advice on how to avoid further trouble. Although this advice should be welcomed and appreciated—after all, a life might be saved or suffering avoided—it is often, almost unimaginably, ignored.

Good intentions

It is probably true that most people value their health and have good intentions to preserve it. When asked about the importance they place on health, it is not surprising that most people rate it very high.[4] Being healthy allows people to do things they want and need to do, such as work, care for their families, and engage in recreation and social affiliation. There is general agreement that being physically ill is undesirable; illness limits a person's autonomy, opportunities, and well-being, and can even challenge their mental and emotional health. But assessing the precise value of health to a person, and determining what they might be willing and able to do to achieve and maintain it, can be difficult because people have different goals and activities, and their physical and social environments might differ greatly.

At the most basic level, a modest amount of exercise, a healthy diet, avoiding the use of tobacco and other harmful substances, getting appropriate vaccinations, and obtaining recommended age-appropriate medical screenings can help a great deal to support an individual's health status. People vary greatly in their approach to these basic behaviors, however. One person might be quite willing to give up alcohol and high fat foods, while another might think such a regimen is absurd. One person might enjoy walking five times a week for exercise, while another finds the task impossible. In addition, even while placing a high value on health and having the best intentions, many people fail at health-related change because they don't know how to regulate their own behavior; and their health professionals might have received little training in how to help them. Without a good understanding of the psychological principles that underlie health behavior change, many patients and providers use techniques that don't work, or they give up in frustration, having never built the communication and motivation necessary to sustain health actions. Further, many individuals are embedded in stressful environments and social systems that make behavioral change very difficult.

A framework for understanding health behavior change and treatment adherence

As we describe in the coming chapters, effective healthcare requires an optimal combination of medical technology and behavioral technology. Throughout this book, we offer evidence to support three simple but profound behavioral principles that have guided our work on adherence, from 1982 with the book *Achieving Patient Compliance*[2] to our more recent work based on the Information-Motivation-Strategy Model[5] (described in more detail in Chapter 2). Three basic principles form an overall framework to understand the complexities of health behavior change and to guide clinical care. They are as follows:

(1) To achieve health behavior change, *people need to know what to do and why*. No one can follow health recommendations that are not clearly communicated to them and that they do not understand or remember.
(2) When it comes to health, *people do mostly what they want to do*. People will not follow behavioral recommendations unless they believe (or are effectively persuaded) that such action is the right thing for them. They may follow recommendations from sources (like health professionals or health authorities) that they trust, but they are unlikely to follow advice from those in whom they have little faith. Their motivation to sustain health action may be difficult to achieve but can be promoted with an understanding of habits and sometimes with the assistance of health behavior technologies.

(3) *People do only what they can do.* Barriers to change (e.g., treatment complexity, challenges to healthcare access) are numerous in most people's lives, and these can impede health behavior change and adherence. Recognition of, and assistance with, the unique environmental conditions that affect their health (sometimes in egregious ways) are essential to help individuals achieve lasting change.

Goals of this book

In this book, we offer evidence-based guidance to healthcare providers in training and in practice, as well as to those who are researching these important issues. We synthesize the results of decades of empirical research and offer health professionals a set of effective, empirically-based strategies to help their patients put long-term behavioral changes into practice. With illustrative composite case studies, we hope to enhance the understanding of why people make the choices they do with respect to their health.

We offer this book to empower current and future health professionals and educators to support their patients with effective communication, collaboration, and partnership. In these chapters, we examine ways to foster patient engagement by developing and maintaining rapport with patients, informing and educating them (while recognizing differences in providers' and patients' perspectives), building patient motivation and commitment in the context of social pressures and persuasion, and keeping a broad focus on the contextual factors that impede health action. We examine the challenges facing population-based health behavior change, and we delve into basic issues that drive acceptance of health messages—whether from a primary care physician advocating cancer prevention or from public health authorities tasked with managing the outbreak of an infectious disease. We strive to understand the psychological factors that underlie resistance to medical recommendations. We hope to convey a comprehensive model of how people come to trust the health messages they receive, and then act upon them. There is a great deal of research available on these issues; our task here is to distill this research and offer its application in the realms of psychology, medical practice, and public health, all of which work to help people change their health behaviors and adhere to what is essential for their own health and that of those around them.

References

1. Hardy MC. Follow-up of medical recommendations; results of a health checkup of a group of well children in Chicago. *J Am Med Assoc.* 1948; 136(1): pp. 20–27. doi: 10.1001/jama.1948.02890180022005
2. DiMatteo MR, DiNicola DD. *Achieving Patient Compliance.* Pergamon; 1982.
3. Malik M, Kumari S, Manalai P. Treatment nonadherence: an epidemic hidden in plain sight. *Psychiatric Times.* 2020; 37(3): pp. 25–26.
4. Lau RR, Hartman KA, Ware JE Jr. Health as a value: methodological and theoretical considerations. *Health Psychol.* 1986; 5(1): pp. 25–43. doi: 10.1037//0278-6133.5.1.25
5. DiMatteo MR, Haskard-Zolnierek KB, Martin LR. Improving patient adherence: a three-factor model to guide practice. *Health Psychol Rev.* 2012; 6(1): pp. 74-91. doi: 10.1080/17437199.2010.537592

Chapter 1
An Overview of Health Behavior Change and Treatment Adherence

This book is about changing behavior to improve health. It seems like a simple enough goal, but as we will see, the achievement of health is anything but simple. People vary a great deal in how they define and view health, and in what they are willing and able to do to realize and preserve it.

In this chapter, we begin with something basic: clarifying what we mean by *health*, and identifying what *behaviors* could and should be enacted to achieve it. Most public health analyses of the concept start with the classic World Health Organization (WHO) definition—that health is "a state of complete physical, mental and social well-being and not merely the absence of disease and infirmity" (p. 1).[1] This definition itself could send us into a flurry of conditionals and "what-ifs." The concept of *well-being* is personal and subjective and depends a great deal on the individual and their context. For example, a 25-year-old without any chronic medical conditions might define it as being able to run a 10k race with friends and then go dancing until 2 a.m. A typical 80-year-old might define it as being able to enjoy an early dinner with friends and an evening walk with the dog. However, a 25-year-old with severe diabetes and a major depressive disorder might describe well-being in much more limited terms because an early dinner and a walk with the dog seem far too difficult to attain. An 80-year-old with no chronic illnesses might insist that personal well-being involves being able to enjoy daily hikes in the local hills and a mountain biking trip in the Rockies.

Despite this variability in perspective, there are some things we can agree on. In this book, for example, we join with the medical and public health communities to argue that health and well-being involve not only current functioning but also preventing illness when possible to do so. Recognizing a developing disease in its early stages, when it can be cured or managed successfully, is better than addressing it later, when serious complications might arise. And although it is challenging to perfectly define the term, it is arguably better if a person's *healthspan*—the length of life they enjoy in good health—involves many years rather than few.[2]

Strategies for prevention, early detection, and treatment really do matter; the leading drivers of both medical costs and mortality are related to behavior.[3] Currently, of the more than 5 million premature deaths from cancer world-wide, 68% could have been prevented through lifestyle changes or efforts aimed at early detection.[4] Chronic conditions, many of which are preventable, represent a substantial illness burden in the United States, affecting 133 million Americans[5] and accounting (depending upon the estimates) for as much as 90%[6] of the $4.1 trillion spent annually on healthcare. Although unhealthy behaviors like smoking and poor eating habits may provide people with rewards in the present, the resulting health complications cause most who experience them to wish that, in the past, they had stopped smoking or had better controlled what they ate. One could argue that behaving in ways that prevent disease from happening at all is ideal, especially if it can be done within the context of what an individual considers a "life worth living."

Of course, health also depends on luck and opportunity, on the options available, and on the constraints faced. Diabetes, cancer, heart disease, and HIV are household words today, but only a few decades ago, they were not well understood and had burdensome (or no) effective treatments. As we will see later in this book, medical advances and treatment options are not equally available to all patients. As we examine the choices that people might make in preventing or managing disease, we will also see that people vary in their access to the information, guidance, motivational support, healthcare, and practical help necessary to benefit from these medical advances.[7]

Levels of health behavior: primary, secondary, and tertiary prevention

Here in Chapter 1, we examine three levels of health behavior related to the prevention, identification, treatment, and long-term management of acute and chronic medical conditions. *Primary prevention* involves actions taken by an individual to prevent disease before it has occurred, and these actions tend to be intercorrelated. That is, healthy habits tend to co-occur, and if individuals engage in health risk behaviors, they generally engage in more than one of them.[8] *Secondary prevention* is the initial interface of the individual with the healthcare system—for example, when they "go for a medical checkup" or follow recommendations for early detection of disease including screening for hypertension or certain cancers. *Tertiary prevention* refers to the health behaviors that are necessary in the treatment of disease, and it addresses the behavioral hurdles that people face in trying to follow recommendations for cure or long-term management. In this book, we examine what happens when patients fail to adhere to treatment, resulting in significant costs to them and to the healthcare system through preventable medical and emergency department visits, hospitalizations, morbidity, missed work days, decreased quality of life, and a shortened lifespan.

In this chapter, and throughout this book, we examine behavioral issues in health with an awareness that social, ecological, economic, and cultural contexts drive personal choices and the opportunities that individuals have to carry out their best behavioral intentions. We show how these contexts can shape outcomes and determine whether health behavior is a true choice or the only viable option.

Primary prevention

Strategies for primary prevention seem straightforward, things your grandmother might have suggested: eat your vegetables, don't smoke, go for a walk, get enough sleep, use condoms (well, maybe not Grandma…). Yet, as we will see, many individuals are poor caretakers of their own bodies. Only a small percentage of U.S. adults meets physical activity guidelines[9] and close to three quarters of the U.S. population is overweight or obese.[10] Tobacco use remains the leading cause of preventable disease, disability, and death; heavy alcohol use can lead to problematic physical and psychological outcomes.[11] Many people engage in several of these behaviors, incurring multiple health risks.[8] The levels of prevention are not exclusive; once a person has a disease, primary prevention behaviors are still central to the management of acute and chronic conditions. Treatment for the long-term management of cancer, diabetes, and many other conditions still requires the primary prevention elements of healthy eating, exercise, and the avoidance of tobacco products and excessive alcohol.

Here we examine the best-understood primary prevention behaviors in the context of some of the more complex socioecological considerations that affect them.

Healthy diet: nutrition, healthy weight, and obesity

A debate about what constitutes healthy eating, movement, and weight sits near the center of this book's address of behaviors related to lifestyle. This debate spans many fields: the psychology of behavior change; the sociology of stigma; the cultural issues in body image; and the medical, surgical, and pharmacological management of body size. New drug treatments for obesity, for example, have recently sparked cultural debate, as many individuals who do not have diabetes use these diabetes medications (which have sometimes been in short supply) to lose weight and conform to cultural values of thinness. This is a potential minefield for those who study and write about health behavior, and we have tried to navigate it here. Because obesity is a significant health risk, it cannot be ignored in a book about health and medicine.[12] It is the case, however, that fashion and weight have been conflated in our diet-focused culture, and "aesthetics" have been known to masquerade as "concerns for health." Sometimes, there are even insinuations of morality, equating "good" with the control of appetite, and elevating one set of cultural preferences over another.[13]

Eating is part of primary prevention, and it is also something we must all do to stay alive. One can steer clear of cigarettes and alcohol forever; but some amount of food has to be eaten to continue living. In this book, we emphasize the notion of "healthy eating," which is defined most broadly to include eating whole foods, avoiding ultra-processed foods, and eating mindfully and not too much. In our discussions of healthy eating, weight management, and obesity prevention, we are *not* talking about "trying to be thin" or "looking good" according to some culturally imposed standard that masquerades as "health behavior."

We start with the basic premise that it is good for a person's health to choose nutritious food and to balance caloric intake with output. The acquisition, preparation, and eating of nutritious food, as well as other actions taken to prevent obesity, form a behavioral goal. Considerable controversy still exists, however, about the measured body weight that results from these actions—what constitutes appropriate measurement and what that measurement means with regard to health. And, if individuals and their healthcare providers are confused about the benchmarks, measurement, and criteria for healthy weight, counseling patients can be challenging. As an example, the American Medical Association (AMA) is now formally discouraging reliance on body mass index (BMI; a ratio involving height and weight) to determine if a person is at a healthy weight, overweight, or obese.[14]

The BMI is overly simplistic, failing to consider other factors such as frame size, bone density, and lean body mass. But BMI *is the exact measure* that the U.S. Centers for Disease Control and Prevention (CDC) uses to classify overweight and obesity, and a measure that researchers employ to identify risk factors for disease. Indeed, as we see in this chapter, overweight and obesity can be significant factors in several chronic diseases. The AMA (in contrast with the CDC) also notes that BMI does not predict disease risk equally well across racial and ethnic groups and argues that BMI is not accurate on its own in predicting health risks at the individual level. The AMA advises physicians that BMI can be one factor used, but that physicians should include other measures such as body composition, belly fat, waist circumference, and genetic factors. The measurement of these latter factors can present some practical challenges, of course, and can allow (for better or worse) subjectivity in assessment of an individual. The AMA position asks doctors to help patients using an individualized approach to weight management, with the goal of attaining a body weight that is the healthiest for that patient.

In this chapter, and throughout this book, we address health issues related to body weight. What are the dangers of obesity? How can it be avoided? How is it treated? We hope to demonstrate the complexity of these issues and to prompt the reader to think in a broader way about the meaning and implications of terms that are often used unthinkingly, such as "diet" and "obesity." We offer some new research findings, ideas to consider, and references to consult. We try to unearth some commonalities. But we do not offer simple answers.

Healthy eating

The American diet is, on average, considerably worse than it should be. In comparison with the Dietary Guidelines for Americans (https://www.dietaryguidelines.gov/), each day people in the United States eat too much dietary fat, saturated fat, sodium, and sugar, and too little fiber, fruits, vegetables, and omega-3 fatty acids. They also tend to eat more food than their energy expenditure requires. Processed foods, which are convenient and often tasty, comprise more than 50% of the calories in an average American diet[15] and are linked to an increased risk of diabetes, obesity, and even cancer.[16,17] The healthiest food choices include fresh fruits and vegetables, legumes and nuts, lean meats, and limited sugar, sodium, and saturated fat.

What people eat depends upon individual food preferences, personal health priorities, time, and the opportunity to acquire and prepare fresh foods; choices tend to be driven by habits and by the socioeconomic and environmental circumstances in which people find themselves.[18] Dietary patterns are influenced by cultural norms, shared meal environments, the frequency of food exposures, and targeted food marketing (which can be quite successful at making a bag of corn chips look much more appealing than an apple and much more convenient than a bowl of steamed vegetables). Some of these factors, as well as food insecurity and stress, can be as important as lack of knowledge and habituation of taste and behavioral patterns.

Obesity

Among adults, overweight is defined as BMI from 25 to <30; BMI of 30 or higher is considered obese. Using the criterion of BMI, 41.9% of U.S. adults age 20 and older are obese, and 9.2% are severely obese, with the highest obesity rates among non-Hispanic Blacks (49.9%).[19] For children and teens, BMI categories are based on sex- and age-specific percentiles; the 95th or higher percentile defines obesity.[20] The prevalence of pediatric obesity is 19.7% (with the highest among Hispanic youth; 26.2%).[21] In both children and adults, obesity can lead to hypertension and high cholesterol (risk factors for heart disease), type 2 diabetes, breathing problems such as asthma and sleep apnea, joint and musculoskeletal problems, and gallbladder disease.[22] Childhood obesity can lead to anxiety and depression, lowered self-esteem, and bullying. Adults with obesity have higher risks for stroke, premature death, clinical depression and anxiety, and some types of cancer.[22]

Many factors can contribute to excess weight gain. What people eat matters a great deal, but obesity results not just from personal behavioral choice but also from additional factors over which the individual might have little control. Genetics and social determinants of health can play a significant role; insufficient sleep affects appetite-regulating hormones and can determine the success or failure of dietary interventions.[23,24] Indeed, the role of dietary change therapy itself has sparked intense debate, because long-term maintenance of weight loss is very difficult.[20] Incorporating physical activity for weight management and maintenance (and for health and well-being) is considered essential but involves yet more behavioral change.

As we examine throughout this book, some strategies for managing weight show success; these combine self-monitoring, self-evaluation, self-reinforcement, problem-solving, stimulus control, social assertion, cognitive strategies, and relapse prevention. Motivational interviewing is a strong factor in counseling for behavior change in weight management, and technologies including mobile apps and virtual health coaching can be helpful. More direct medical approaches including pharmacology (weight-loss drugs) and bariatric surgery can help reduce obesity-related comorbidities like type 2 diabetes, hypertension, sleep apnea, stroke, and some cancers; but even these require considerable health behavior change and treatment adherence to bring about long-term weight control.[25]

Smoking, alcohol use, substance use, and sexual risk behaviors

While not exactly like "sex, drugs, and rock 'n' roll," these health risk behaviors do tend to go together; they intercorrelate across populations and they often comprise a pattern of co-occurring health risk behaviors known as a person's "multiple-risk behavior profile."[8]

Jake is a great example. He usually smokes at least a pack of cigarettes a day, sometimes more, and he enjoys two or three beers most evenings with his friends. On weekends, when there is no work the next day, he drinks quite a bit more. Jake says he is not interested in what he calls "mind altering drugs," but on occasion he uses amphetamines when he must drive long distances to make deliveries for his work. And when his back hurts, he buys some oxycodone from a friend.

Shaylene is another good example. She loves to go to clubs with her friends on Friday and Saturday nights. They dose "lightly" with ecstasy/MDMA or a benzodiazepine, and they drink a significant number of tequila shots over the course of the evening. One thing Shaylene would like to change is her habit of having unprotected sex; she knows that she risks contracting sexually transmitted infections, but her judgment is impaired when she is "high."

Both Jake and Shaylene think their use of "substances" is well within normal limits for people their age. They might be right, although the commonality of a behavior does not make it the best choice.

Despite decades of public health warnings about the dangers of using tobacco and cigarettes, at least one quarter of U.S. adults smoke cigarettes, vape, or chew tobacco. The popularity of e-cigarettes and vaping continues to grow worldwide, with lifetime prevalence rates ranging from 15% (Asia) to 26% (Europe), placing the global lifetime prevalence rate at 23%.[26] These products facilitate the intake of nicotine, a drug that is both powerful and addicting.[27] The health dangers of tobacco are legion, ranging from cardiovascular disease, to emphysema, to many forms of cancer; most prominent among them is lung cancer.[8,11,27] Considerable progress has been made toward tobacco use prevention in the public health realm, with successful interventions that involve media campaigns, images on cigarette packs, and financial incentives to quit in the workplace or on health and life insurance plans.[11]

In the realm of alcohol use, Jake and Shaylene are also not alone. Alcohol use is the sixth biggest risk factor for disability and premature death in high income countries and the most significant health risk factor among young people. A recent meta-analytic review (a statistical technique used to combine the results of multiple studies that address the same research question) showed that the consequences of alcohol consumption (in years 2000–2019) cost 2.6% of global GDP, with about 39% being direct healthcare costs and 61% being productivity losses.[28] In the United States it is estimated that alcohol problems cost $249 billion/year. Excessive alcohol use leads to a repeated pattern of risky behaviors and of physical and/or psychological problems. As with weight, positions on the safe use of alcohol and other substances vary, making across-the-board recommendations from health professionals challenging, and highlighting the need for an individualized approach. The moderate use of alcohol is endorsed by many healthcare providers in practice, although recent evidence suggests that light or no use of alcohol may promote greater longevity, longer healthspan, and most effective prevention of cardiovascular disease, diabetes, and many cancers. In the United States, about 80% of adults use alcohol, suggesting that its moderate use, not complete abstinence, is probably a more realistic goal.[29,30]

While alcohol treatment programs focus on targeting the most severe alcohol dependencies, it is the case that episodic binge drinking causes significant problems, among them risky sexual behaviors and traffic collisions. The management of alcohol use plays a major part in chronic disease care. In research on alcohol use among cancer patients, for example, it has been found that despite recommendations to avoid alcohol, 80% of cancer patients continue to drink, and of those who drink, 40% drink to excess or binge drink. Heavy alcohol use, in addition to its usual detrimental health effects, can jeopardize the effectiveness of some cancer treatments, raise the risk of recurrence or progression, and increase the toxicity of many medicines used to treat cancer.[31] Interventions that target alcohol-related behavior can be quite effective and involve many of the components we examine in this book: knowledge, beliefs, attitudes, perceptions, and cultural and contextual factors. These interventions can include educational, technological, and psychological approaches such as motivational communication, habit management, and cognitive behavior therapy, among others.[32]

With alcohol, "percentage alcohol content" is just that; and an ounce is an ounce. But, with substances, dosages can be difficult or impossible to measure, especially in the case of "party drugs" or "street drugs." In addition, the likelihood of a provider obtaining truthful answers from a patient to questions about substance use is low, especially when the substance is not legal. Many people use substances to self-manage conditions that might be best managed by a health professional. Often, these involve anxiety, depression, bipolar disease symptoms, and other forms of serious mental health challenges. Considering the critical shortage of mental health professionals in the United States, the large number of people with inadequate insurance coverage for mental health, and the ready availability of online advice and remedies offered by social media, it is no surprise that suffering individuals sometimes try to self-medicate. Providers' nonjudgment and empathy are crucial to address the underlying personal and societal factors that contribute to the initiation and maintenance of substance use as well as the complex landscape of treatment and intervention as it exists today. In every provider-patient conversation, questions about the patient's use of alcohol, tobacco, and substances—and the reasons for it—need to be part of the dialogue.

Sexual behavior, while very personal, is a subject that doctors and patients discuss and public health officials address because of its health implications. High-risk sexual behavior involves unprotected sex with a person or persons who could be infected with a sexually transmitted infection (STI), and/or sex without a means of preventing unwanted pregnancy.[33] These behaviors can lead to an increased incidence of STIs and to unintended pregnancies, which can have a significant effect on an individual's quality of life and that of others with whom they are close. Myriad statistics on sexual risk behaviors are available for various age groups,[33] although researchers warn of the importance of interpreting their relative risk in context. What might seem high-risk in one situation (e.g., unprotected sex with a new partner whose disease status is unknown) may be considered "safe" in another (e.g., unprotected sex with a long-term partner in a monogamous relationship). This issue is of central importance, especially in the healthcare of teens and emerging adults.[34] Our goal here is to include sexual behavior as a set of health-related actions that make up an individual's life choices. We contextualize the complex nature of sexual behavior as an element of personal risk assessment and personal choice, specifically in the realm of infectious disease management. Doing so requires us also to think about the broader picture of nonsexual individual health behaviors that also affect the health of others.

Communicable respiratory disease prevention
At various points in the past several years, there has been high or very high transmission of Respiratory Syncytial Virus (RSV) and influenza in some states, and waves of the SARS-CoV-2 virus (COVID-19) activity in the United States and across the globe. These diseases draw our attention to many behavioral issues, including masking, testing, social distancing, and acceptance of vaccinations and boosters. While the risk of dying or becoming hospitalized with one of these respiratory viruses tends to be relatively low in many age groups, those who are very young or very old, or who have preexisting medical conditions, remain at higher risk.

Primary prevention actions to check the spread of influenza and other respiratory illnesses are simple. They include obtaining vaccinations and boosters, avoiding others when one is contagious, and wearing a well-fitting N95 or KN95 mask if one is ill or caring for individuals who are sick (see Case Study 1.1). Yet, despite its simplicity, many people regularly refuse the annual flu shot;[35] the same is anticipated for the RSV vaccine. During the pandemic, refusal to be vaccinated against COVID-19, or to follow other recommendations (e.g., masking, social distancing), merged in not-so-subtle ways with political ideologies and underlying values.[36,37] And social media played a significant role in vaccine hesitancy.

Case Study 1.1 Celia

Celia works in a large chain store that sells discount home goods; the store is often packed with shoppers who have "decided" that COVID-19 is a thing of the past. Celia's manager prefers that she not wear her N95 mask in the store because he wants his customers to see her smiling face and feel carefree and welcome. Celia doesn't like wearing the mask either,

> because it is stuffy and uncomfortable, but she is just barely recovering her energy after a cold, the flu, and two bouts with COVID-19 this season alone. She doesn't want to get sick again, and it seems like every shopper she encounters is coughing and sneezing, sometimes directly in front of her as she rings up their items. Celia wishes that people who are sick would at least wear a mask, so they don't transfer their germs to others.

If Celia lived and worked in Japan, Taiwan, or Korea, she would experience the norm for public behavior, which involves protecting others from communicable illness. Wearing a mask in this situation would be expected. Public health experts cite this issue as one of "13 takeaways" from the COVID-19 public health emergency; many Americans refused to wear masks to protect themselves and others, even when it made rational sense to do so.[38,39] These experts have noted that *we know how* to reduce the spread of airborne viruses. While the designation in 2020 of the SARS-CoV-2 virus as one that could spread by airborne transmission was somewhat late in coming from the WHO and CDC, it eventually became clear that quality N95 or KN95 respirators (aka effective "masks") could reduce transmission. But public health officials had to rely on political figures and media personalities to help create social norms of mask-wearing, distancing, and even vaccinating. Unfortunately, the messages sometimes worked at cross purposes, with some influencers supporting, and others rejecting these measures.

Physical activity and exercise

Of all the effective health behaviors that doctors might encourage in their patients, avoiding a sedentary lifestyle is at the top of the list. Physical activity is a well-documented and powerful health-promotion tool, available to everyone. Humans evolved to move a lot to survive, but in modern industrial society, survival usually depends not on moving, but on sitting still at work.[40]

There are significant health risks of prolonged sedentary behavior.[41] Even sleeping is better than sitting.[42] A fascinating study showed that if moderate-to-vigorous activity is not an option, an individual can still experience health benefits by replacing sitting with *any* other activity, including walking, standing, or sleeping. This latter finding might be both amusing and puzzling, until we consider that people cannot snack or have stressful conversations when they are sleeping—something they might do while sitting. Furthermore, there are additional health advantages to adequate sleep, such as more effective glucose metabolism. Changing one's behavior to replace 30 minutes of sitting each day with equal time sleeping could improve markers of obesity like body weight and waist circumference, according to this research. While higher-intensity activities would confer even more benefits sooner, sitting less could improve one's health over time.

Exercise offers the greatest disease prevention benefit for population health among all of the primary prevention actions people could take.[43,44] In a meta-analysis of meta-analyses, the effectiveness of exercise was as high as that of medications in preventing death from coronary heart disease; exercise was better than drugs in preventing death from stroke.[45] In a large systematic review of more than 45 studies and several million participants, researchers found strong evidence that exercise can reduce the risk of several cancers—including bladder, breast, colorectal, and gastric cancers—by up to 20%.[46] Immune cells that attack cancer cells were found to be more active in individuals who exercised.[47] One ten-year prospective study found that adhering to the CDC-recommended level of physical activity was associated with significant reductions in cardiovascular disease mortality risk, and that higher-than-recommended levels of moderate to vigorous physical activity lowered cancer risk and all-cause mortality even more.[48]

In many ways, physical activity functions as a "wonder drug" for many chronic medical conditions. A huge meta-analysis examined the effectiveness of exercise and showed that after a heart attack, exercise therapy significantly reduced mortality from all causes, and reduced cardiac disease mortality by almost a third.[49] Exercise lowers blood pressure in patients with hypertension, and improves cholesterol and triglyceride levels in those who are at risk for heart disease. In patients with COPD, exercise improves functioning and the distance a person can walk; for people with Parkinson's disease, exercise improves mobility and physical functioning. Diabetics who exercise have lower blood sugar levels and a reduced risk of complications. Movement boosts pain tolerance in those with osteoarthritis, allowing additional movement which in turn lowers pain, improves muscle strength, and improves mood.[50,51] Exercise also decreases symptoms of depression and chronic fatigue syndrome, and decreases fatigue in patients who are having cancer therapy. Exercise is indeed a "wonder drug."

Given all these potential benefits, one would think that most people would spend as much time as they can moving. Most people in the United States, however, don't come close to the level of physical activity that the CDC recommends,[41] which, for adults, is 150 minutes per week of movement that increases aerobic capacity (e.g., 30 minutes, five days a week), with two of those days per week doing some overall muscle-strengthening exercise.[52] Plenty of activities do both at the same time (e.g., swimming laps, brisk walking or running, weight lifting, dancing, aerobics classes, calisthenics, bicycle riding, and hiking, to name a few). With some variation depending on measurement method and criteria used, at most only about 28% of Americans meet these physical activity guidelines.[53] Doing *no physical activity at all* outside of work was reported by 25.3% in one survey.[9] In another, a nationwide 10-year prospective study of a half-million U.S. adults, roughly 35% followed *none* of the CDC guidelines—no aerobic and no muscle strengthening activity. In this study, only 11.7% did as much as the CDC recommends.[41]

Most people say they don't have the time, interest, or energy to exercise. But even moving a small amount is better than nothing; even modest increases in physical activity can be beneficial.[42] For example, short activity bouts of a few minutes a day can lower the risk for heart attack, stroke, and early death. Regular walking at brisk pace lowers the risk of type 2 diabetes.[54] Any amount of physical exercise reduces the risk for diabetic neuropathy and nephropathy (kidney disease) by between one fifth and one third.[55] Even brief periods of movement can offer some important health benefits.

The reasons that people remain sedentary are varied. First, except in specific locations, physical activity may not be a significant part of the local culture; even in places where the weather is excellent much of the time, the most common mode of transportation might be the automobile. Ideally, one could get exercise going back and forth to work, and some more densely populated downtown areas encourage walking and provide safe and reliable public transportation. But, as a rule in the United States, movement is not the norm; in only four states are adult inactivity rates below 20%. Regions do vary significantly. For example, Colorado has the highest proportion of active adults; only 17.7% are inactive and don't participate in any physical activities outside of work. In the territory of Puerto Rico, the adult inactivity rate is 49.4%.[56]

Second, information about the value of exercise may not be readily available to everyone. Some educational campaigns have been helpful. For instance, "Active People, Healthy Nation" is a national initiative led by the

CDC. Its goal is to increase regular physical activity to reduce the risk of developing at least 20 chronic diseases, improve health and quality of life, and reduce healthcare costs for those with chronic disease.[57]

Third, most doctors tend not to prescribe exercise to their patients; they mostly don't even talk about it. For many diseases that are associated with physical inactivity (hypertension, heart disease, type 2 diabetes), physicians readily prescribe medication. But research suggests that they feel uncomfortable talking about exercise with their patients, often believing they don't have the expertise to do so and that their patients lack the motivation to make such discussions worthwhile.[58] There tends to be little or no training in medical school on educating, persuading, and/or motivating patients and in helping them to develop healthy habits.[59] Doctors, particularly those who have good rapport with their patients, are in a unique position to counsel them about exercise and make a difference in their patients' success (see Case Study 1.2). Studies show that patients *want* counseling, support, help, and advice about exercise; they want their physicians to prescribe exercise to them, and to guide them in becoming more physically active.[60]

Case Study 1.2 Elders and Exercise

Marlene is 68 years old. Like many her age, she is moderately overweight, but she has no chronic disease conditions beyond arthritis. She says, however, that the arthritis limits her mobility and her quality of life. She has knee pain and stiffness, as well as aching joints and occasional loss of balance. Her doctor has found nothing wrong except that she does not move very much. Marlene sits for a good portion of her day; she reads, knits, talks on the phone, and watches TV. Marlene is like more than 75% of individuals aged 65 to 74 who fail to get any regular exercise. Even though she has the time in retirement, Marlene feels too out-of-shape to do even the simplest and potentially most beneficial exercise—taking regular walks.

Dr. Hansen made it clear to Marlene that there exist excellent data on the importance of moving throughout the lifespan, and especially into older age. She told Marlene that many of the symptoms associated with older age are actually symptoms of inactivity and not of aging, and that studies show a significant decrease in osteoarthritis pain with movement.

> Exercise can help prevent bone loss and cardiovascular disease and can elevate mood. It can reduce the chances of falling by improving strength, balance, and coordination, and it can assist in avoiding medications and surgical interventions for many conditions (including knee osteoarthritis in overweight older adults).
>
> Marlene can enjoy the benefits of moving at modest or no cost; her senior center (like most) has fitness classes, and many TV channels offer exercise demonstrations. Elders with chronic medical conditions may be eligible through Medicare for sessions with a physical or occupational therapist, and many health insurers cover all or part of the cost of gym membership for those over 65. Although working out at a gym can be intimidating to many older people, some gyms have a welcoming atmosphere. In the town where Marlene lives, there is a facility with a very broad age range of members and an environment that fosters strong social connections; it functions like a community center, with organized activities, trainers, and staff who are supportive and encouraging. The shuttle from her senior center could take her there if she'd like to go. Offering a fitness center with social support and respect for all is an excellent business decision. The U.S. population is aging, and the benefits of exercise are increasingly recognized by those who pay the medical bills—insurance companies, medical plans, and patients themselves.

Secondary prevention: disease screening

Secondary prevention focuses on early detection of subclinical disease and requires an interface with some element of the healthcare system, including a private physician, a community clinic, or a public health department. The U.S. Preventive Services Task Force (USPSTF) and other reputable professional organizations such as the American Cancer Society, the American Heart Association, and the American Medical Association make recommendations for patient screenings (e.g., for breast cancer, gestational diabetes, hypertension). Some also offer recommendations regarding talking with patients to screen for anxiety, depression, and suicide risk, underscoring the central role played by providers in intervening before disease develops, or identifying it early when treatment can be successful. It is interesting to note that recommendations from various entities are not always identical.[61] Although these guidelines can be very helpful to physicians, populations with limited access to a regular physician may struggle to have their screening needs met.

Tertiary prevention: adherence to medical treatments

In recent years, complex and impressive medical technologies, medications, and treatments have become available which, if adhered to, can successfully manage diseases that once caused significant morbidity and mortality.

In an ideal world, patient adherence would be perfect. Diabetics would test their blood glucose levels and confidently take their medications in doses congruent with their food intake and exercise.[62,63] Those with high blood pressure and heart disease would cope effectively with "polypharmacy," remembering to take several different medications per day on their various schedules. Patients with celiac disease would follow restrictive diets and those with musculoskeletal conditions would regularly attend physical therapy and perform daily exercises.

But many don't. Some don't fill their medication prescriptions or begin their treatment regimens such as a restricted diet or a program of exercise. This is *primary nonadherence* or *nonfulfillment*. Some carry out the regimen incorrectly or inconsistently, and some give it up entirely; this is called *nonpersistence*. Although adherence to a health regimen is always important, it is especially vital once a disease has gained momentum, and vigilance and persistence are needed to slow its progression.

Unintentional and intentional nonadherence

Many people *unintentionally* fail to follow their treatments correctly.[64] For example, a patient might fully intend to take their medications in the morning before work, but become distracted by their children's needs before they have a chance to swallow their pills. Because of memory lapses or a disorganized schedule, another patient might time their medication doses too close or too far apart, taking fewer or more pills than prescribed, or even skipping entire days of medication. Unintentional failures to adhere are also caused by poor communication with their provider. The patient might have an incomplete understanding of the necessity of their medication treatment or may have misunderstood how to use their medical device or carry out their prescribed exercises. The individual might engage in proscribed behaviors, such as eating certain prohibited foods or ingredients, not realizing what should be avoided. Or the patient may not have the skills or the resources they need to follow their regimen. They might miss treatment appointments because of a lack of transportation or unreliable internet service, having planned to follow the treatment but being unable to do so.

On the other hand, *intentional* nonadherence results when a patient intends not to follow treatment. The patient might believe that their prescribed medication is unsafe or ineffective, or make a conscious choice to ignore the recommendation because their friends or family members say they should. Patients might simply think they know better than their doctor (e.g., "I don't think I need this much medication; I'll just cut these pills in half") or have a competing value (e.g., "I'll save the rest of this antibiotic until the next time I need it—that's the most frugal approach"). Intentional nonadherence can also result when patients distrust medicine or public health officials (perhaps in response to the online proliferation of misleading medical misinformation). Patients could also experience "motivated forgetting" because they do not really believe that the medication is worth taking; or they might cease the medication or necessary health behavior activity because they are simply tired of it all.

The prevalence of nonadherence

There have been tens of thousands of studies published on adherence. While researchers do not know the precise extent of the problem for every treatment and every condition, or even all the reasons why, they *do* know that a disturbingly high percentage of people with chronic disease don't do a very good job of adhering to treatment. At least 25% of patients (and for many chronic diseases closer to 50%), leave the medical office and fail to adhere to the recommendations given during the visit.[65]

Many new prescriptions are never filled. In a recent, major meta-analysis, the pooled average primary nonadherence rate for four chronic disease medications was 14.6%.[66] Primary medication nonadherence in North America was twice that of Europe and was highest for lipid-lowering medications (20.8%). Adherence to treatment, once it has been started, is usually defined as taking 80% or more of a prescribed medication dose or following 80% or more of a behavioral directive; after six months of treatment have passed, more than half of people with a chronic condition are nonadherent. Many feel overwhelmed or get bored or become frustrated with the demands of the regimen and just give up.[65]

Not surprisingly, adherence to lifestyle change and to complex medication regimens can be difficult. Adherence is lower for medication regimens that are complex (such as multiple medications with different dosing schedules) and for treatments that require more behavioral management. This is true for a variety of chronic medical conditions including asthma, cardiovascular disease, cystic fibrosis, inflammatory bowel disease (IBD), arthritis, and transplant care.[67] In the treatment of IBD, it might seem that any intervention that would reduce troublesome symptoms might have high adherence, but this is not always true. Between 43% and 60% of adults with IBD are nonadherent to prescribed oral medication, despite the fact that they are more likely to experience flare-ups in their disease condition.[68] Adherence in osteoarthritis (OA) and rheumatoid arthritis (RA) care tends to be low when lifestyle changes, such as weight reduction, exercise, sleep management, smoking cessation, and pacing of physical activity are required.[69] Finally, medication nonadherence rates post-transplant are also high, despite the significant danger of organ rejection, morbidity, and even mortality.[70]

In a comprehensive meta-analysis of 569 studies reporting adherence to medical treatment prescribed by a nonpsychiatrist physician, the average nonadherence rate was 25%. Adherence overall was highest (around 80%) for HIV and cancer, and lowest (around 65%) for complex treatments that did not improve current quality of life by relieving bothersome symptoms. Adherence was found to vary considerably by the type of regimen: medication adherence was higher than adherence to lifestyle alteration, and higher among patients with greater resources (such as education and income). It did not, however, vary simply as a function of illness severity or the demographic characteristics of age and gender.[71]

Providers are generally unaware of their patients' nonadherence; it has been said that medication nonadherence is "barely on the radar" of most practicing physicians.[72,73] Clinicians tend to overestimate the degree to which their own patients are adherent, and as a result much treatment nonadherence goes unrecognized. Many providers cannot accurately identify which of their patients are having adherence difficulties, and they often fail to inquire if patients are following their treatment regimens at all. Patients typically do not volunteer information about their nonadherence, and they may try to get through the medical visit without revealing their adherence difficulties. Furthermore, adherence may not be consistent across regimens;

a patient might be highly adherent to one regimen, but nonadherent to another, making nonadherence less obvious than if patients were consistent.

Costs and consequences of nonadherence

Does it matter if people adhere? Can health behavior change and treatment adherence actually contribute to longevity and health outcomes? Can adherence lengthen the healthspan and offer advantages in survival and quality of life? The answer is a resounding "yes." More to the point, health outcomes among individuals who adhere to treatment well, versus poorly, are overall 26% better; for many diseases, adherence offers an even greater outcome advantage.[74,75] The most comprehensive investigation to date of the value of adherence is a review of 771 adherence-promoting intervention studies.[76] This review found a standardized mean difference effect size of 0.29 when comparing treatment and control groups, showing that interventions to improve adherence really do improve health outcomes.

Financial costs

Chronic disease conditions are common; over one-third of the U.S. population lives with at least one chronic disease and 81 million people have multiple chronic illnesses. Increases are forecast for virtually every common chronic condition, mostly because of an aging population combined with a rise in disease-specific risk factors such as obesity.

With many diseases, the long-term costs resulting from nonadherence can be very high. For example, if HIV patients fail to take medications regularly and correctly, they may experience many expensive hospitalizations. If diabetics do not properly test their glucose levels, self-administer insulin, and follow appropriate diet and exercise regimens, the costs of care for resulting heart disease, amputations, vision impairment, and kidney failure can be very high. Rising rates of obesity and poorly managed type 2 diabetes are already contributing to rapidly rising healthcare expenditures in the United States.

Nonadherence costs the U.S. healthcare system more than 300 billion dollars annually in preventable hospitalizations and emergency room visits, poor outcomes, and avoidable complications.[77] It is estimated that every year at least 275 million medical visits for prevention or treatment of chronic conditions may be wasted (or are less than optimal) because the advice that the physician gives to the patient is misunderstood, forgotten, or ignored and the result is nonadherence.[77] It is likely that if there existed a blockbuster drug that would save the U.S. healthcare system these losses *and* improve healthcare outcomes, many would jump at the chance to use it.[78] Methods for improving adherence may offer the same benefits.

Human costs
The human costs of nonadherence are many. Nonadherence to medication for hypertension, for example, may result in 89,000 premature deaths in the United States annually.[79] Among the hundreds of thousands of individuals who die of heart disease prematurely, many do so because of nonadherence. Nonadherence fosters the development and exacerbation of the complications of diabetes, such as loss of limbs and eyesight, resulting in suffering among patients and frustration among providers.[78] The accuracy of scientific research and clinical conclusions can also be threatened by nonadherence to treatment protocols.[78]

Potential threats to other people might also derive from nonadherence. Failure to take antibiotics correctly can result in drug-resistant strains of bacteria that can make many people sick and jeopardize future treatments.[80] Failure to adhere to strategies to mitigate a communicable disease raises the risk of illness for everyone, not just the nonadherent individual.[81] The COVID-19 pandemic reminded us that communicable diseases are of concern to everyone in a population, and that the behavior of some can increase risk to all.

Why health behavior change and adherence sometimes fail

Human behavior has been described as the "wild-card"—an unknown or unpredictable factor—in healthcare. As can sometimes happen when a consequential, but not fully understood, element exists in a system, myths can arise about its causes. These myths are common beliefs that seem intuitively right but are not correct and are not supported by evidence. In this book, we will examine these myths, and offer readers a chance to look beyond what they think they know about health behavior. We will see some surprising statistics and some challenges to myths about what people do and why. As we will see, health behavior change and treatment adherence are not simple, but they can be understood by relying on literally thousands of empirical studies—if we "trust the science." Let's take a look at some of the "myths" and science-based realities in Table 1.1.

Table 1.1 Myths and Realities About Patient Adherence and Health Behavior Change

Myth	Research-Based Reality
If a physician tells a patient something, that patient will understand and remember it.	Somewhere between 40% and 80% of what is said in a medical visit is forgotten by the patient by the time they leave the office.
Costs solely drive nonadherence.	In systems and countries with zero copay for medications, nonadherence drops by only about 10%, on average. Patients do operate within the limitations of their resources, but resources are not the only factors that drive nonadherence.
Motivation for health is personal and primarily internal.	Cognitive factors, such as beliefs and attitudes, combine with habits and motivational, social, cultural, and contextual factors to drive health behavior.
It is always a bad idea (or a good idea, depending upon your perspective) for patients to consult the internet.	The wisdom of internet searching depends upon the websites chosen and patients' level of health literacy. If patients consult reliable sources such as universities or respected medical institutions or associations, the information is very likely accurate and framed to help patients understand and seek appropriate medical care when necessary. But many patients (46% of U.S. adults) have low to marginal health literacy and cannot evaluate the quality of information they find. Less reliable sources might provide misinformation, and personally trusted sources such as online "influencers" and social media "friends" might simply be wrong in the advice they offer.
Social support is always good for health.	Support from family, friends, and coworkers can be helpful *if* they favor an effective health behavior and if the relationships are strong and positive. A lack of family support can work against health behavior change, however, reducing it by 20% or more. Of course, coercive relationships can be quite problematic, and family conflict can be a strong inhibitor of adherence; a social support system might push a patient to ignore their physician's advice.

A social-ecological perspective on health behavior and adherence

As we have seen in this chapter, the costs of illness and chronic disease are considerable, not only in financial terms but also in lost productivity, absence from work and education, and the presence of pain, suffering, and loss. Health behaviors and the social conditions that influence them are central to the development, treatment, and management of most causes of disease. Throughout this book, we examine health behavior change and adherence from both an individual (social-psychological) and a social-ecological perspective.[82] In this framework, the human being is, in many ways, the last step on the health behavior pathway. What seem to be personal choices, such as to consume ultra-processed foods or to smoke cigarettes, are actions that rest on a multitude of influences including: personal beliefs, social norms, culture, family, and environmental pressures such as poverty, chronic environmental stress, and neighborhood saturation with fast food, tobacco products, and alcohol. As sociologists Bruce Link and Jo Phelan have noted,[83] a person might make the choice to light a cigarette, but there are multiple determinants that cause that behavior. These fundamental causes explain the association between mortality and socioeconomic status, which embodies not only financial resources but also health information, knowledge, social power, and social connections that protect or threaten health.

Throughout this book, we offer a look at the complexity of individual behavioral choices for health promotion, disease prevention, and illness management. We view choice as it occurs within the social-ecological-economic-cultural context that surrounds the individual, as well as the opportunities they have to carry out their best behavioral intentions. Throughout the chapters that follow, we examine how the social-ecological context in which the individual is functioning provides them with opportunities, or limits their choices, for health action. We consider how this context can drive resistance to clinical implementations of care through treatment nonadherence. We assess the social and psychological factors that have challenged health policy, and we offer insights into the management of currently widespread (some say epidemic levels of) chronic diseases.

In the context of a social-ecological perspective, in Chapter 2 we will consider the many theoretical models that formalize our understanding of multiple determinants of health behavior and treatment adherence. In Chapter 3, we will center our attention on the role of the therapeutic relationship and examine the foundational elements of trust and empathy, personalized care, and the social and psychological well-being of patients in interpersonal communication with their medical providers. In Chapter 4, we will examine essential elements of communication that patients and providers need in order to assess health risks and make joint medical decisions. We will also explore the formulation of effective health messages that successfully teach and guide patients. In Chapter 5, we will consider the content and framing of persuasive health messages and characteristics of effective messengers, as well as the role of reasoning and emotion, self-efficacy and competence, personal motivation, and resistance to authority as we focus on ways to help patients make simple but important behavioral changes in their lives. In Chapter 6, we will focus on daily habits and the psychology of behavior change in the science of habit formation, acquisition, maintenance, demotivation, and behavioral avoidance. Then in Chapter 7, we will consider the individual's sociocultural context as it drives their health behavior and treatment adherence; this context includes "networks" broadly defined to include social media, family norms, cultural habits, and social expectations that can boost sustained commitment to health promotion and disease prevention activities, or stridently reject them and prohibit the individual's adherence. We will also address the socioeconomic determinants of health, including inequalities and disparities in healthcare, environmental risks and health challenges in vulnerable populations, and the increasing recognition of the role of trauma and mental health in health vulnerabilities. In Chapter 8, we will examine the valuable role played by healthcare teams and offer an analysis of the expanding role of and options for technology in medicine. We will examine the management of medical information available to patients, artificial intelligence–based tools, virtual medical visits, technologies in medical interactions, and technological aids for behavioral self-management. Finally, in Chapter 9, we will examine the role of systems and public policies that relate to health behavior change and treatment adherence, viewing individual behavioral choice within a complex network of stakeholders in healthcare. We will examine the delivery of care in integrated health systems. Finally, we will examine the broader context of laws and public policies, and the potential for managing the health behavior and adherence of populations in the face of future communicable disease threats.

Summary

In Chapter 1, we examine the concept of "health" and the three levels of prevention (primary, secondary, and tertiary) that facilitate health promotion and maintenance. We approach behavioral issues in health with an awareness that the social-ecological-economic-cultural context surrounding each person drives their choices as well as the opportunities they have to carry out their best behavioral intentions toward the goal of health. We consider several important primary prevention behaviors, those that are strongly linked to health outcomes and are most likely to be of concern to providers in the care of their patients. These include healthy diet, obesity prevention, alcohol and substance use, tobacco use, sexual risk behavior, and physical activity. We consider why these basic health behaviors may be difficult to achieve and why, in the context of medical care delivery, they can be difficult to address. We examine secondary prevention in the form of disease screening, and tertiary prevention involving the treatment of acute and chronic medical conditions. We consider intentional and unintentional nonadherence to medical recommendations, and the prevalence of its various types, and we describe some of the financial and human costs and consequences of nonadherence, addressing some common myths about why health behavior change and adherence sometimes fail. Finally, we emphasize the role of a social-ecological perspective and introduce the ways in which this perspective guides the topics covered in this book.

Tools for instruction and self-study

Learning objectives

By the end of this chapter, readers should be able to

1. Differentiate primary, secondary, and tertiary levels of prevention.
2. Explain the complexities in defining obesity, and the potential health consequences of obesity.
3. Discuss the meaning of multiple-risk behavior profile.
4. Describe psychological factors that may be helpful in understanding and preventing substance use and in changing substance use behaviors.
5. Demonstrate how primary prevention plays a role in reducing the spread of communicable disease.
6. Discuss how physical activity is important in chronic disease prevention and management.
7. Explain reasons why people maintain a sedentary lifestyle.
8. Identify different types of recommended disease screening.
9. Contrast primary nonadherence and non-persistence.
10. Summarize the financial and human costs of nonadherence.

Review questions

1. List and briefly describe the three levels of prevention.
2. Why might it be that sleeping is better for you than just sitting?
3. What makes food consumption such a difficult aspect of lifestyle to change?
4. Define, and give one example of, unintentional nonadherence and intentional nonadherence.
5. What is meant by the term "social-ecological" in the context of health and health behavior?

Prompts for discussion and further study

1. How might we best view the challenges of weight management, healthy eating, and obesity prevention? What are some of the issues we should consider?
2. How might one navigate one's relationships with people whose health behaviors are inconsistent with (or even a threat to) one's own? For example, how can one balance needs for social support and companionship with needs for encouragement of one's own health-related goals?
3. All things considered, do you think the internet is a benefit or a detriment when it comes to maintaining health? Why?

Suggested reading

1. Hotez P. *The Deadly Rise of Anti-Science.* Johns Hopkins University Press; 2023.
2. Offit PA. *Deadly Choices: How the Anti-Vaccine Movement Threatens Us All.* Basic Books; 2015.
3. Walker P. *The Miracle Pill.* Simon & Schuster; 2021.
4. Miller T. *What Doesn't Kill You: A Life with Chronic Illness—Lessons from a Body in Revolt.* Henry Holt and Company; 2021.
5. Gawande A. *Being Mortal: Illness, Medicine, and What Matters in the End.* Henry Holt & Company; 2014.

References

1. *Basic Documents*. 49th ed. Geneva: World Health Organization; 2020.
2. Kaeberlein M. How healthy is the healthspan concept? *Geroscience*. 2018; 40(4): pp. 361–364.
3. Glanz K, Kahan S. Conceptual framework for behavior change. In: Kahan S, Gielen AC, Fagan PJ, Green LW, eds. *Health Behavior Change in Populations*. Johns Hopkins University Press; 2014; pp. 9–25.
4. Frick C, Rumgay H, Vignat J, et al. Quantitative estimates of preventable and treatable deaths from 36 cancers worldwide: a population-based study. *Lancet Glob Health*. 2023; 11(11): e1700–e1712. doi: 10.1016/S2214-109X(23)00406-0
5. Health for life: focus on wellness. American Hospital Association website. Retrieved January 21, 2024. https://www.aha.org/system/files/content/00-10/071204_H4L_FocusonWellness.pdf
6. Health and economic costs of chronic disease. National Center for Chronic Disease Prevention and Health promotion. Centers for Disease Control and Prevention website. Retrieved January 21, 2024. https://www.cdc.gov/chronicdisease/about/costs/index.htm
7. Hesse BW, Beckjord E, Ahern DK. Role of technology in behavior change to expand reach and impact of public health. In: Hilliard ME, Riekert KA, Ockene JK, Pbert L, eds. *The Handbook of Health Behavior Change*. 5th ed. Springer; 2018; pp. 525–544.
8. Prochaska JJ, Prochaska JM, Prochaska JO. Building a science for multiple-risk behavior change. In: Hilliard ME, Riekert KA, Ockene JK, Pbert L, eds. *The Handbook of Health Behavior Change*. 5th ed. Springer; 2018; pp. 265–288.
9. Adult physical inactivity prevalence maps by race/ethnicity. National Center for Chronic Disease Prevention and Health Promotion. Centers for Disease Control and Prevention website. Retrieved January 21, 2024. https://www.cdc.gov/physicalactivity/data/inactivity-prevalence-maps/index.html
10. Adult obesity prevalence remains high; support for prevention and treatment needed. Centers for Disease Control and Prevention website. Retrieved January 21, 2024. https://www.cdc.gov/media/releases/2023/p0922-adult-obesity.html
11. Mukherjea A, Green LW. Tobacco and behavior change. In: Kahan S, Gielen AC, Fagan PJ, Green LW, eds. *Health Behavior Change in Populations*. Johns Hopkins University Press; 2014; pp. 153–187.
12. Kahan S, Cheskin LJ. Obesity and eating behavior and behavior change. In: Kahan S, Gielen AC, Fagan PJ, Green LW, eds. *Health Behavior Change in Populations*. Johns Hopkins University Press; 2014; pp. 233–261.
13. Sole-Smith V. *Fat Talk: Parenting in the Age of Diet Culture*. Henry Holt and Co; 2023.
14. AMA adopts new policy clarifying BMI as a measure in medicine. American Medical Association website. Retrieved March 10, 2024. https://www.ama-assn.org/press-center/press-releases/ama-adopts-new-policy-clarifying-role-bmi-measure-medicine
15. Martínez Steele E, Baraldi LG, Louzada ML, Moubarac JC, Mozaffarian D, Monteiro CA. Ultra-processed foods and added sugars in the US diet: evidence from a nationally representative cross-sectional study. *BMJ Open*. 2016; 6(3):e009892. doi: 10.1136/bmjopen-2015-009892

16. Isaksen IM, Dankel SN. Ultra-processed food consumption and cancer risk: a systematic review and meta-analysis. *Clin Nutr.* 2023; 42(6): pp. 919–928. doi: 10.1016/j.clnu.2023.03.018
17. Pagliai G, Dinu M, Madarena MP, Bonaccio M, Iacoviello L, Sofi F. Consumption of ultra-processed foods and health status: a systematic review and meta-analysis. *Br J Nutr.* 2021; 125(3): pp. 308–318. doi: 10.1017/S0007114520002688
18. Thomson CA, Johnston C. Dietary behavior change. In: Hilliard ME, Riekert KA, Ockene JK, Pbert L, eds. *The Handbook of Health Behavior Change.* 5th ed. Springer; 2018. pp. 134–152.
19. Adult obesity facts. Centers for Disease Control and Prevention website. Retrieved March 10, 2024. https://www.cdc.gov/obesity/data/adult.html
20. Goode, RW, Yu, Y, Burke, LE. Obesity. In: Hilliard ME, Riekert KA, Ockene JK, Pbert L, eds. *The Handbook of Health Behavior Change.* 5th ed. Springer; 2018. pp. 381–400.
21. Childhood obesity facts. Centers for Disease Control and Prevention website. Retrieved March 10, 2024. https://www.cdc.gov/obesity/data/childhood.html
22. Rubino F, Batterham RL, Koch M, et al. Lancet Diabetes & Endocrinology Commission on the Definition and Diagnosis of Clinical Obesity. *Lancet Diabetes Endocrinol.* 2023; 11(4): pp. 226–228. doi: 10.1016/S2213-8587(23)00058-X.
23. Jean-Louis G, Williams NJ, Sarpong D, et al. Associations between inadequate sleep and obesity in the US adult population: analysis of the national health interview survey (1977–2009). *BMC Public Health.* 2014; 14: p. 290. doi: 10.1186/1471-2458-14-290
24. Wu Y, Gong Q, Zou Z, Li H, Zhang X. Short sleep duration and obesity among children: a systematic review and meta-analysis of prospective studies. *Obes Res Clin Pract.* 2017; 11(2): pp. 140–150. doi: 10.1016/j.orcp.2016.05.005
25. Ditez WH. Foreword. In: Kahan S, Gielen AC, Fagan PJ, Green LRW, eds. *Health Behavior Change in Populations.* Johns Hopkins University Press; 2014. pp. xi–xii.
26. Tehrani H, Rajabi A, Ghelichi-Ghojogh M, Nejatian M, Jafari A. The prevalence of electronic cigarettes vaping globally: a systematic review and meta-analysis. *Arch Public Health.* 2022; 80(1): p. 240. doi: 10.1186/s13690-022-00998-w
27. Pbert L, Jolicoeur D, Haskins BL, Ockene JK. Addressing tobacco use and dependence. In: Hilliard ME, Riekert KA, Ockene JK, Pbert L, eds. *The Handbook of Health Behavior Change.* 5th ed. Springer; 2018. pp. 197–221.
28. Manthey J, Hassan SA, Carr S, Kilian C, Kuitunen-Paul S, Rehm J. What are the economic costs to society attributable to alcohol use? A systematic review and modelling study. *Pharmacoeconomics.* 2021; 39(7): pp. 809–822. doi: 10.1007/s40273-021-01031-8
29. Geijer-Simpson E, McGovern R, Kaner E. Alcohol prevention and treatment: interventions for hazardous, harmful, and dependent drinkers. In: Hilliard ME, Riekert KA, Ockene JK, Pbert L, eds. *The Handbook of Health Behavior Change.* 5th ed. Springer; 2018. pp. 223–242.
30. Holder H. Alcohol and behavior change. In: Kahan S, Gielen AC, Fagan PJ, Green LW, eds. *Health Behavior Change in Populations.* Johns Hopkins University Press; 2014. pp. 188–206.

31. Shi M, Luo C, Oduyale OK, Zong X, LoConte NK, Cao Y. Alcohol consumption Among adults with a cancer diagnosis in the All of Us research program. *JAMA Netw Open.* 2023; Aug 1;6(8):e2328328. doi: 10.1001/jamanetworkopen.2023.28328
32. Strain EC, Tompkins DA. Substance use and behavior change. In: Kahan S, Gielen AC, Fagan PJ, Green LW, eds. *Health Behavior Change in Populations.* Johns Hopkins University Press; 2014. pp. 207–232.
33. Koenig HC, Holtgrave D. Sexual risk and behavior change. In: Kahan S, Gielen AC, Fagan PJ, Green LW, eds. *Health Behavior Change in Populations.* Johns Hopkins University Press; 2014. pp. 259–387.
34. Lim CS, Schneider EM, Janicke DM. Developmental influences on behavior change: Children, adolescents, emerging adults, and the elderly. In: Hilliard ME, Riekert KA, Ockene JK, Pbert L, eds. *The Handbook of Health Behavior Change.* 5th ed. Springer; 2018. pp. 75–101.
35. Flu vaccination coverage, United States, 2022-2023 influenza season. Centers for Disease Control and Prevention website. Retrieved March 10, 2024. https://www.cdc.gov/flu/fluvaxview/coverage-2223estimates.htm
36. Albrecht D. Vaccination, politics and COVID-19 impacts. *BMC Public Health.* 2022; 22(1): p. 96. doi: 10.1186/s12889-021-12432-x.
37. Young DG, Rasheed H, Bleakley A, Langbaum JB. The politics of mask-wearing: political preferences, reactance, and conflict aversion during COVID. *Soc Sci Med.* 2022; 298: p. 114836. doi: 10.1016/j.socscimed.2022.114836
38. Thaweethai T, Jolley SE, Karlson EW, et al. RECOVER Consortium. Development of a definition of post-acute sequelae of SARS-CoV-2 Infection. *JAMA.* 2023; 329(22): pp.1934–1946. doi: 10.1001/jama.2023.8823.
39. We worked on the U.S. pandemic response: here are 13 takeaways for the next health emergency. *New York Times* website. Retrieved March 10, 2024. https://www.nytimes.com/2023/05/11/opinion/covid-pandemic-lessons.html
40. Cradock AL. The role of the built environment in supporting health behavior change. In: Hilliard ME, Riekert KA, Ockene JK, Pbert L, eds. *The Handbook of Health Behavior Change.* 5th ed. Springer; 2018. pp. 481–504.
41. López-Bueno R, Ahmadi M, Stamatakis E, Yang L, Del Pozo Cruz B. Prospective associations of different combinations of aerobic and muscle-strengthening activity with all-cause, cardiovascular, and cancer mortality. *JAMA Intern Med.* 2023; 183(9): pp. 982–990. doi: 10.1001/jamainternmed.2023.3093.
42. Blodgett JM, Ahmadi MN, Atkin AJ, et al; ProPASS Collaboration. Device-measured physical activity and cardiometabolic health: the Prospective Physical Activity, Sitting, and Sleep (ProPASS) consortium. *Eur Heart J.* 2024; 45(6): pp. 458–471. doi: 10.1093/eurheartj/ehad717.
43. MacAuley D, Bauman A, Frémont P. Exercise: not a miracle cure, just good medicine. *Br J Sports Med.* 2016; 50(18): pp. 1107–1108. doi: 10.1136/bmj.h1416.
44. Posadzki P, Pieper D, Bajpai R, et al. Exercise/physical activity and health outcomes: an overview of Cochrane systematic reviews. *BMC Public Health.* 2020; 20(1): p. 1724. doi: 10.1186/s12889-020-09855-3.
45. Naci H, Ioannidis JP. Comparative effectiveness of exercise and drug interventions on mortality outcomes: metaepidemiological study. *Br J Sports Med.* 2015; 49(21): pp. 1414–1422. doi: 10.1136/bjsports-2015-f5577rep

46. McTiernan A, Friedenreich CM, Katzmarzyk PT, et al; 2018 Physical Activity Guidelines Advisory Committee*. Physical activity in cancer prevention and survival: a systematic review. *Med Sci Sports Exerc.* 2019; 51(6): pp. 1252–1261. doi: 10.1249/MSS.0000000000001937
47. Deng N, Reyes-Uribe L, Fahrmann JF, et al. Exercise training reduces the inflammatory response and promotes intestinal mucosa-associated immunity in Lynch Syndrome. *Clin Cancer Res.* 2023; 29(21): pp. 4361–4372. doi: 10.1158/1078-0432.CCR-23-0088.
48. Blair SN, Kohl HW 3rd, Paffenbarger RS Jr, Clark DG, Cooper KH, Gibbons LW. Physical fitness and all-cause mortality. A prospective study of healthy men and women. *JAMA.* 1989; 262(17): pp. 2395–2401. doi: 10.1001/jama.262.17.2395.
49. Valkeinen H, Aaltonen S, Kujala UM. Effects of exercise training on oxygen uptake in coronary heart disease: a systematic review and meta-analysis. *Scand J Med Sci Sports.* 2010; 20(4): pp. 545–555. doi: 10.1111/j
50. Feehan L, Westby M. Patients with rheumatoid arthritis should exercise more, sit less. *The Rheumatologist.* November 1, 2014. https://www.the-rheumatologist.org/article/patients-with-rheumatoid-arthritis-should-exercise-more-sit-less/2/
51. Wilkes C, Kydd R, Sagar M, Broadbent E. Upright posture improves affect and fatigue in people with depressive symptoms. *J Behav Ther Exp Psychiatry.* 2017; 54: pp. 143–149. doi: 10.1016/j.jbtep.2016.07.015
52. Physical activity for different groups. Centers for Disease Control and Prevention website. Retrieved March 10, 2024. https://www.cdc.gov/physicalactivity/basics/age-chart.html
53. Abildso CG, Daily SM, Umstattd Meyer MR, Perry CK, Eyler A. Prevalence of meeting aerobic, muscle-strengthening, and combined physical activity guidelines during leisure time among adults, by rural-Urban Classification and Region - United States, 2020. *Am J Transplant.* 2023; 23(3): pp. 443–446. doi: 10.1016/j.ajt.2023.01.021
54. Jayedi A, Zargar M, Emadi A, et al. Walking speed and the risk of type 2 diabetes: a systematic review and meta-analysis. *Br J Sports Med.* 2024; 58: pp. 334–342.
55. Kristensen FPB, Sanchez-Lastra MA, Dalene KE, et al. Leisure-time physical activity and risk of microvascular complications in individuals with type 2 diabetes: a UK biobank study. *Diab Care.* 2023; 46(10): pp. 1816–1824. doi: 10.2337/dc23-0937.
56. CDC releases updated maps of America's high levels of inactivity. Centers for Disease Control and Prevention website. Retrieved March 10, 2024. https://www.cdc.gov/media/releases/2022/p0120-inactivity-map.html
57. Active people, healthy nation. Centers for Disease Control and Prevention website. Retrieved March 10, 2024. https://www.cdc.gov/physicalactivity/activepeoplehealthynation/index.html
58. Din NU, Moore GF, Murphy S, Wilkinson C, Williams NH. Health professionals' perspectives on exercise referral and physical activity promotion in primary care: findings from a process evaluation of the National Exercise Referral Scheme in Wales. *Health Educ J.* 2015; 74(6): pp. 743–757. doi: 10.1177/0017896914559785.
59. Cinal BJ, Park EA, Kim M, Cardinal MK. If exercise is medicine, where is exercise in medicine? Review of U.S. medical education curricula for physical activity-related content. *J Phys Act Health.* 2015; 12(9): pp. 1336–1343. doi: 10.1123/jpah.2014-0316.
60. Falskog F, Landsem AM, Meland E, Bjorvatn B, Hjelle OP, Mildestvedt T. Patients want their doctors' help to increase physical activity: a cross-sectional

study in general practice. *Scand J Prim Health Care.* 2021; 39(2): pp. 131–138. doi: 10.1080/02813432.2021.1910670.
61. American Cancer Society recommendations for the early detection of breast cancer. American Cancer Society website. Retrieved March 10, 2024. https://www.cancer.org/cancer/types/breast-cancer/screening-tests-and-early-detection/american-cancer-society-recommendations-for-the-early-detection-of-breast-cancer.html
62. Fagan PJ, Dunbar L. Chronic conditions and population health management for health care systems. In: Kahan S, Gielen AC, Fagan PJ, Green LW, eds. *Health Behavior Change in Populations.* Johns Hopkins University Press; 2014. pp. 497.
63. Hood KK, Raymond JK, Adams RN, Tanenbaum ML, Harris MA. Diabetes management behaviors: The key to optimal health and quality of life outcomes. In: Hilliard ME, Riekert KA, Ockene JK, Pbert L, eds. *The Handbook of Health Behavior Change.* 5th ed. Springer; 2018. pp. 309–328.
64. Lindquist LA, Go L, Fleisher J, Jain N, Friesema E, Baker DW. Relationship of health literacy to intentional and unintentional non-adherence of hospital discharge medications. *J Gen Intern Med.* 2012; 27(2): pp. 173–178.
65. DiMatteo MR. Variations in patients' adherence to medical recommendations: a quantitative review of 50 years of research. *Med Care.* 2004; 42(3): pp. 200–209. doi: 10.1097/01.mlr.0000114908.90348.f9
66. Lemstra M, Nwankwo C, Bird Y, Moraros J. Primary nonadherence to chronic disease medications: a meta-analysis. *Patient Prefer Adherence.* 2018; 12: pp. 721–731. doi: 10.2147/PPA.S161151.
67. Le TT, Bilderback A, Bender B, et al. Do asthma medication beliefs mediate the relationship between minority status and adherence to therapy? *J Asthma.* 2008; 45(1): pp. 33–37. doi: 10.1080/02770900701815552.
68. Greenley RN, Kunz JH, Walter J, Hommel KA. Practical strategies for enhancing adherence to treatment regimen in inflammatory bowel disease. *Inflamm Bowel Dis.* 2013; 19(7): pp. 1534–1545. doi: 10.1097/MIB.0b013e3182813482
69. Knittle K, De Gucht V, Maes S. Lifestyle- and behaviour-change interventions in musculoskeletal conditions. *Best Pract Res Clin Rheumatol.* 2012; 26(3): pp. 293–304. doi: 10.1016/j.berh.2012.05.002.
70. Low JK, Williams A, Manias E, Crawford K. Interventions to improve medication adherence in adult kidney transplant recipients: a systematic review. *Nephrology Dialysis Transplantation.* 2015; 30(5): pp. 752–761. doi: 10.1093/ndt/gfu204.
71. Foley L, Larkin J, Lombard-Vance R, et al. Prevalence and predictors of medication non-adherence among people living with multimorbidity: a systematic review and meta-analysis. *BMJ Open.* 2021; 11(9):e044987. doi: 10.1136/bmjopen-2020-044987. Erratum in: BMJ Open. 2022; 12(7): e044987corr1
72. Malik M, Kumari S, Manalai P. Treatment nonadherence: an epidemic hidden in plain sight. *Psychiatric Times.* 2020; 37(3): pp. 25–26.
73. Kleinsinger F. The unmet challenge of medication nonadherence. *Perm J.* 2018; 22: pp. 18–33. doi: 10.7812/TPP/18 033.
74. DiMatteo MR, Giordani PJ, Lepper HS, Croghan TW. Patient adherence and medical treatment outcomes: a meta-analysis. *Med Care.* 2002; 40(9): pp. 794–811. doi: 10.1097/00005650-200209000-00009.
75. Simpson SH, Eurich DT, Majumdar SR, et al. A meta-analysis of the association between adherence to drug therapy and mortality. *BMJ.* 2006; 333(7557): p. 15. doi: 10.1136/bmj.38875.675486.55.

76. Conn VS, Ruppar TM. Medication adherence outcomes of 771 intervention trials: systematic review and meta-analysis. *Prev Med.* 2017; 99: pp. 269–276. doi: 10.1016/j.ypmed.2017.03.008.
77. Iuga AO, McGuire MJ. Adherence and health care costs. *Risk Manag Healthc Policy.* 2014; 7: pp. 35–44. doi: 10.2147/RMHP.S19801
78. DiMatteo MR, Haskard-Zolnierek KB, Martin LR. Improving patient adherence: a three-factor model to guide practice. *Health Psychol Rev.* 2011; pp. 1–18.
79. Cutler DM, Long G, Berndt ER, et al. The value of antihypertensive drugs: a perspective on medical innovation. *Health Aff (Millwood).* 2007; 26(1): pp. 97–110. doi: 10.1377/hlthaff.26.1.97.
80. Singh R, Dwivedi SP, Gaharwar US, Meena R, Rajamani P, Prasad T. Recent updates on drug resistance in Mycobacterium tuberculosis. *J Appl Microbiol.* 2020; 128(6): pp. 1547–1567. doi: 10.1111/jam.14478
81. Scalera A, Bayoumi AM, Oh P, Risebrough N, Shear N, Lin-in Tseng A. Clinical and economic implications of non-adherence to HAART in HIV infection. *Disease Management and Health Outcomes.* 2002; 10: pp. 85–91.
82. Green LW, Gielen AC. Evidence and ecological theory in two public health successes for health behavior change. In: Kahan S, Gielen AC, Fagan PJ, Green LW, eds. *Health Behavior Change in Populations.* Johns Hopkins University Press; 2014. pp. 26–43.
83. Phelan JC, Link BG, Tehranifar P. Social conditions as fundamental causes of health inequalities: theory, evidence, and policy implications. *J Health Soc Behav.* 2010; 51 Suppl:S28–40. doi: 10.1177/0022146510383498.

Chapter 2
Models of Health Behavior Change and Treatment Adherence

Being sick is not easy. Illness can cut to the heart of who a person is; it can threaten so much about them: their livelihood, their sense of self, their valued activities, their self-presentation, their unique creative expression, their relationships with others, and their plans and hopes for the future.

Many illnesses can leave a person feeling terrible—restless, exhausted, and in pain.[1] Acute conditions can be bad enough, consuming time and resources, adding fear and worry. These experiences are temporary; acute conditions might not get better immediately, but they will get better. The fractured limb is rested for six weeks, or the medicine is taken for eight, and the patient is grateful that modern medicine makes them well once again.

As we have already seen in Chapter 1, however, this is not true for chronic conditions. More than six in 10 adults in the United States have at least one chronic illness.[2] These are serious ailments which, if not managed properly, can cause significant long-term suffering and even death. They include such conditions as heart disease, chronic lung disease, stroke, diabetes, and chronic kidney disease, just to name a few.

Chronic illness, by definition, remains with the person for the rest of their life. There is no opportunity to be completely well again; there is only the possibility of managing the condition and being grateful for a halt or slowing of its progression. Chronic illness can make many people depressed. Rates of depression are two to three times higher among chronically ill patients compared with age- and gender-matched controls.[2-4] Chronic illness also predicts future depressive episodes.[5] Comorbid depression can propel individuals into pessimism, cause them to withdraw from others, and interfere with their cognitive processes. Case Study 2.1 illustrates how chronic illness affects Carl's life.

> **Case Study 2.1 Carl**
>
> Carl is only 54 years old, an age that seems ancient to his 16-year-old son Jamal; according to the U.S. actuarial life table,[6] Carl's life expectancy is another 25 years. There is a lot that he would like to experience and enjoy, but Carl smokes cigarettes. His doctors have warned that his lungs are being damaged, and Carl has been diagnosed with emphysema. He used to enjoy playing baseball and running on the beach with his son, but now they opt for sedentary activities together, like playing video games. Some evenings Carl doesn't feel much like bowling with his league, and he misses the great group of friends he has had since high school. Everything takes more effort than it used to. He often feels lethargic and uses caffeine and the nicotine from cigarettes to get himself up and moving for work every day. Carl's doctor said that if he stops smoking, uses his medications properly, and follows a program of graduated aerobic exercise, Carl can slow the progression of damage to his lungs. If he doesn't, his quality of life will probably get much worse and his life expectancy will be reduced.
>
> Carl wishes he could turn back the clock and never start smoking in the first place. He wishes he had understood what the consequences of smoking might be. Back then, he imagined that smoking might lead to a slightly shorter life, but one filled with adventures and a sense of vigor. That is not how it is turning out for him.

Understanding irrational health-related behaviors

We might expect that people would be more interested in preventing chronic illness than they apparently are. On the surface, the most rational choice is to *prevent* things like emphysema from smoking, liver disease from alcohol abuse, stroke from uncontrolled hypertension, or retinopathy and amputations from unmanaged diabetes. In Chapter 1, we saw that preventive health behaviors and treatment adherence can significantly improve longevity and quality of life and can help avoid some medical problems entirely. But we also saw some rather grim statistics on the prevalence of unhealthy behaviors that contribute to the development and exacerbation of many chronic disease conditions.

How can we understand this disconnection between the most rational choices and what people are actually doing? This is essentially the topic of this entire book. Why, when information is available to people about how to protect their health, do so many forego preventive health behaviors and adherence to treatment? Why do so many still smoke?[7] Why do many people who are overweight or obese consume large amounts of high fat foods and lead sedentary lives?[8] Why don't people (including 30% of health professionals working in hospitals) wash their hands properly to prevent illness?[9,10] Why did vaccination efforts to prevent hospitalization and death from COVID-19 meet with such resistance?[11]

Failing to engage in preventive health behaviors and adherence seems irrational, especially in the face of potentially serious chronic disease. Researchers have been trying to understand this seeming irrationality for decades, and they have built a number of theoretical models to explain what people are thinking and why they make the choices they do. Many researchers have concluded, not surprisingly, that the factors driving health behavior are *complicated*. These factors involve what people are thinking, believing, feeling, and concluding, as well as the environments in which people are embedded, the constraints on their resources, and the social pressures they face. The theoretical models built to explain health behavior and treatment adherence vary in their level of complexity; in this chapter, we examine their development, application, effectiveness, and limitations.

Theoretical models of health behavior and treatment adherence

Health professionals and researchers have developed a number of useful theoretical models for understanding health actions and the strategies people use to maintain behavioral change. While some explanatory models have received more empirical evaluation than others, each can be helpful in some contexts and can provide a useful organizational structure to help us address the maintenance of health behavior change and adherence to treatment plans.

Prominent in these models are the constructs of "beliefs" and "attitudes." Beliefs involve conclusions about the truth of something and are *cognitive* elements in the picture of how people evaluate and respond to ideas. Attitudes include affective (emotional) elements and involve *evaluative states* based on the individual's personal feelings and emotions regarding a belief. In other words, attitudes subsume beliefs. For example, if Devin believes that exercise is unpleasant, his attitude toward exercise will likely be negative, even if he is willing to admit (i.e., he believes) that exercise is important.

Two psychologists, Icek Ajzen and Martin Fishbein, first proposed in the 1970s that beliefs precede attitudes and, further, that attitudes are the precursors for (and driving forces behind) individuals' intentions to perform behavior as well as the actual performance.[12] Others have built upon these foundational ideas. In this chapter, we examine the best-known models of health behavior along with the contributions they have made to our understanding of behavior change and adherence. We provide explanations of the use and effectiveness of each model as well as a summary of problems or weaknesses in each of the approaches.

Health Belief Model

The Health Belief Model was originally developed to explain engagement in preventive health behaviors.[13] In the early 1950s, researchers at the U.S. Public Health Service were specifically interested in why people were willing, or not willing, to undergo x-ray screening for tuberculosis, and why some people would refuse to obtain needed immunizations. More research studies have been based on this model than on any other. The Health Belief Model focuses primarily on beliefs as the motivators of health behavior. These include: (1) beliefs about how susceptible or at-risk a person is to a particular disease or other negative health outcome, (2) beliefs about how severe an illness or negative health outcome might be, if the person did develop it, (3) beliefs about whether recommended treatments are effective or whether health behavior change is feasible and beneficial, and (4) beliefs about how well-equipped one is to confront the challenges of achieving and maintaining health. These challenges include such potential barriers as the inability to regulate one's own behavior, the financial cost associated with treatment, and the time constraints of health behavior.

Additional factors that have been added to the model over the years include demographic characteristics (e.g., age, gender) and environmental cues (e.g., a doctor's recommendation, a friend's heart attack) that might motivate a person to take action.[14] These additions highlight the fact that while individual perceptions, beliefs, and attitudes are critically important, they are not sufficient to predict actual health behaviors. One must look to the individual's life to understand the role of additional idiosyncratic factors.

As do all models, the Health Belief Model has limitations. Over the years, for example, elements have been added to its original form; in research, however, these elements are loosely connected to underlying theory and tend to be suboptimal in their measurement and linkage with behavioral outcomes. Further, in some research studies, the outcomes assessed are behavioral *intentions* rather than behaviors, limiting the utility of the Health Belief Model as a template for designing effective health behavior interventions. Nonetheless, the Health Belief Model is one of the best-known theories and it makes important contributions to understanding health behavior partly because it emphasizes the crucial role of the individual's *perceptions* in choosing and carrying out health behaviors.

After 1988, self-efficacy (the belief that one is capable of enacting change) was formally added to the Health Belief Model, making a theoretically valuable (although empirically modest) contribution of this model to predicting behavioral outcomes.[15] Incorporating efficacy-expectations (i.e., belief in one's ability to change) and outcome-expectancies (i.e., expectations for what will happen following a behavior) makes the model even more useful in developing effective interventions for behavior change. Addressing efficacy expectations has clearly enhanced our understanding of the role of beliefs in changing health behaviors. Figure 2.1 depicts the elements of the Health Belief Model.

The body of research involving the Health Belief Model has become quite substantial. In a classic 1984 review, Janz and Becker examined 46 studies conducted between 1956 and 1984.[16] Twenty-four of these focused on preventive health behaviors, 19 involved seeking and following treatment, and three examined healthcare utilization (e.g., clinic visits, appointment-keeping). Each of the dimensions of the Health Belief Model was significantly associated with health behavior, and perceptions of the barriers to change figured most prominently. Barriers were followed closely by perceived susceptibility, perceived benefits associated with change, and perceived severity of the disease or negative health outcome. It has been hypothesized that perceptions of disease severity might be relatively less important to individuals who are contemplating primary prevention behaviors and more important to those who already have a diagnosis and want to prevent disease progression.

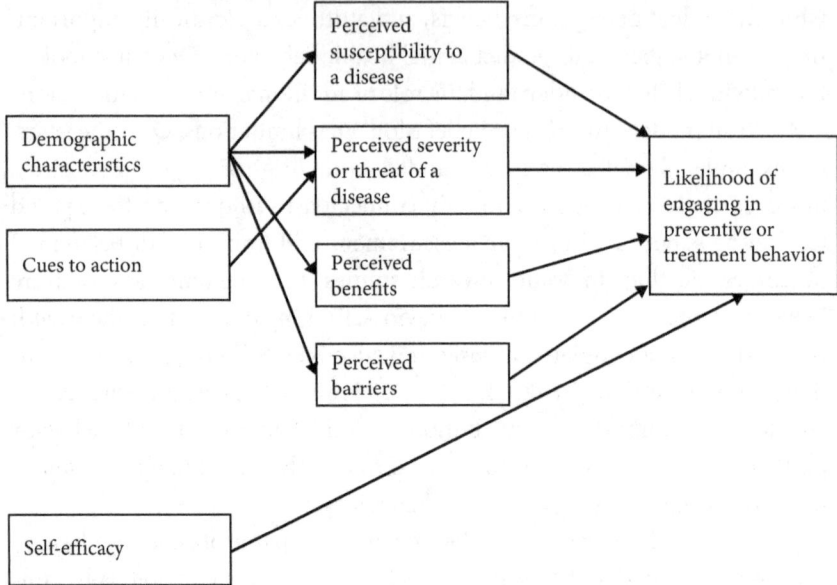

Figure 2.1 Health Belief Model

Later studies on the Health Belief Model are generally consistent with findings from the 1984 large-scale review, although they emphasize the variability in predictive success of the model's components depending on the population or health outcome studied. For instance, Wallace's research on college women's engagement in weight-bearing exercise and intake of calcium to prevent osteoporosis found that self-efficacy, perceived barriers, and perceived susceptibility were the strongest predictors of these health actions.[17] On the other hand, recent meta-analyses of diabetes management,[18] mammography screening,[19] COVID-19 vaccination intention,[20] and general health behavior[21] found that perceived benefits, cues to action, and combinations of perceived benefits and cues to action, and perceived benefits and barriers were the best predictors.

In these studies of the Health Belief Model, perceptions about the severity of a disease did not emerge as the most important element in predicting behavior; in some cases, though, severity perceptions can still be quite meaningful. Beliefs about severity appear to play a larger role for those already diagnosed with a disease than they do for primary prevention. A meta-analysis of the relationship between perceived disease severity and adherence behaviors found that if patients believe that their disease is serious and threatening, they are almost 2.5 times more likely to adhere to their treatment recommendations than if they view the disease as less ominous.[22] When findings from meta-analyses are considered in the aggregate, they clearly indicate that the adoption and maintenance of good health behaviors require health messages and recommendations (particularly from healthcare professionals) that are compelling and persuasive.[16,18–23] If individuals are well informed about the potential dangers of unhealthy behavior, they are more likely (but of course, not certain) to follow recommendations for health behavior change.

Theory of Reasoned Action

In the mid-to late-1970's, researchers formalized the theory that behavior is driven by *intentions* that derive from attitudes toward, and social norms about, those behaviors.[12,24] According to this formulation, attitudes involve an overlay of feeling and emotion on specific beliefs that the individual holds. When this idea was first proposed, however, it represented a distinct divergence from earlier social-psychological thought, which viewed attitudes as the "readiness" to respond in a particular way to environmental stimuli. Many studies had demonstrated, however, that attitudes were not always very closely tied to actual behaviors. These findings necessitated the development of a more complex model to explain the attitude–behavior relationship, and the Theory of Reasoned Action was born.

Two elements of the Theory of Reasoned Action are particularly noteworthy. The first is that changes in belief are necessary to effect changes in behavior because all behavioral choices are ultimately based on beliefs of one sort or another. Second, an individual's behavioral intention (which is the best predictor of the behavior itself) is governed by the relative importance of personal *attitudes* toward the behavior and *subjective norms* (i.e., the person's beliefs about what others think about the behavior and whether the person *cares* what others think).

Thus, for any specific behavior, personal attitudes may be more or less important depending on the weight carried by the subjective norms. For example, Devin's attitude toward quitting smoking will be partly determined by his beliefs about the link between smoking and lung cancer but may also be influenced by the opinions of his family and friends. Having a group of close friends who also smoke and are not willing to quit might make Devin less inclined to commit himself to quitting, even if he personally believes that smoking leads to lung cancer and is worried about this prospect for himself. Figure 2.2 illustrates the components of the Theory of Reasoned Action.

According to the Theory of Reasoned Action, effective health behavior interventions will take into account the degree to which a particular behavioral intention is influenced by social norms and personal attitudes. Strategies designed to modify beliefs can then be appropriately targeted to the area that most influences behavior.

A great deal of research has focused on testing the tenets of this model, although in many cases, researchers have interpreted the model rather loosely by measuring behavioral outcomes that are not completely under the individual's control, or by assessing and using behavioral predictors while various intentions are still somewhat in flux for the individual. Also, just as with the Health Belief Model, research studies have often used behavioral *intentions* as the measured outcome, instead of actual behaviors. Intentions are most proximal and a necessary precursor to health-related decisions, but they are not actual *behavior*. Despite these caveats, the predictive utility of the Theory of Reasoned Action is robust across a variety of behavioral outcomes.[25] A meta-analysis of studies on condom use, for example, found that this safer sex behavior was related to intentions based on subjective norms and attitudes, and that these attitudes were, in turn, based on normative and behavioral beliefs.[26] Indeed, as predicted by the model, the thoughts and actions of others helped to influence individuals' own condom use. In predicting engagement in physical activity, meta-analyses confirm the importance of a person's intentions, as well as the links between intentions, attitudes, and beliefs.[27,28] The Theory of Reasoned Action also predicts a wide range of other health behaviors including contraception, sunscreen use, screenings, weight loss, smoking cessation, and AIDS-related risk behaviors.[25,29-34]

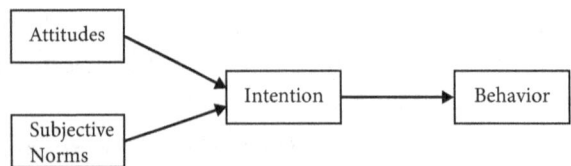

Figure 2.2 Theory of Reasoned Action

Theory of Planned Behavior

The Theory of Planned Behavior is an extension of the Theory of Reasoned Action that was formulated in the 1980s, and is specifically targeted at situations in which individuals do not have full control over the behavior in question.[35,36] As in the Theory of Reasoned Action, an individual's intention is of central importance, but here it is influenced not only by attitudes and subjective norms but also by perceived behavioral control (which is an individual's belief about the amount of control they have over a given behavior). Perceived behavioral control is very similar to the concept of self-efficacy, described as part of the expanded Health Belief Model, and it involves the individual's confidence that they *can* enact change. This already-complex model is made even more complicated by the fact that the relative importance of each of these three elements (attitudes, subjective norms, and perceived behavioral control) varies according to the situation. This added complexity does provide flexibility, and it emphasizes the individualized role of each component when attempting to understand behavior change for a specific person.

Research models typically cannot be applied to individual people using a simple recipe-book approach, however; outcomes cannot be expected to be equivalent for everyone or across different situations. As is often true, a model's intricacy can make it a better representation of reality but can also make it more difficult to test. Despite this, comparisons of the Theory of Reasoned Action with the Theory of Planned Behavior have shown that, for a variety of behaviors, the inclusion of perceptions of behavioral control allows for better prediction of both intentions and behaviors, especially when behaviors are clearly under a person's volitional control.[28,34,37,38] For example, a 2001 meta-analysis of 185 studies published between 1985 and 1997 found that including perceived behavioral control significantly improved the predictive ability of the model; perceptions of control influence intentions, perhaps because a person's belief that they "can do it" prompts them to try.[39] Thus, research suggests that an individual is more likely to attempt a behavior if success seems likely. In fact, even when accomplishment of an aim is not clearly under their control, the *perception that it is* can still be valuable. Thus, if a young man, Devin, can come to believe that he indeed has the willpower to quit smoking, he is more likely to take on the challenge of trying to quit. Figure 2.3 shows the elements of the Theory of Planned Behavior.

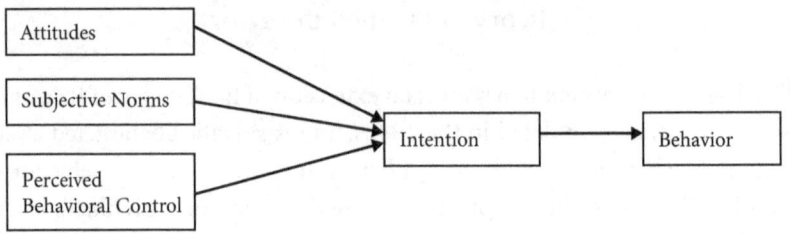

Figure 2.3 Theory of Planned Behavior

The 185-study meta-analysis also showed that the link between subjective norms and intentions may be less robust than other connections in the model; that is, subjective norms appear to be poorer predictors of behavioral intentions. Typically, these norms are assessed with only a single item; therefore, weaknesses in measurement may account for the more limited predictive power of social norms.

This apparent methodological weakness highlights the importance of examining subjective norms carefully and with powerful assessment tools. For example, it has been suggested that the social pressure of subjective norms is moderated by the degree to which an individual identifies with a group of people whose health behavior is relevant to the individual.[40] A good measurement tool will, therefore, assess not only the norm itself but also the degree to which the individual identifies with those who create the norm (even if the norming group is via social media). A person might, for example, identify strongly with work colleagues who are all committed to maintaining a healthy lifestyle. This identification makes subjective norms much more powerful than if there is little connection to the reference group. We will look at social norms and social influence in much more detail in Chapter 7, where we examine sociocultural influences on health behavior, including through social media.

Transtheoretical Model

The Transtheoretical Model grew out of an effort to understand change within a psychotherapeutic setting.[41] In the initial stages of developing this model, during the late 1970s and early 1980s, several processes were defined, including the following: *(1) Consciousness raising*, which involves techniques aimed at increasing a person's awareness (e.g., about the health risks associated with smoking); *(2) Choosing among options*, which allows an individual to see or create more possibilities for action and take personal responsibility for subsequent behavior; and *(3) Contingency control*, which involves providing resources to help a person change their environment and create a system of rewards and punishments that maximize their behavior-change success.

In ongoing work with these concepts, researchers Prochaska and DiClemente suggested that whether individuals are in psychotherapy or using other approaches to behavior change, they progress through stages.[42] These stages involve first thinking about changing a behavior, then becoming determined to enact the change, then actively modifying habits and/or environments, and finally, finding ways to maintain the change. These researchers also found that thinking through and verbalizing different options could be especially important when individuals were just becoming determined to take action. Controlling contingencies (rewards and punishments) tended to work only when the individual reached the stage of actively modifying their habits.

One very useful aspect of this model (indeed, of change models in general) is the recognition that what will most effectively move a person toward their ultimate behavioral goal may vary depending on the individual's current stage. The best strategies for one stage may not be effective at another. For instance, when Devin is giving no serious thought to changing his lifestyle, he likely will ignore any efforts to devise a reward system for him; he probably will not stick to a behavioral change regimen designed by someone else. If he *did* want to change, however, he likely would be motivated to work *with* a health professional to create a personalized and effective plan and stick to it. When a person is trying to change (or to help others change), various tools, interventions, and strategies are available, but they are only likely to work if they are matched to the individual's stage in the change process.

The Transtheoretical Model of Change was formalized in 1983 with five stages that subsumed ten separate proposed "processes for change."[43] These five stages were later revised (based on reevaluations of the statistical models, and more attention to cluster analyses) and were labeled as follows: precontemplation, contemplation, preparation, action, and maintenance.[44] "Relapse" is viewed as a "slide backwards" to restart the cycle at one of the earlier stages.[45] Figure 2.4 depicts the stages of the Transtheoretical Model.

Regarding smoking, Devin is at the first stage (*precontemplation*) and he provides a good model for illustrating each of the stages in the

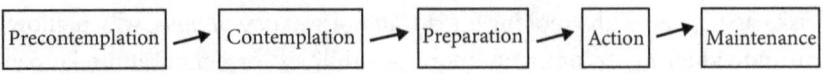

Figure 2.4 Transtheoretical Model

Transtheoretical Model of Change. As we meet him, he is not considering or even contemplating quitting smoking. He is minimally aware of his health risks (primarily lung cancer and heart disease) and he doesn't view them as particularly important. If an event increases the salience of these health risks (e.g., a fellow smoker at work develops lung cancer), Devin might move into the *contemplation* stage, where he would be more fully aware of the issues and would begin contemplating various risk-reduction strategies. In the third stage, *preparation*, Devin would solidify a plan for action and possibly seek advice or help from family, peers, or members of a healthcare team. Devin might use a nicotine patch or gum, ask others to encourage and support him, take on new activities to distract him from his desire to smoke, and avoid places where other people are smoking. Then, in the fourth stage (*action*), Devin would begin to actually give up cigarettes entirely. During the last stage, called *maintenance*, Devin would continue his "action" plan, avoiding pitfalls that might cause him to lapse or relapse, working to build habits that are fully integrated into his lifestyle, and modifying his behavior as his life changes.

Devin's example is simplified above, as we consider the fairly well-defined behavior of smoking. In fact, smoking and its cessation can occur in varying degrees. Devin could reduce but not eliminate his smoking, and utilize cigarettes in varying quantities for varying periods of time. People seldom proceed linearly through the changes described above. Instead, they typically *cycle* through the stages, showing progress and then regression, through various indicators of success or failure. A valuable goal would be to exhibit a general trend toward greater success over time,[44] such as by cutting back on the number of cigarettes per day and maintaining the lower level. Devin's health professional could offer vitally important support by encouraging his progress.

Much of the research literature on the stages-of-change model addresses addictive behaviors like smoking. It is not entirely clear that all of the lower-order constructs in the model (e.g., consciousness-raising, reinforcement management) have the same meaning when other types of behavior change are the focus. For example, in a meta-analysis applying the Transtheoretical Model of Change in 71 published studies on physical activity, researchers attempted to differentiate between processes of change that were experiential (consciousness-raising) and those that were behavioral (reinforcement management). They found that this distinction was not meaningful in the exercise domain, and that in understanding exercise, the stage-by-process interactions were less clear than they have been in studies of psychotherapy and addictive behavior.[46] For some primary prevention behaviors like exercise, the most active behavior change steps occur during the transition from precontemplation to contemplation, suggesting that the most difficult part of changing individuals' exercise behavior (or making other lifestyle changes aimed at prevention) might be getting them to even consider increasing their physical activity. This differs from our smoking example where the risks and benefits of quitting may be more obvious, but the challenges associated with planning and implementation may be greater.

The Transtheoretical Model serves to highlight two very important concepts about health behavior change. First, verbal communication and cognitive processing in the early stages of change are important. What people think, and the things that they say about their health, really do matter. Second, Prochaska and DiClemente hypothesized that if a health professional's focus and direction are very different from that of the patient, or if the two are working at different levels of the change process, the patient can become quite resistant to change.[42] People are particularly likely to drop out of psychotherapy, or to quit behavior change efforts, when their expectations and those of their practitioners are quite disparate. Thus, effective communication is not only an important facilitator of early-stage change, it may be *the key* to establishing an appropriate level at which patient and clinician can target their common efforts.

Social Cognitive Models

The concepts of classical conditioning[47] and operant conditioning (behavior modification)[48] combine with an emphasis on cognitive processing to form the foundation for Social Cognitive Models. Sometimes labeled Social Learning Theories,[49,50] these approaches posit that both personal expectancies and environmental factors (e.g., reinforcements) determine behavior, and that modifying *either* of these can result in behavioral change.

Expectancies may be of several kinds. Individuals might expect that certain events are related to each other *causally* (i.e., in terms of cause and effect). They might have "outcome expectations" about the *consequences* of personal action. Or individuals might have expectancies of the likelihood of their own personal success (the *self-efficacy* we introduced previously). In all of these cases, expectations about what is likely to "happen next" can influence attitudes, intentions, and behaviors.

Similarly, the environments in which a person lives, works, and plays provide feedback to the individual. Some behaviors are met with praise or other rewards, while other behaviors result in less positive outcomes, serving to encourage or discourage similar behaviors in the future. Thus, managing behavioral consequences is one way of influencing the behaviors themselves. Figure 2.5 illustrates the components of the Social Cognitive Theory.

There are some similarities between Social Cognitive Models and the Health Belief Model.[15] As a group, Social Cognitive Models hold as crucially important the inclusion of cognitive elements such as self-efficacy (also an important component of the HBM). Other cognitive factors, including beliefs about the causes of various outcomes and the sense that they can be controlled, also warrant attention according to Social Cognitive Models.

Self-regulation (which includes self-reflection and observational learning) provides an additional mechanism for achieving desired outcomes and maintaining changes over time. Strategies such as learning through observation and reflecting on one's successes and failures, along with a good understanding of other cognitive processes (such as how we see causes and effects) represent a set of tools that can be quite useful when working toward health behavior change and treatment adherence.

An individual's own unique experiences, beliefs, and personal attributes influence their responses to new information, to environmental reinforcements, to motivational messages, and to other potential triggers for behavioral change. In every application of theoretical models to the motivation and management of real people, we must pay close attention to the ways in which personal characteristics can alter the meaning of environmental

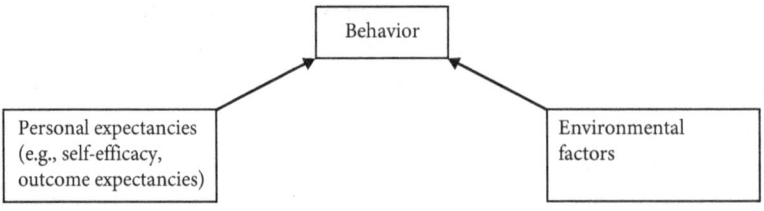

Figure 2.5 Social Cognitive Theory

factors for an individual. Close attention to the "person by environment interaction" allows us to tailor behavior change strategies to the individual, optimizing the likelihood of successful change. Failure to attend to this interaction prevents us from accurately reflecting the individual's views, beliefs, motivations, and expectations. Such interventions are less likely to succeed, even if they seem to be well conceived. We consider these issues in more detail in Chapter 4, where we examine the interplay between personal characteristics and external factors. And in Chapter 7, we consider social cognitive models in further detail, and examine how social comparison, social media, social influences, and the individual's sociocultural context affect health behavior and treatment adherence.

Precaution Adoption Process Model

Like the Transtheoretical Model of Change, the Precaution Adoption Process Model is a stage model which, rather than predicting levels of behavior across individuals, focuses on an individual's change over time. It is aimed specifically at understanding reactions to health hazards and the initiation of new or more complex precautionary health behaviors. This model, formally proposed in 1988, presumes seven specific stages, some of which are similar to those described in the Transtheoretical Model of Change. In the Precaution Adoption Process Model, the individual is first unaware, then aware but disengaged, then engaged and deciding what action to take, then deciding to act (or not to act, at least not yet), then acting, and finally maintaining the adopted behavior.[51,52] Just as optimal strategies are proposed to vary by stage, barriers to change have also been found, in several studies, to differ according to stage.[52-54]

For example, in 1992 researchers[52] applied this theory to precautions taken to mitigate lung cancer risk by reducing radon gas exposure in the home. In the first stages of this model, a person is not aware of radon gas and its associated risks. Once radon gas is learned about, the individual's initial reaction may depend upon their sense that it is personally relevant. The next stages involve the individual recognizing that they are indeed at risk, then identifying precautionary steps that might be taken (such as increasing ventilation in the home to reduce radon exposure), and, finally, following through and implementing those precautionary measures. Figure 2.6 depicts the stages of the Precaution Adoption Process Model.

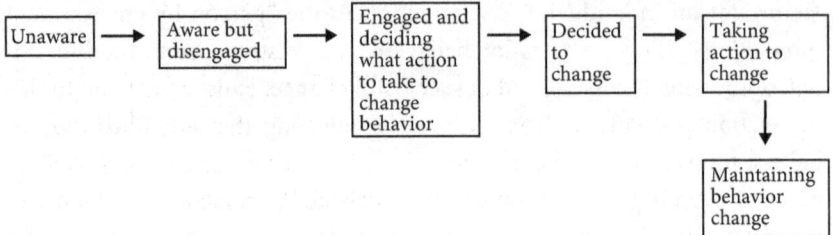

Figure 2.6 Precaution Adoption Process Model

Studies have also demonstrated that with some health hazards, individuals do not progress beyond the early stages of awareness; they believe that the problem may exist for others but that they are not personally vulnerable. Recommended "precautions" in the absence of an obvious and immediate threat may not sufficiently motivate an individual to act and change their relevant behaviors. Someone with hypertension, for example, might never adopt a low-sodium diet because they have no symptoms and believe that they are in no danger of having a stroke.[51]

Tests of the Precaution Adoption Process Model have not unequivocally demonstrated that the sequence of stages proposed by the model is the "right" sequence, but studies to date are promising. Some have yielded surprisingly large effect sizes (i.e., measures of the strength of the relationship between two variables). It does seem clear, though, that when we know which stage an individual is in, we can more easily identify barriers to change and find ways to encourage them to take precautions.

While stage models can be very useful, it is important to keep in mind that they are descriptive (rather than explanatory) and that stages can vary widely along various dimensions (e.g., time frame, intensity). Stages can also differ between people and can fluctuate over time for the same person, as research has found with parents' intentions for children's HPV vaccinations. Fluctuation was more likely, of course, for parents whose initial hesitancy was more "flexible" compared with those showing more "rigid" hesitancy.[55]

Information-Motivation-Strategy Model

This final model is a conceptual approach to guiding adherence and health behavior change, designed to simplify and consolidate many components of the previous models, while including a broader range of health-related behaviors.[56] This model is based on the design recommended by DiMatteo and DiNicola.[57] The Information-Motivation-Strategy Model states that before a person can achieve health behavior change, that person must: *(1)* know what change is necessary (*information*); *(2)* have the desire to change (*motivation*); and *(3)* have the necessary tools to achieve and then maintain the change (*strategy*). A great deal of evidence links each of these components to positive patient outcomes including health behavior change and treatment adherence. Figure 2.7 shows the components of the Information-Motivation-Strategy Model.

Due to the flexible nature of this model, it easily incorporates new techniques and strategies while remaining consistent with many of the cornerstones present in the other models and theories already described in this chapter. For instance, the information component of the model includes health literacy, beliefs, knowledge, memory or recall of what to do, and other related factors. Motivation involves attitudes, feelings, confidence, and expectations, among other elements. Finally, the strategies to create and maintain change include physical tools such as monetary resources, practical tools such as time, and social tools such as support of friends and loved ones. Some of these factors have been discussed in this chapter, and others will be detailed in later chapters.

Throughout this book we will refer to components of each of the models and theories presented in this chapter, and we will especially emphasize the concepts of informing, motivating, and strategizing. For an individual making personal health behavior changes and for healthcare professionals trying to help their patients change, the theoretical models of health behavior, along with the research evidence supporting them, provide a sturdy foundation for understanding. In this book we delve further into the complexities of individual behavior change. We describe how information and motivation

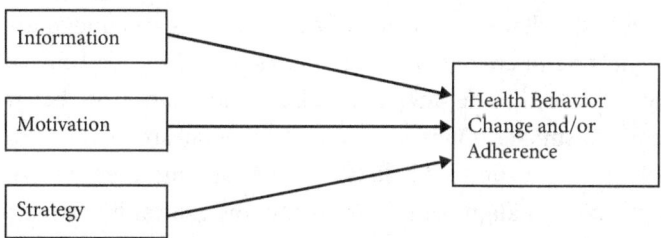

Figure 2.7 Information-Motivation-Strategy Model

are crucial elements of the behavior change process and recognize that even if people have a good idea of *what* should be done, they may have no clear sense of *how* to do it effectively. We focus intensively on the strategy component, offering tools that, when carefully selected and implemented, can help create and maintain lasting change.

Cognitive dissonance reduction and behavior change

The Theory of Cognitive Dissonance,[58] a foundational concept in the field of social psychology, argues that a discordance between two beliefs, or between one's beliefs and one's behavior, leads to a sense of discomfort. This discomfort can motivate people to change either their behavior or their beliefs in order to reduce it. Case Study 2.2 examines how Martine experiences cognitive dissonance regarding the management of his chronic illness.

> **Case Study 2.2 Martine**
>
> Martine has diabetes, and he believes in the importance of preparing and eating whole foods to manage his blood sugar levels; he is rarely able to do so, however. He eats mostly processed foods because of the time and energy required to shop for and cook healthy meals. He knows all about the dangers of cigarette smoking, and he really wants to quit completely, but he still smokes nearly every day. Martine recognizes that there is a significant disconnection between what he says he believes about health behavior, and what he actually does. It is in this disconnection that there may be an opportunity for change.

The Theory of Cognitive Dissonance predicts that believing smoking is dangerous while simultaneously being a smoker will create enough discomfort to push Martine to change one of these. He could decide (unwisely) that smoking is perfectly safe after all, or he could change his behavior and become a nonsmoker. Once a person is made aware of the inconsistencies between their expressed beliefs and their actions, they are likely to try to bring these into alignment.[59] Regarding his unhealthy eating patterns, Martine is unlikely to argue that healthy eating is not desirable, or that managing his diabetes is not necessary. Instead, to achieve cognitive dissonance reduction, he would be likely to change his behavior (with some helpful strategies) to bring it into line with his beliefs. In the absence of something like diabetes, however, a person might decide that dietary changes are too difficult and instead rationalize that eating healthfully isn't very important so long as one takes a multivitamin regularly.

A multilevel determinants approach

Many individual, interpersonal, sociocultural, and contextual environmental factors can affect the ability of an individual to change. These include psychological factors (cognitions, emotions), demographics, interpersonal (social) factors, and characteristics of the target behavior or regimen. They also include financial and cost factors, characteristics of the disease as a target for prevention or management, variables in the treatment context such as the relationship between provider and patient, unique elements of the health delivery system, and contextual factors that affect the individual's thinking and functioning in relation to ongoing challenges.[60] With a multiple determinants model approach, researchers strive to understand not only behavior change but also how these factors affect health, health risks, functioning, and quality of life.[61] Case Study 2.3 shows the multiple levels of factors that drive Rosalie's health behavior as she manages her chronic illness.

Case Study 2.3 Rosalie

Rosalie is a full-time nursing student and a full-time care manager at a nursing home. She is also a single mom to her 5-year-old son, Max. Rosalie considers herself very lucky to have her sister, who lives nearby and has two children of her own, provide the childcare she needs for Max when he is not in school. Financial stresses definitely occupy her mind, as tuition, rent, food, and transportation costs keep rising. Rosalie has type 2 diabetes; she has difficulty managing her weight, and she has hypertension. Sometimes she struggles with the symptoms of depression, when the challenges of her life feel overwhelming to her.

Lately, Rosalie has faced a few unique stresses as a single working parent who is also a student. The internet in her apartment building has become unreliable and this interferes with her online classes and research as well as her communication with professors and other students. Rosalie commutes to school and work by subway and bus, and although she had hoped to use her commuting time to study, the crowded spaces make that difficult. Rosalie is often deprived of adequate sleep, forcing herself to get up in the middle of the night to study when it is quiet. To boost her energy to get through her day, Rosalie depends on coffee, simple carbohydrates, and processed foods that are high in sugar, fat, and salt. Now and then, she smokes a cigarette to keep herself going. Rosalie wants so much to be a good role model for healthy eating for Max, but her neighborhood has little fresh produce available to purchase, and Rosalie does not have the funds or the time to buy and prepare it. She wants to avoid cigarettes completely because she knows what a danger they are to her health, and she wants to exercise but she does not feel completely safe walking in her neighborhood.

Fortunately, Rosalie has resisted the temptation to use alcohol, even when she feels overwhelmed and anxious about the precarity of her situation. She is careful to take her anti-hypertensive and diabetes medications correctly and consistently, and regularly checks her blood pressure. Rosalie's diet, though, is not conducive to the weight loss her doctor hopes for her, nor does it support the management of her blood glucose levels, which she tends to test sporadically and not nearly often enough.

In terms of some of our earlier models above, Rosalie holds attitudes and beliefs that are very much in line with treatment adherence and necessary behavior change. As a future nurse, she believes wholeheartedly in the importance of medication, and she wants very much to have consistently positive health behaviors. She knows what she needs to do behaviorally, although in practice taking medication is so much easier than the many lifestyle changes required. So, in Rosalie's case, her beliefs, plans, expectations, and hopes all align to point to behavior change. In practice, however, it is all just too difficult in the context of the many, sometimes crushing, responsibilities she faces as she tries to better her own life and that of her son.

The Social Determinants of Health (SDOH) approach is a social-ecological framework stating that conditions in people's physical and social environments can often work to constrain the range of health behaviors and quality-of-life outcomes that are open to them.[62] Rosalie's case reminds us that we must broaden our perspective beyond the models we examined earlier to ensure that we carefully consider the individual's context. Rosalie believes in the importance of eating whole foods, not smoking, getting regular exercise, and effectively managing her diabetes with glucose monitoring and medications. However, she faces contextual challenges that could easily discourage even the most dedicated health-behavior enthusiast. In order to understand and support Rosalie toward her goal of improving her health and that of her son, we must remain aware of the bigger picture of Rosalie's life and circumstances. She is doing her best in the face of limited options and opportunities; she faces pressures that, despite her best intentions, get in the way of her optimal health behavior.

Throughout this book, we focus on a multilevel approach to health behavior and treatment adherence, including the social determinants of health. We examine how the challenges of achieving health are driven by a complex combination of many forces: individual determinants (such as beliefs and attitudes), interpersonal determinants (such as families, social networks, and online communities), sociocultural determinants (including ethnic background and socioeconomic environments), and structural and policy determinants (such as healthcare delivery systems, health policies, and the built environment). Dr. William H. Dietz, a prominent researcher on obesity prevention, nutrition, and physical activity, has emphasized the important role of context in understanding and improving health behaviors as follows: "An individual cannot be expected to make healthful choices unless there are healthful choices to make (p. xi)."[62] This multilevel determinants approach serves to guide us clinically, as a template to explore each person's unique circumstances with an eye toward helping with some of them, and perhaps offering a better perspective on others. In our research and in our clinical work, we must use this bigger picture to better understand the complexity of each individual's behavior in health and illness and help them to achieve their best possible health outcomes.

Summary

This chapter reviews the theoretical models that have guided thinking and research on health behavior change, providing an historical perspective on major developments in this field of study. Included in this chapter's overview are the Health Belief Model, Theory of Reasoned Action, Theory of Planned

Behavior, Transtheoretical Model of Change, Social-Cognitive Models, Precaution Adoption Process Model, and the Information-Motivation-Strategy Model. We examine the Theory of Cognitive Dissonance in understanding how an individual's cognitions and beliefs relate to their health behaviors, and we consider ways in which all of these models contribute to understanding behavior change both in clinical medical practice and at the population level.

In this chapter, we also adjust our perspective to consider, within a social-ecological framework, a multilevel contextual approach to individual, interpersonal, sociocultural, and contextual environmental factors as we examine health behavior change and treatment adherence. This multilevel approach allows for analysis of the complexity of many factors in the full context of the patient's life that drive and/or constrain his or her adherence and health behavior change. These include individual factors (cognitions, emotions, attitudes, beliefs), demographics and socioeconomic factors, interpersonal (family, social network) and cultural/sociocultural factors, regimen factors, as well as environmental, organizational, and policy determinants. We examine the contexts in which health behavior models have been tested, along with their effectiveness as demonstrated by the empirical literature. Examples for practical application are also provided, as are caveats and information about contexts in which these models (or portions thereof) are not well supported.

Tools for instruction and self-study

Learning objectives

By the end of this chapter, readers should be able to

1. Describe the difference between beliefs and attitudes.
2. List the components of the Health Belief Model.
3. Differentiate the Theory of Reasoned Action from the Theory of Planned Behavior.
4. Explain the stages of the Transtheoretical Model.
5. Discuss the concept of self-efficacy.
6. Compare and contrast the Precaution Adoption Process Model and the Transtheoretical Model.
7. Describe the components of the Information-Motivation-Strategy Model.

8. Examine how a multilevel determinants approach may be important for researchers and clinicians to consider in understanding challenges to individual health behavior change.

Review questions

1. In the Health Belief Model, what is a "cue to action" and how does it affect health behavior?
2. How is the Theory of Planned Behavior different from the Theory of Reasoned Action? What do the data suggest about the utility of one over the other?
3. What are the five stages of the Transtheoretical Model of Change? How is "relapse" currently understood in this model?
4. How might one describe the social cognitive theories (or models) as a group?
5. Briefly, describe what is meant by each of the elements of the Information-Motivation-Strategy Model.
6. What is cognitive dissonance? Why does it sometimes lead to behavior change and sometimes to changes in beliefs or attitudes?
7. What is meant by a "multilevel determinants approach" to understanding health behavior?

Prompts for discussion and further study

1. What strategies might a healthcare provider use to ensure that a patient experiencing cognitive dissonance about his food choices actually shifts toward healthier eating rather than adjusting his attitudes to be less interested in a nutritious diet?
2. Describe how the Transtheoretical Model of Change might help a physician understand her patient's reluctant response to her recommendations for exercise. How might the concept of "relapse" play out in this patient's efforts to exercise?
3. Select a health-related challenge (e.g., sedentary lifestyle, excessive alcohol consumption, heart disease) and one of the models described in this chapter. Then, describe how a clinician could use the model most effectively to interact with a patient to improve their health behaviors in this area.

Suggested reading

1. Poldrack RA. *Hard to Break: Why Our Brains Make Habits Stick.* Princeton University Press; 2021.
2. O'Rourke M. *The Invisible Kingdom: Reimagining Chronic Illness.* Riverhead Books; 2022.
3. Fajgenbaum D. *Chasing My Cure: A Doctor's Race to Turn Hope into Action; A Memoir.* Ballantine Books; 2019.
4. Jaouad S. *Between Two Kingdoms: A Memoir of a Life Interrupted.* Random House; 2021.

References

1. Strauss AL. *Chronic Illness and the Quality of Life.* Saint Louis, MO: Mosby; 1975.
2. Chronic diseases in America. Centers for Disease Control and Prevention website. December 13, 2022. https://www.cdc.gov/chronic-disease/
3. Ali S, Stone MA, Peters JL, Davies MJ, Khunti K. The prevalence of co-morbid depression in adults with Type 2 diabetes: a systematic review and meta-analysis. *Diabet Med.* 2006; 23(11): pp. 1165–1173. doi: 10.1111/j.1464-5491.2006.01943.x
4. Spijkerman T, de Jonge P, van den Brink RH, et al. Depression following myocardial infarction: first-ever versus ongoing and recurrent episodes. *Gen Hosp Psychiatry.* 2005; 27(6): pp. 411–417. doi: 10.1016/j.genhosppsych.2005.05.007
5. Turvey CL, Schultz SK, Beglinger L, Klein DM. A longitudinal community-based study of chronic illness, cognitive and physical function, and depression. *Am J Geriatr Psychiatry.* 2009; 17(8): pp. 632–641.
6. Actuarial life table, 2020. Social Security Administration website. Retrieved December 17, 2023. https://www.ssa.gov/oact/STATS/table4c6.html
7. Tong EK, Strouse R, Hall J, Kovac M, Schroeder SA. National survey of U.S. health professionals' smoking prevalence, cessation practices, and beliefs. *Nicotine Tob Res.* 2010; 12(7): pp. 724–733. doi: 10.1093/ntr/ntq071
8. Sturm R. Increases in morbid obesity in the USA: 2000–2005. *Public Health.* 2007; 121(7): pp. 492–496. doi: 10.1016/j.puhe.2007.01.006
9. Measuring hand hygiene adherence: overcoming the challenges. Joint Commission, 2009. Retrieved December 17, 2023. https://www.jointcommission.org//media/tjc/documents/resources/hai/hh_monograph.pdf
10. Tousman S, Arnold D, Helland W, et al. Evaluation of a hand washing program for 2nd-graders. *Journal of School Nursing.* 2007; 23: pp. 342–348.
11. Fitzpatrick MC, Moghadas SM, Pandey A, Galvani AP. Two years of U.S. COVID-19 vaccines have prevented millions of hospitalizations and deaths. *To the Point* (blog), Commonwealth Fund. December 13, 2022. https://doi.org/10.26099/whsf-fp90; https://www.commonwealthfund.org/blog/2022/two-years-covid-vaccines-prevented-millions-deaths-hospitalizations
12. Ajzen I, Fishbein M. *Understanding Attitudes and Predicting Social Behavior.* Englewood Cliffs, NJ: Prentice Hall; 1980.

13. Rosenstock IM. Historical origins of the Health Belief Model. *Health Education Monographs.* 1974; 2(4).
14. Becker MH, Maiman LA. Sociobehavioral determinants of compliance with health and medical care recommendations. *Med Care.* 1975; 13(1): pp. 10–24.
15. Rosenstock IM, Strecher VJ, Becker MH. Social learning theory and the Health Belief Model. *Health Educ Q.* 1988; 15(2): pp. 175–183.
16. Janz NK, Becker MH. The Health Belief Model: a decade later. *Health Educ Behav.* 1984; 11(1): pp. 1–47.
17. Wallace LS. Osteoporosis prevention in college women: application of the expanded Health Belief Model. *Am J Health Behav.* 2002; 26(3): pp. 163–172.
18. Khosravizadeh O, Ahadinezhad B, Maleki A, Vosoughi P, Najafpour Z. Applying the health belief model and behavior of diabetic patients: a systematic review and meta-analysis. *Clinical Diabetology.* 2021; 10(2): pp. 209–220.
19. Ritchie D, Van den Broucke S, Van Hal G. The health belief model and theory of planned behavior applied to mammography screening: a systematic review and meta-analysis. *Public Health Nurs.* 2021; 38(3): pp. 482–492. doi: 10.1111/phn.12842
20. Yenew C, Dessie AM, Gebeyehu AA, Genet A. Intention to receive COVID-19 vaccine and its health belief model (HBM)-based predictors: a systematic review and meta-analysis. *Hum Vaccin Immunother.* 2023; 19(1): 2207442. doi: 10.1080/21645515.2023.2207442
21. Carpenter CJ. A meta-analysis of the effectiveness of health belief model variables in predicting behavior. *Health Commun.* 2010; 25(8): pp. 661–669. doi: 10.1080/10410236.2010.521906
22. DiMatteo MR, Haskard KB, Williams SL. Health beliefs, disease severity, and patient adherence: a meta-analysis. *Med Care.* 2007; 45(6): pp. 521–528.
23. Harrison JA, Mullen PD, Green LW. A meta-analysis of studies of the Health Belief Model with adults. *Health Educ Res.* 1992; 7(1): pp. 107–116.
24. Fishbein M, Ajzen, I. *Belief, Attitude, Intention, and Behavior: An Introduction to Theory and Research.* Reading, MA: Addison-Wesley; 1975.
25. Sheppard BH, Hartwick, J, Warshaw, PL. The theory of reasoned action: a meta-analysis of past research with recommendations of modifications and future research. *J Consum Res.* 1988; 15: pp. 325–343.
26. Albarracin D, Johnson BT, Fishbein M, Muellerleile PA. Theories of Reasoned Action and Planned Behavior as models of condom use: a meta-analysis. *Psychol Bull.* 2001; 127(1): pp. 142–161.
27. Hagger MS, Chatzisarantis NL, Biddle SJ. The influence of autonomous and controlling motives on physical activity intentions within the Theory of Planned Behaviour. *Br J Health Psychol.* 2002; 7(Part 3): pp. 283–297.
28. Downs DS, Hausenblas HA. The theories of reasoned action and planned behavior applied to exercise: a meta-analytic update. *Journal of Physical Activity and Health.* 2005; 2(1), pp. 76–97.
29. Doll J, Orth B. The Fishbein and Ajzen Theory of Reasoned Action applied to contraceptive behavior: model variants and meaningfulness. *J Appl Soc Psychol.* 1993; 23(5): pp. 395–415.
30. Fisher WA, Fisher JD, Rye BJ. Understanding and promoting AIDS-preventive behavior: insights from the Theory of Reasoned Action. *Health Psychol.* 1995; 14(3): pp. 255–264.

31. Godin G, Kok G. The Theory of Planned Behavior: a review of its applications to health-related behaviors. *Am J Health Promot*. 1996; 11(2): pp. 87–98.
32. Hillhouse JJ, Stair AW, 3rd, Adler CM. Predictors of sunbathing and sunscreen use in college undergraduates. *J Behav Med*. 1996; 19(6): pp. 543–561.
33. Montano DE, Taplin SH. A test of an expanded Theory of Reasoned Action to predict mammography participation. *Soc Sci Med*. 1991; 32(6): pp. 733–741.
34. Cooke R, French DP. How well do the theory of reasoned action and theory of planned behaviour predict intentions and attendance at screening programmes? A meta-analysis. *Psychol Health*. 2008; 23(7): pp. 745–765. doi: 10.1080/08870440701544437
35. Ajzen I. From intentions to actions: a Theory of Planned Behavior. In: Beckman JKJ, ed. *Action-control: From Cognition to Behavior*. Heidelberg: Springer; 1985. pp. 11–39.
36. Ajzen I. The Theory of Planned Behavior. *Organizational Behavior and Human Decision Processes*. 1991; 50: pp. 179–211.
37. Hausenblas HA, Carron AV, Mack DE. Application of the Theories of Reasoned Action and Planned Behavior to exercise behavior: a meta-analysis. *J Sport Exercise Psychol*. 1997; 19(1): pp. 36–51.
38. Madden TJ, Ellen PS, Ajzen I. A comparison of the Theory of Planned Behavior and the Theory of Reasoned Action. *Pers Soc Psychol Bull*. 1992; 18(1): pp. 3–9.
39. Armitage CJ, Conner M. Efficacy of the Theory of Planned Behaviour: a meta-analytic review. *Br J Soc Psychol*. 2001; 40(Pt 4): pp. 471–499. doi: 10.1348/014466601164939.
40. Terry DJ, Hogg MA. Group norms and the attitude-behavior relationship: a role for group identification. *Pers Soc Psychol Bull*. 1996; 22(8): pp. 776–793.
41. Prochaska J. *Systems of Psychotherapy: A Transtheoretical Analysis*. Homewood, IL: Dorsey Press; 1979.
42. Prochaska JO, DiClemente CC. Transtheoretical therapy: toward a more integrative model of change. *Psychotherapy: Theory, Research and Practice*. 1982; 19(3): pp. 276–288.
43. Prochaska JO, DiClemente CC. Stages and processes of self-change of smoking: toward an integrative model of change. *J Consult Clin Psychol*. 1983; 51(3): pp. 390–395.
44. Prochaska JO, DiClemente CC, Norcross JC. In search of how people change. Applications to addictive behaviors. *Am Psychol*. 1992; 47(9): pp. 1102–1114.
45. DiClemente CC, Prochaska JO, Fairhurst SK, Velicer WF, Velasquez MM, Rossi JS. The process of smoking cessation: an analysis of precontemplation, contemplation, and preparation stages of change. *J Consult Clin Psychol*. 1991; 59(2): pp. 295–304.
46. Marshall SJ, Biddle SJ. The Transtheoretical Model of behavior change: a meta-analysis of applications to physical activity and exercise. *Ann Behav Med*. 2001; 23(4): pp. 229–246.
47. Pavlov I. *Conditioned Reflexes: An Investigation of the Physiological Activity of the Cerebral Cortex*. London: Oxford University Press; 1927.
48. Bandura A. *Principles of Behavior Modification*. New York: Holt, Rinehart, & Winston; 1969.
49. Bandura A. *Social Learning Theory*. Englewood Cliffs, NJ: Prentice Hall; 1977.
50. Rotter JB. *Social Learning and Clinical Psychology*. New York: Prentice Hall; 1954.

51. Weinstein ND. The Precaution Adoption Process. *Health Psychol.* 1988; 7(4): 355–386.
52. Weinstein ND, Sandman PM. A model of the Precaution Adoption Process: evidence from home radon testing. *Health Psychol.* 1992; 11(3): pp. 170–180.
53. Blalock SJ, DeVellis RF, Giorgino KB, DeVellis BM, Gold DT, Dooley MA, Anderson JJ, Smith SL. Osteoporosis prevention in premenopausal women: using a stage model approach to examine the predictors of behavior. *Health Psychol.* 1996; 15(2): pp. 84–93.
54. Weinstein ND, Lyon JE, Sandman PM, Cuite CL. Experimental evidence for stages of health behavior change: the precaution adoption process model applied to home radon testing. *Health Psychol.* 1998; 17(5): pp. 445–453.
55. Tatar O, Shapiro GK, Perez S, Wade K, Rosberger Z. Using the precaution adoption process model to clarify human papillomavirus vaccine hesitancy in Canadian parents of girls and parents of boys. *Hum Vaccin Immunother.* 2019; 15(7–8): pp. 1803–1814. doi: 10.1080/21645515.2019.1575711
56. DiMatteo MR, Haskard-Zolnierek KB, Martin LR. Improving patient adherence: a three-factor model to guide practice. *Health Psychology Review.* 2012; 6(1), pp. 74–91. doi: 10.1080/17437199.2010.537592
57. DiMatteo MR, DiNicola DD. *Achieving Patient Compliance.* New York: Pergamon Press; 1982.
58. Festinger L. *A Theory of Cognitive Dissonance.* Stanford University Press; 1957.
59. Spangenberg ER, Kareklas I, Devezer B, Sprott DE. A meta-analytic synthesis of the question–behavior effect. *Journal of Consumer Behavior.* 2016; 26(3): pp. 441–458.
60. Williams SL, Haskard Zolnierek KB. Psychosocial predictors of behavior change. In: Hilliard ME, Riekert KA, Ockene JK, Pbert L, eds. *The Handbook of Health Behavior Change.* 5th ed. New York, NY: Springer; 2018; pp. 51–73.
61. Social determinants of health. Healthy People 2030, U.S. Department of Health and Human Services, Office of Disease Prevention and Health Promotion. Retrieved December 17, 2023. https://health.gov/healthypeople/priority-areas/social-determinants-health
62. Dietz WH. Foreword. In: Kahan S, Gielen AC, Fagan PJ, Green LW, eds. *Health Behavior Change in Populations.* Baltimore, MD: Johns Hopkins Press; 2014; p. xi.

Chapter 3
Trust and Interpersonal Communication in the Provider-Patient Relationship

Trust and effective interpersonal communication in the provider-patient relationship are essential to promoting health behavior change and to assessing and managing adherence to treatment. Patients do not tell their doctors the truth if they don't trust or particularly like them. While this might seem obvious to us now, the notion that it is clinically beneficial for patients to like and trust their providers is fairly new. Early theories of medical communication held that doctors' and patients' behaviors should be highly scripted—with the doctor in charge and the patient being submissive. The doctor's role embodied social power, and patients, having no power at all, were expected to comply. While this model made sense theoretically, it turns out that, in reality, patients often took power into their own hands by hiding their noncompliance, just as Damien does in Case Study 3.1.

> **Case Study 3.1 Damien**
>
> Damien is athletic, strong, agile, and always up for a game of basketball. He eats healthfully, and doesn't drink alcohol, smoke, vape, or use any other drugs. His friends sometimes tease him because, for a young man of 25, he is surprisingly adherent to most recommended health behaviors. He is not, however, adherent to his prescription medications for hypertension and hypercholesterolemia. Despite a lot of exercise and eating mostly whole foods, Damien's blood pressure and cholesterol levels are concerning, and his primary care physician has told him that he absolutely *must* take his medication.
>
> During one of his recent follow-up visits with Dr. Lowell, a pleasant clinician who believes "the doctor knows best," Damien spent the 8-minute visit (as he told a friend later) trying "not to get busted." Damien

didn't tell Dr. Lowell that he'd failed to refill his prescriptions, and that he'd left the bottles at home for two weeks when traveling with friends. Dr. Lowell spent most of their visit listening to his heart and lungs and filling in the electronic medical record, so Damien was able to hide these facts. His reasons for nonadherence were simple. The medications made Damien feel tired, and because he had no symptoms from his conditions, the pills did not seem necessary. The co-payments for clinic visits and medications were also higher than he could comfortably afford. Knowing nothing of these issues, Dr. Lowell pressed on, assuming that Damien had been following "doctor's orders."

Fortunately, before abandoning treatment entirely and becoming "lost to follow-up" (as the clinic would have labeled him), Damien came back one more time. Dr. Johnson was filling in for Dr. Lowell; he and Damien quickly fell into an easy conversation about Damien's first love, basketball. They talked about the previous day's college game, and about Damien's basketball league, his work, and his junior college classes. Dr. Johnson was clearly interested in Damien as a person, and asked for his thoughts about hypertension, high cholesterol, and the medications prescribed to manage them. Damien explained his position, and Dr. Johnson listened with attention and respect to Damien's descriptions of side effects and financial costs. He responded to Damien with nonjudgmental concern, caring, and empathy. Damien really liked him, and so he told Dr. Johnson the truth.

Throughout this chapter, we review the importance of interpersonal factors in health behavior change and treatment adherence. We consider the roles of familiarity, trust, empathy, and patients' satisfaction with their medical care. And we see that health professionals typically have the chance, just as Dr. Johnson did with Damien, to build partnerships that recognize patients' beliefs and practical circumstances, respect the emotional challenges of their illnesses, and help ease the burdens of carrying out their care.

The roles of provider and patient

The physician-patient relationship was first examined in the mid-20th century by sociologists who viewed it in terms of highly scripted social roles which participants were expected to enact.[1,2] The physician, in the role of healer, was to maintain "nonjudgmental neutrality," always calm, confident, and unmoved by the characteristics or behavior of the patient. The patient was expected to be both obedient and grateful for the physician's competence and dedication to eradicating their common enemy—the disease. Indeed, the "sick role" (the behavior expected of a person too sick to be productive) required that the patient be adherent to "orders" from the physician. Society was believed to function best if people acceded to the power of the physician who told them what to do in order to get well.[1] Doctors and patients were believed to engage in a "social contract" in which the patient, who at that time had very limited access to information about their health, was expected to defer not to the *person of the physician* but to the *social role of the physician*, who had a fiduciary responsibility to operate in the patient's best interest.

Empirical evidence began to emerge that many patients contradicted the script and did not comply with medical advice. Noncompliance was especially likely if patients did not trust their doctor as a person and did not feel that their doctor cared about them.[3,4] Researchers argued that medicine involved the art of care and that "rapport" was essential to remedy distrust. This rapport was built on mutual understanding and emotional affinity,[5] although the theoretical frameworks guiding the analyses varied. Sociologist Eliot Freidson grounded the concept of rapport in a "mutuality of hope" in which the patient seeks a provider's aid, believing that the provider can help alleviate their suffering (p. 263).[6] Physician Eric Cassell viewed rapport as being firmly rooted in the mutual sharing of health-related values (i.e., health promotion, disease prevention, treatment management).[7] Sociologist Judith Lorber argued that rapport depended upon such interpersonal factors as communication skills and a similarity of culture and background.[8]

The early empirical research deriving from these theories found that patients indeed wanted their providers to understand and care for them as people[9] and to provide them with information, guidance, education, and advocacy in the context of their treatment. If these elements were absent, many patients failed to keep their medical appointments and were generally dissatisfied with their medical care.[10] When patients did not feel cared for, they ignored medical advice; without a two-way commitment to mutual communication, patients hid their noncompliance. Extensive reviews and meta-analyses have confirmed that patient satisfaction, adherence (i.e., compliance) to medical treatment, and resultant healthcare outcomes are significantly better in the context of more solid provider-patient rapport and effective communication.[11,12]

Of course, not all patients want exactly the same interpersonal behavior from their physicians. In the example in Case Study 3.2, the physician's behavior is consistent over time. He demonstrates an active concern for his patients and tries to collaborate with them in the process of their medical care. Yet these two patients react quite differently to what Dr. Brenton probably views as an "ideal" interactional style.

Case Study 3.2 Sylvia and Alvin

Dr. Brenton cheerily greets his longtime patient. "It's good to see you, Sylvia," he says. "How have things been since I saw you three months ago?" After a quick glance at the chart, Dr. Brenton leans against the examining table where Sylvia sits and meets her gaze before asking, "Do you think we made the right decision in switching your pain meds? Have your side effects gone away?" Sylvia launches into her reply, conversing easily with her physician. She feels cared for, empowered, and comfortable being honest about her experiences with her treatment plan. Sylvia believes that Dr. Brenton is concerned for her health and well-being, and that her opinions and perceptions about her own health matter a great deal. She likes that Dr. Brenton doesn't shy away from difficult topics, such as the challenge of managing her chronic pain, and he doesn't treat her like she's abnormal or imagining her symptoms. She views Dr. Brenton not only as a good physician but also as her friend.

After finishing his visit with Sylvia, Dr. Brenton goes down the hall to the examining room where Alvin waits. Just as before, Dr. Brenton's greeting is friendly and almost immediately he asks Alvin for input about his heartburn and accompanying symptoms. Dr. Brenton sincerely wants to know whether Alvin thinks medication or lifestyle change is the best possible strategy for managing them. Dr. Brenton stands close to Alvin and maintains eye contact, indicating active listening and true interest in what Alvin is saying. But unlike Sylvia, Alvin feels uncomfortable with what he considers to be Dr. Brenton's violation of his personal space. He also wonders why Dr. Brenton is asking for his opinion; after all, *he* doesn't have a medical degree—that's why he's here!

As do many, these patients differ in their preferences for the process of care and the behavior of their providers.[13–15] These differences are important to understand because health behavior change and treatment adherence can be heavily influenced by the *context of the therapeutic relationship* in which health messages and behavioral recommendations are communicated. Several basic models of the patient-practitioner relationship have been identified and examined in terms of how they influence adherence and behavior change.

Models of the practitioner-patient relationship

Different labels can be applied to clinician-patient interactions; these labels often describe how power, control, and decision-making are shared (or not) in the relationship. Although the labels may vary and the underlying concepts differ somewhat, there are four commonly encountered categorical distinctions that represent types of practitioner-patient relationships. These are: *paternalism, consumerism, expertise,* and *mutuality*.

Paternalism

A "paternalistic" relationship is one in which the patient is acquiescent and unassertive, providing information only when asked and following instructions without much question or discussion.[16,17] Paternalism is viewed as similar to the relationship between a parent and child,[1] with one party (clinician) holding most of the status, decision-making power, and information, and the other party (patient) following along, guided by medical expertise. This framework views the healthcare provider as trustworthy and beneficent, relying on the best medical practices and caring for the patient as would a loving parent; correspondingly, paternalism permits the medical professional to compel obedience. Of course, such an approach casts aside the patient's concerns and opinions.[18] Consider the following excerpt translated from the first aphorism of Hippocrates, which illustrates the paternalistic model: "The physician must not only be prepared to do what is right himself, but also to make the patient, the attendants, and the externals cooperate."

Prior to the 1980s, a paternalistic relationship between physician and patient occurred more commonly than any other.[19] As some argued, however, paternalism was bound to foster an unhealthy level of patient dependency, even counter to the patient's true best interests.[20] And, although some patients do at times prefer a paternalistic approach, especially when they are quite ill,[21,22] a "consumerist" style has grown in popularity over the past decades,[17] as the provision of healthcare in the United States has changed and technology has taken a prominent role (as we will see in Chapter 8).

Consumerism

A consumerist view of the patient's role arose from a more general concern for protecting individuals from overzealous providers of medical products and services.[23] As such, consumerism came to view patients as purchasers of a product (i.e., their healthcare) with an overriding philosophy of *caveat emptor* (buyer beware). This approach emphasizes the rights of patients as consumers of medical information and medical care, and highlights accountability on the part of those who provide that information and care.[18] In 1991, the Patient Self-Determination Act mandated, among other things, that patients must be made aware of their rights to participate in making medical decisions. This law formalized the elements of a consumerist approach in which the patient holds a good deal of power because decisions to continue or discontinue care lie with the patient as the purchaser of that care. Thus, a consumerist encounter is ideally characterized by considerable information exchange, as well as questions and directions from the patient to the provider.[24] More recently the consumerist approach has been encouraged by the availability of massive amounts of medical information on the internet and by direct-to-consumer advertising from pharmaceutical companies, as well as by the growing recognition that patients' beliefs and preferences may clash with the recommendations of their providers and of scientific medical experts.[25,26]

Expertise

The "expert" model of the physician-patient relationship falls between the paternalistic and the consumerist styles. It emerged when medicine became more professionalized in the 1920s, and while it shared the paternalistic model's emphasis on the principles of beneficence, fidelity, non-malfeasance, and confidentiality, this model was based less on guardianship (which was foundational in the paternalistic model) and more on professional competence. As a result, it became less expected of physicians to make personal sacrifices for patients, and patients were increasingly expected to take some responsibility for decisions about their own care. This approach set the stage for the consumerist model that characterizes much of modern healthcare today.[27]

Mutuality

The fourth type of patient-practitioner relationship is one of mutual participation and collaboration, often referred to as "mutuality."[17] Here, both patient and clinician are viewed as experts; the patient is an expert about their symptoms, medical history, lifestyle, and preferences; and the physician or allied health professional is an expert about medical matters. With mutual participation, power is shared between the two parties as they work together to make decisions that will result in the best possible outcomes for the patient.[28-30] In this type of relationship, an active exchange of ideas and open negotiation of differences facilitate the patient's ability to make personal healthcare decisions, taking into account their needs and abilities while also being fully informed by the knowledge and experience of the medical expert.[31] The mutuality model relies heavily on each member of the healthcare partnership but is nonetheless patient-centered.[32] The relationship is mutual in its *focus* because the patient's best interest is paramount, and in its *effort* because both parties are fully engaged in the patient's care. Table 3.1 summarizes situational contexts in which different models of physician-patient relationships might be most appropriate; these have been adapted from a commentary by Lussier and Richard[33] in which the "expert-in-charge" approach is analogous to "paternalism" above. The "partner" approach reflects "mutuality." The "facilitator" approach is

Table 3.1 Repertoire of Doctor-Patient Relationships and Their Appropriate Contexts[33]

Role of Physician	Goal of Physician	Example Context
Expert-in-Charge	Make decisions and carry them out.	Emergency situation (e.g., heart attack)
Expert-Guide	Give the patient information, make recommendations, and provide treatment.	Less serious situations (e.g., simple fracture, laceration)
Partner	Build a partnership with the patient; provide information, and guide decision-making; motivate the patient to follow treatment.	Chronic illnesses (e.g., diabetes)
Facilitator	Motivate the patient; facilitate treatment; follow the patient's lead.	Well-controlled chronic illness (e.g., asthma)

similar though not equivalent to the "consumerist" model presented here. The "expert-guide" approach falls between paternalism and mutuality.

Trust

The American Heritage Dictionary defines trust[34] as a "firm belief in the integrity, ability, or character of a person or thing"; when one has trust in an entity, one has confidence in it. When we trust another person or group, we believe that we can rely on their support and perhaps their affection or caring; we believe that the trusted entity has our well-being and best interest at heart, and that the information they provide is reliable (as further discussed in Chapter 5 when we examine persuasion).

In the relationship between provider and patient, trust is built when the patient truthfully discloses information, problems, feelings, attitudes, beliefs, and behaviors, and when the provider responds nonjudgmentally with warmth, acceptance, understanding, and expressions of cooperative intent. Trust is damaged when the patient feels judged, criticized, or rejected. Trust requires verbal and nonverbal communications of reassurance, and it is essential for helping patients make health behavior changes even when doing so demands considerable personal cost in time and resources.[35] Trust in an authority, such as a public health department, is essential for adherence to directives from that authority and requires belief in the competence and good will of its representatives.

In the remainder of this chapter, we examine the elements that promote interpersonal trust including the provider's affective communication of warmth and caring, sensitivity to individuals' concerns and emotions, and understanding of their psychological state. As we will see, these interpersonal aspects of patient care comprise a set of skills that can be taught, practiced, and improved by providers and incorporated into their care of patients.[36]

The elements of interpersonal communication

The relationship between a patient and their medical provider is limited in time compared to most other relationships in a patient's life, and yet this relationship can assume great personal importance. People usually remember much about the emotional and interpersonal tone of the encounters with their medical professionals, whether good or bad.[37,38] Patients tend to be very sensitive to subtle cues, partly because of the emotional uncertainty they feel when facing the challenges of illness, separation from the comfort and support of loved ones, and the unfamiliar nature of medical treatment (with its jargon and scientific terms, strange procedures, and peculiar surroundings). Provider conduct is a key factor in patients' evaluation of, and satisfaction with, health services.[39,40] Optimal relationships are characterized by provider warmth, empathy, genuineness, and sensitivity to patients' feelings and emotional reactions to their disease and treatment.[40–42]

Practitioner-patient communication

Within the context of the practitioner-patient relationship, communication comprises both a primary task and a useful tool.[43,44] As early as 1899, Sir William Osler taught that if physicians would listen, patients would reveal the diagnosis. Today, some would argue that communication is *the* most important ingredient in medical care.[17] The *Accreditation Council for Graduate Medical Education* (www.acgme.org) and the *Association of American Medical Colleges* (www.aamc.org) both recognize the crucial role that communication plays; they require competency in interpersonal communication as a *core skill* in medical practice.

The vast body of research that exists on this topic shows that provider-patient communication is complex and uniquely tied to the characteristics of the individuals involved. There is consistency across encounters (e.g., history-taking, physical exam[45]), but characteristics like patient age and socioeconomic status have proven to be strong predictors of the ways in which patients and clinicians communicate with each other during the medical encounter.[17] There are also many differences from one individual encounter to another, such as in the amount and type of humor that is used.[46–48] Further, the parties' personalities and past experiences are unique factors that each brings to the interaction.[17]

In the next section we will address many of the factors that influence the quality and content of communication (both verbal and nonverbal) in medical settings. As we see in the following analysis, aspects of the physical environment and the events that happen prior to the visit can set the stage for communication between clinician and patient, influencing things like patient participation and later recall. These factors, in turn, influence the individual's commitment to carry out treatment plans as well as their success in doing so.

Physical environment
Research in business and marketing is rich with studies showing how the physical environment (such as the layout of a shop or the décor in a restaurant) creates an image and affects customers' initial impressions. A physical space can affect moods, behaviors, and satisfaction with services.[49–51] In medical settings, as well, it is increasingly recognized that aspects of the physical environment play an important role. The design and layout of a waiting area and an exam room, including the colors and furnishings, the temperature, the noise, and other aspects can affect patients' perceptions of, and satisfaction with, care.[52–54] Characteristics of the medical setting have been linked to patients' increased blood pressure[55] and higher levels of anxiety, which can have detrimental effects on patients' abilities to report, process, and remember information from the medical encounter.

Incorporating a "homelike" design—one that feels familiar—can make patients more comfortable,[56,57] reduce their anxiety, and improve attention and recall. Some evidence of this comes from a study in which patients on a specially-designed hospital ward learned more about their illness and self-care and were more satisfied than patients on the standard ward (although after discharge no behavioral differences were found).[58] Scenery has been shown to decrease patient anxiety and physiological reactions such as heightened blood pressure. A beautiful view from a window, realistic and appropriately lighted pieces of art (especially water scenes),[59–61] on-site gardens, live plants, and structural features that allow in natural light can be healing;[55,62] and music has a calming effect on patients.[63]

Privacy is important to patients; the design of a counseling area can influence communication with their practitioners.[64] Most meetings with doctors, nurses, dentists, and physician's assistants take place in private examination or procedure rooms, so privacy is likely. More and more frequently, though, pharmacists are expected to take on educational roles once filled by other medical professionals. Lengthy discussion, fielding of patient questions, and even demonstrations of medication administration require private (but not confining) space to prevent embarrassment and encourage patients to ask necessary questions and commit fully to their medication regimens.

Lighting and color can influence mood. Walls that are reddish-colored trigger more depressed moods in office workers compared with a blue-green color scheme.[65] In other research, darker indoor lighting led to low moods, which improved when light was increased to "just right" and then decreased again as the room became overly bright. When illumination was measured objectively there was no association with mood, however; all associations were based on subjective perceptions.[50] Preferences for levels of light were personal and idiosyncratic, suggesting the importance of individual variation, and possibly of environmental control on the part of the individual.

As we will see in more detail in Chapter 8, electronic handheld, laptop, or desktop devices in the exam room have become ubiquitous and may affect patients in some important ways. Surveys show that although patients are generally accepting of the use and incorporation of digital devices in the medical environment, they prefer doctor-patient encounters in which these devices are absent.[66] In addition, patients may be negatively impacted when their clinicians are less experienced and less proficient at using these devices.[66-68] Patients do seem to prefer architecture that conveys a modern "high tech" image, perhaps instilling confidence that the technical aspects of medical care will be "top-notch."[57] Sensitivity to patients' experiences of technology, especially if they feel threatened or distressed by it, can be important to consider. While the technological elements that enhance accuracy and effectiveness of care are essential parts of medicine today, their incorporation need not interfere with the interpersonal elements of provider-patient communication. The ways in which digital devices are used (for instance, whether the clinician must turn their back to the patient in order to access computerized records, and whether they clearly explain the purpose for use of the device) may be quite important in setting the tone for a medical encounter.

Studies like these suggest that some flexibility might be ideal, so that environments can be tailored to fit the preferences of each patient, ensuring that they are comfortable and relaxed and have control, choice, and active participation whenever possible.[69]

Verbal communication
Patient-centered care is a popular research topic, although exactly what is meant by "patient-centered" varies from study to study.[70] Most researchers agree that a patient-centered approach is responsive to the patient's preferences and views health from a biopsychosocial perspective rather than from a more narrow, biomedical one.[71,72] It is impossible to know a patient's

preferences and psychosocial context without hearing their story. Thus, the verbal communication that takes place between patients and their healthcare providers is crucial.

Open-ended questions

Patients often complain that their medical practitioners don't listen to them[73] and don't ask questions in a way that encourages them to talk. Listening to the patient, understanding the meaning of their symptoms, and knowing the story of their illness experience are essential, however, to making a correct diagnosis, finding a treatment plan the patient can adhere to, and connecting with the patient in a meaningful way.[74-76]

Clinical training in medicine emphasizes *differential diagnosis*, in which various possibilities about the causes of symptoms are considered and eliminated, eventually leaving only one, which is then settled on as the diagnosis. Particularly when supplemented with the results of medical tests, this method can be effective in leading to an appropriate diagnosis, but it can also lead the physician to *premature closure*[77]—making a decision before all the relevant information is gathered. Using a series of closed-ended questions makes premature closure more likely because the questioner may follow only one path of reasoning and miss important information. An all-too-familiar complaint from clinicians is that their patients suddenly introduce additional symptoms or queries just as the medical visit is nearing completion.[77] The constraints imposed by over-reliance on closed-ended questions from the health professional make this more likely to happen; it may be avoided if patients are allowed to describe their illness experience fully.[78] Open-ended questions invite patients to tell their stories. These questions are broad and rely on the patient to provide details that inform the practitioner. "What does the pain feel like to you?" will offer descriptive material from which more pointed follow-up questions can be asked. With open-ended questions, patients provide a more complete picture of their experience within their psychosocial context.[79,80]

Imagine, for example, that a patient is struggling unsuccessfully to incorporate exercise into their daily schedule. They might have the time, but they describe feeling constantly fatigued. What should the clinician make of this? Is the patient simply lazy? Are they suffering from some medical syndrome? Through telling their story, the patient might reveal difficulties getting a good night's sleep. The reasons for that challenge might then be addressed. The open narrative approach makes patient-centered care much easier. In Case Study 3.3 we find illustrations of clinician-patient exchanges that vary in terms of the clinician's questioning style and the resultant types of information that are shared. These dialogues illustrate the things that may be missed when health professionals rely heavily on closed-ended questions, and the richness of communication that often results when patients are invited to share what they have experienced.

Case Study 3.3 Simplified Illustrations of Medical Interviews Using Closed-Ended versus Open-Ended Questions

Medical Problem: Chronic Headaches
Closed-Ended Question Dialogue

Physician's Assistant:	"So, let's discuss these headaches.... Would you describe the pain as a stabbing?"
Patient:	"Yes."
Physician's Assistant:	"Is the pain worse in the evening?"
Patient:	"Um, sometimes."
Physician's Assistant:	"Have you tried over-the-counter pain relievers?"
Patient:	"Yeah."
Physician's Assistant:	"Which ones have you tried?"
Patient:	"Um, I've tried aspirin, and also some 'multi-symptom' relief things."
Physician's Assistant:	"Have you found these helpful?"
Patient:	"No, not really."
Physician's Assistant:	"Well, maybe you need something stronger. Let's talk about some prescription options, okay?"

Open-ended Question Dialogue

Physician's Assistant:	"So, let's discuss these headaches.... Can you describe them to me?"
Patient:	"Well, I get them two to four times per week. I'm usually fine in the morning but by mid-afternoon I can start to feel them coming on. They get pretty severe by late afternoon or evening."

Physician's Assistant:	"Describe the pain to me."
Patient:	"I'd say that initially it's just a dull ache but as the pain gets worse it starts to throb. It feels like the throbbing almost matches my heartbeat or something. By that point it's not a dull pain anymore, it's much more intense. But it's not sharp."
Physician's Assistant:	"And how have you tried to get rid of them?"
Patient:	"Well, I've tried about every pill they have at the drugstore. None of those seem to work very well. Sometimes, if I can distract myself when I first start to feel the pain, the headache will go away. I usually can't do that though. But two weeks ago, I started getting one just as I was packing up to go hiking in the mountains. I would have stayed home but one of my friends was riding with me so I figured I'd give her a ride up, and maybe hike just a little with the group, and make it home before the pain got too bad. But the funny thing was that we were talking in the car, and laughing, and it wasn't until we got up there that I realized the pain was completely gone!"
Physician's Assistant:	"Hmmm... it almost sounds like they might be stress-related. You were pretty relaxed when you were driving up to the mountains, right?"
Patient:	"Yeah."
Physician's Assistant:	"Since over-the-counter pain medications don't seem to work for you, I think that you might need something stronger for those times when you can't control the pain. I also think you might find a few stress-management techniques useful. Wouldn't it be great to only have to resort to medications once in a while?"

Refraining from interruption

Many clinicians seem to have difficulty letting their patients finish what they are saying. One study[77] found that patients were allowed to complete their initial statement about what had brought them to the doctor's office in less than a quarter of the cases studied (23%). In addition, in more than half the cases, physicians interrupted and directed questions toward one of the specifics the patient had mentioned; typically, this happened within the first 18 seconds of the patient's speech. A follow-up study found similar results—that only 28% of patients were allowed to complete their initial statements of concern, and patients were interrupted after, on average, about 23 seconds.[81]

Failure to listen to a patient's narrative likely communicates the following: "I'm in a rush, so please hurry up," or "That second thing you said was important, but the rest of this is not." Interruptions, directions, and failures to listen in medical interviews tell the patient that the health professional has all the control; this imbalance of power, research suggests, can lead to poorer health outcomes and greater dissatisfaction.[82]

As we noted earlier, if providers interrupt or direct the medical interview too much, important information can be overlooked, and the failure to note certain pieces of data from a patient might lead to misdiagnoses and medical errors. The information might reemerge near the end of the medical encounter, reopening the discussion, delaying the rest of the clinical schedule, or putting off a potentially valuable discussion until a future visit.[77]

One obvious question is, "Will allowing the patient to finish their whole story take up too much time?" Probably not, according to research by Marvel et al.,[81] who found that when patients were allowed to complete their opening statements, the medical interaction took, on average, only about six seconds longer.

Providing clear information

The medical visit involves an *exchange* of information. Healthcare providers must elicit information *from* their patients and convey information *to* them. Communicating effectively with patients requires that verbalizations be thorough and precise, and that patients understand what is presented to them. Thus, it is important that the patient's level of *health literacy* be accurately targeted. In Chapter 4, we examine health literacy and the factors influencing a patient's ability to understand and remember health information. In general, though, health professionals should consistently use simple and clear language with all patients, avoid technical terms, and explain and build on patients' existing knowledge and understanding.[83] Age, gender, level of education, anxiety, and the content of communication can influence what patients receive and understand.[84] Targeting communications appropriately can promote partnership with patients.[85]

Patients' verbalizations

When given the chance to talk, what factors influence what a patient says? How can providers best understand what their patients say to them?

In Chapter 2, we discussed how a patient's health behaviors are influenced by their beliefs about health and by a variety of sociocultural factors that affect those beliefs. These same variables can influence a patient's behavior within the medical interaction. Eliciting their explanations for symptoms and illness can be crucial to effective communication about health management—not only to help with diagnosis but also to frame health information and interventions most effectively for the individual.[86,87] For example, a clinician might ask questions about what the patient thinks might have caused the medical problem, why it might have started at the time it did, or what kind of treatment might be desired. The patient's answers can provide insight to possible causes for the problem (as we saw in Case Study 3.3) and might help predict the patient's ultimate adherence. For a patient who states that they "do not take medication," the choice of non-pharmacological remedies (if available) might better address patient preferences and improve patient adherence. If medications must be used, additional time in discussion might increase adherence.

Another important clue to understanding a patient involves the narrative they tell of their illness. Somaticizers (also called somatizers), are patients whose symptoms tend not to be directly linked to an identifiable organic cause, or who tend to "convert" their emotional distress to the report of solely physical experience. Somaticizers have been found to describe their symptoms using the same terms and with the same degree of emotion as other patients, but they tend *not* to tell a chronological story of their experience.[88] Case Study 3.4 illustrates the differences with two hypothetical descriptions from patients, one of them a somaticizer. Therefore, in addition to health-related details, the way the narrative is told can provide additional help to the clinician in understanding the patient's symptoms and their surrounding context, offering leverage in considering treatment options. One study, for example, showed that patients who come to the doctor's office with somatic symptoms of psychological distress usually *will* talk about their psychological experience *if they are asked*.[89] This is very important because knowing about psychological comorbidities allows the clinician to help (or refer) the patient and/or design medical interventions to take these into account.[90,91] A psychologist in the medical practice or a Patient-Centered Medical Home (as will be discussed in Chapter 8) would be ideal for helping patients with psychological comorbidities.

> ### Case Study 3.4 Chronological Story Development in Two Patients
>
> Consider the responses of Mark and Renee to the following question, posed by their physical therapist, "How has your back been since your last visit?"
>
> Mark: "I've still been in a lot of pain. My back feels tight and it's like the pain radiates out from about waist-level. It's kind of a tight, squeezing sensation. Sometimes it's not too bad and I can just take my meds and go on with life, but other times I feel like I can't even do my stretches or my exercises. It's just too painful to even start. At that point I just lie down, take a couple of extra pills, and hope that it goes away."
>
> Renee: "I've still been in a lot of pain. After our last session I felt better for a couple of days, but then on about the third day I noticed that the pain was significantly worse. It starts out with just some stiffness in the morning but throughout the day a kind of tight, squeezing sensation begins and it gets more and more intense throughout the day. By evening it's radiating out from my lower back, about waist-level, and it's so painful that I can't even do the stretches and exercises I'm supposed to do. Each day it seems like the pinnacle of pain is a little worse. Yesterday and the day before I just had to lie down and take some extra pills."

Both Mark and Renee describe almost identical symptoms. Renee describes her back pain symptoms chronologically, according to the time frame in which they were experienced. Mark, however, focuses his description of symptoms on the theme, and not on any timeline. The lack of chronological development in Mark's description of his symptoms suggests that they might be interwoven with emotional issues.[88] This important clue suggests that the route to successful symptom management may be different for these two patients.

Nonverbal cues, of course, can also be quite helpful in identifying patients' unstated emotional distress as well as other medically relevant issues. They are the topic of the next section.

Nonverbal communication

Much of what is communicated in medical interaction involves no words. Instead, facial expressions, postures, body movements, voice tone, and other *non*verbal cues convey messages between clinician and patient. The sending of these messages is referred to as "encoding," whereas the detection and interpretation of nonverbal signals is called "decoding." For most nonverbal cues, however, there is no clear and unambiguous meaning. Although used constantly in our social interactions, nonverbal language, just like verbal communication, is subject to misunderstanding and errors.

Sometimes nonverbal messages supplement what is said verbally; at other times, verbal and nonverbal messages contradict each other. Take, for example, the case of the patient Julia. When Tiana, the office nurse, enters the examining room to ask a few questions and take vital signs, Julia smiles and cheerfully assures her that everything is just fine and that this should be nothing more than a quick, routine check-up. Tiana observes, however, that Julia's movements seem tentative, and when she raises her arm for the blood pressure cuff, Julia winces. "Did I pinch you?" Tiana asks. Julia shakes her head and intensifies her smile saying, "Oh no, not at all!" Nevertheless, Tiana makes a brief notation in the chart so that the physician can follow up during her visit with Julia. What Julia is not reporting (but her body is) may be important.

Unlike Julia, Miles reports to his physician a long list of side effects of his new antidepressant medication; he seems anxious to include everything. Although she is listening intently to his narrative, Dr. Trask also notes several things that Miles hasn't mentioned, including his dilated pupils and a slight tremor in his hands. After asking some follow-up questions and coupling Miles's responses with what she has observed in his nonverbal behavior, Dr. Trask is able to rule out several possible diagnoses and orders some tests to narrow down the possibilities. In this case, nonverbal cues provide additional, complementary information to what Miles is reporting to his physician. Julia's nonverbal cues provide a cautionary indicator that Julia is not being entirely candid about the symptoms she is experiencing, and this lack of candor might provide a useful hint about Julia's psychosocial context. Conclusions based on verbal messages alone would be different for each

Indicators of distress

Often, patients are reluctant to express emotional discomfort or anxiety about their medical experiences. Some feel intimidated or think there is not enough time to share their concerns with their healthcare professionals. In such situations, patients often express their feelings and emotional experience through nonverbal channels.[27] For example, a patient might say, "I understand," or, "No, I can't think of any questions," but display a confused facial expression or fail to meet the provider's gaze.[92] A clinician who is alert to nonverbal cues will be better prepared to probe further and offer necessary information and reassurances to benefit the patient.

Physical pain and sensitivity cues

A patient's level of pain might be best determined by observing nonverbal cues.[93] This is especially true for populations that have difficulty with verbal expression (such as infants, preverbal children, and cognitively impaired individuals) and those stoically hiding their discomfort.[94] For people of all ages, nonverbal pain behaviors usually include grimaces, moans, sighs, or clenching of teeth, jaw, and/or hands. In particular, facial expressions can be useful indicators of physical pain.[95] Although some of our facial expressions can be controlled and manipulated quite well,[96] the cortical pathways that control purposeful facial expressions are different from the subcortical areas that govern spontaneous expressions.[97] Thus, even when consciously trying to "present" certain facial expressions, others are likely to "leak" or slip through unintentionally. An astute observer of facial expressions can often obtain a more accurate picture of an individual's pain experience than one who relies only on the individual's words.

Can skill at decoding nonverbal messages be improved? To some degree, yes. Although there is variability in the degree to which individuals are naturally attentive to, and accurate in reading nonverbal cues, there is also evidence that practice increases accuracy. Some measurement tools exist that can highlight areas of strength and weakness regarding nonverbal communication. The Profile of Nonverbal Sensitivity (PONS)[98] provides subscale scores indicating whether, for example, an individual is skilled at understanding (decoding) facial expressions, body movements, and/or tone and inflection in voices. The Facial Action Coding System[99] measures individual abilities to "read" facial expressions but does not address other aspects of nonverbal communication (e.g., bodily or extralinguistic cues).

Communication training programs[100–102] typically include both verbal and nonverbal components; nonverbal skills are essential elements in teaching empathy.[103,104]

Empathy

"A pair of kidneys will never come to the physician for diagnosis and treatment. They will be contained within an anxious, fearful, wondering person, asking puzzled questions about an obscure future, weighed down by the responsibilities of a loved family, and with a job to be held, and with bills to be paid.... the clinician must learn the facts about it all, and comprehend it all, and have a feeling for it all, and develop a plan of management for it all." (p. 21)[105]

Empathy describes what happens when one understands, on a deep level and without judgment, the experience of another. (Note that this is different from sympathy, which denotes that one feels sorry for another.) It is a central concept for all healthcare providers, including counselors and psychologists in therapeutic settings.[100] The clinician's goal, as noted in the above quote, is to understand the entire being of the patient, and to offer treatments based on experiencing empathy for the whole person.

Conveying empathy can be challenging; verbal expressions such as that one "feels what they are feeling" or can "identify with" their experience are not helpful. Empathy is better conveyed through nonverbal means.[106,107] The medical professional's first task—to correctly perceive the patient's inner experience expressed in their verbal and nonverbal cues—needs to be followed up with communication that helps the patient feel valued and cared for (such as through cues of attentiveness like forward lean, open posture, appropriate eye contact, and nodding).[108] Touch, when welcomed and appropriate, is also a common way of reassuring patients and conveying comfort and caring.[109]

Empathy can also be conveyed through paralinguistic cues—those that accompany spoken language—such as voice tone and cues to active listening such as the use of "back-channel" communications, which are extraverbal utterances that facilitate a narrative but do not interfere with it.[110] For example, as a patient describes the symptoms they've experienced over the past week, a nurse may periodically say things like, "Mm-hm," "Oh, I see," or "Ah," which indicate to the patient that they are being heard and understood. These utterances are also referred to in the linguistics literature as "continuers." They encourage patients to continue speaking and indicate interest on the part of the listener. By demonstrating concern and connection, the clinician can show *empathy* for the patient.

Voice tone is also important in conveying empathy.[111] Voice tones rated as "warm" are associated with higher degrees of patient satisfaction,[112] whereas physicians' positive *words* coupled with nonverbal vocal indicators of anxiety are also related positively to patient satisfaction; anxiety may convey concern for and investment in the patient.[113] Voice tone is also related to a number of other healthcare outcomes. One of the earliest studies conducted in a medical care setting examined how physicians' voice tone was related to their ability to appropriately refer alcoholic patients for further treatment; specifically, physicians with angry voice tone were less likely to be successful in their referrals.[114] Another study involving ratings of surgeons' voices found that those whose voice tones were judged to be more dominant and less concerned were more likely to have a history of malpractice claims than those who sounded more concerned and collaborative.[115]

Individuals differ somewhat in their natural abilities to understand and express nonverbal information, and research suggests that many health professionals are not as empathic as they might ideally be. For instance, one study showed that *most* cues given by patients indicating that they needed empathic understanding (in this study, a total of 384 cues) went unnoticed by physicians, who responded to only 10% of them.[116] In family medicine, where patient education and counseling are strong components of training, physician empathy tends to be higher than in other specialties.[117]

It is indeed possible to measure empathic abilities and, with training and effort, to enhance empathic skills.[118,119] Empathy assessment tools come in different forms; the simplest to use are brief questionnaires. For example, the Jefferson Scale of Physician Empathy is both brief (20 self-report items) and psychometrically sound, and predicts empathy in the clinical setting three years later.[120] Those desiring to improve their empathy skills might consider a training program.[119,121] These programs typically highlight three components: *(1) cognitive* (learning to observe and understand the meaning, at least intellectually, of what is observed in a patient's communication); *(2) affective*, or emotional (learning to relate observed patient emotions to one's own emotional experience, as a way to connect better with the patient); and *(3) communicative* (learning to effectively convey this cognitive and emotional understanding to the patient).

Empathy and the actor-observer asymmetry

The "actor-observer asymmetry" (known in social psychology as the fundamental attribution error) offers some insights into understanding empathy.[122] Based on an extensive body of research, this phenomenon finds that when viewing our own behavior, we tend to acknowledge, and explain our actions in terms of, situational constraints.[123] For example, we explain that we are late because the traffic was unusually heavy. We are not trying to avoid responsibility for our actions or offer excuses; it is just that the traffic we faced is salient to us. We tend to explain other people's behavior, on the other hand, in dispositional terms (i.e., as a characteristic of the person). We might "explain" another person's tardiness as reflecting their tendency to fail to budget time and properly plan ahead. We see them as "the kind of person who tends to be late." This asymmetry, then, involves the tendency for people to place undue emphasis on the internal characteristics (e.g., temperament or intentions) of another when explaining their actions, but to explain their own behavior in terms of more situational factors. In physician-patient communication, a patient might see the physician's rushed demeanor as reflecting the physician's abruptness or insensitivity, unaware of the fact that the physician has just been paged to the emergency department. The physician might view the patient's limited adherence as caused by the patient's resistant personality or laziness, while the patient could list five pressing family problems they must deal with before they can follow their treatment.

These differences in attributions for behavior tend to exist because we are more aware of our own situational constraints, whereas the pressures on others are typically not visible to us. Having empathy allows us to look beyond the surface and try to understand the pressures that another person is facing. With empathy, we try to see the world through that person's eyes.

Social psychologists have extensively studied the complexities of this "actor-observer" phenomenon, which is more or less likely to occur in certain contexts than in others (including whether actor and observer are from the same or different cultural backgrounds).[124] They have found that it takes effort to overcome our tendency to minimize the situations that affect other people; it takes empathy to see the barriers that people face in trying to change their health behavior and adhere to treatment. This is especially true in having empathy for vulnerable populations including: individuals who are poor, have limited education and low or marginal health literacy, or have perceptual and/or cognitive deficits, mental health challenges, and/or language and culture not accommodated effectively by the healthcare institutions they access. In many care settings, most patients fall into at least one of these categories. Case Study 3.5 demonstrates how a health professional can show empathy when asking about adherence to treatment.

Case Study 3.5 Asking about Adherence

Nurse practitioner Carla Estrada has been thinking about the best way to ask her patients if they really are taking their medications as directed. She suspects that some might not be following her prescriptions correctly, or even at all, but asking about their behavior seems too confrontational. Fellow nurse practitioners in her integrated healthcare system have some suggestions for Carla. They recommend always asking about adherence in a nonjudgmental way. Carla might disclose that she herself (or a friend) has difficulty remembering to take medication; targeted disclosure can build a bridge to the patient's experience. Carla might ask her patient to bring in pill bottles so they can talk about the various medications—how they are taken and how they affect the patient. While prescription databases such as pharmacy records can provide indirect measures of adherence (prescription refills and on-time pickup), they don't record whether the patient actually takes the medication. In research, patients' self-reports have been the most consistently studied method of assessment;[125] in the context of rapport and empathic communication, they can most accurately reflect the patient's medication adherence and further the therapeutic communication about the patient's goals and health behaviors.[125]

Carla tries to implement these suggestions. "Mr. Rios, we can see here on your test results that your cholesterol level is higher than we had hoped. How have things been going for you with the new medication we decided on in our last visit?" Carla's goal is to use these discussions not

> only to find out about adherence, but also to build trust and rapport; she wants her patient to feel comfortable asking for help. She is working on being empathic, attentive, and sensitive to her patients' verbal and nonverbal communications. So far, her new strategy seems to be working. As she discusses adherence challenges with her patients, she notices that they work together to solve adherence challenges; she is already seeing some improvement.

Empathy involves seeing the constraints that so many individuals face in trying to better their health, and their need for assistance in overcoming challenges. Empathy involves listening to patients' reasons for their nonadherence, and avoiding judgment; it requires recognizing that, under the circumstances, a person may be doing the best they can.[101,126,127]

Summary

In this chapter, we explore the practitioner-patient relationship and the ways in which effective interpersonal communication can enhance treatment adherence and improve the outcomes of patient care. We offer an historical perspective on the models that have scripted provider-patient interactions over the past seven decades, and consider the implications of paternalism, consumerism, expertise, and mutuality. We examine partnership, the roles of acceptance and reassurance, and the meaning, building, and maintenance of trust. We explore providers' sensitivity to patients' emotional expressions as well as providers' verbal and nonverbal communications of understanding and cooperative intent. In examining the elements of communication, we consider the physical environment in which the interaction takes place, as well as verbal nuances in communication including nonjudgmental questioning, the use of open-ended inquiries, and the management of interruptions. We explore nonverbal communications such as facial expressions, body movements, and voice tone as indicators of both emotional and physical experience in the clinician-patient relationship. We examine empathy and the ways in which medical professionals can strive to understand their patients' perspectives; and we consider the fundamental attribution error, or "actor-observer asymmetry" (a concept in social psychology) as a driver of challenges to empathy.

Tools for instruction and self-study

Learning objectives

By the end of this chapter, readers should be able to

1. Compare and contrast paternalism, consumerism, expertise, and mutuality, in the provider-patient relationship.
2. Define trust and describe elements of trust in the healthcare professional-patient relationship.
3. Explain the meaning of a patient-centered approach to medical visit communication.
4. Write examples of open-ended and closed-ended questions in medical interviews.
5. Explain factors that promote provider understanding of patients in the medical visit.
6. Describe the role of nonverbal communication in the medical visit.
7. Discuss how empathy is conveyed to patients in medical visits.

Review questions

1. List and briefly describe two of the different perspectives regarding the foundations of rapport between clinicians and patients.
2. What are the four clinician-patient relationship styles described in this chapter?
3. Name three things about the physical environment that have been shown, in research studies, to impact patients in the clinical setting.
4. What is the benefit to using open-ended (vs. closed-ended) questions when conducting a medical interview?
5. What is nonverbal encoding? What is nonverbal decoding? What are paralinguistic cues?
6. How prevalent are interruptions and redirections in medical encounters? Why might these be problematic?
7. What is empathy? What components are ideally included in an empathy-training program?

Prompts for discussion and further study

1. Think of someone you know who does not experience mutuality in communication with their physician (or other healthcare provider). What are some of the barriers to active engagement for this person, and how might they be overcome?
2. After considering what we know about physical space in relation to various patient outcomes, design a clinic or medical office setting. What elements would you want to incorporate in your design? How would you leverage the physical space to maximize positive outcomes?
3. A clinician cares deeply about patients and endeavors to follow the practices outlined in this book. This clinician has a patient, however, who loves to talk—making it very difficult to aspire to never interrupt. What might be going on here? How would you handle this situation?

Suggested reading

1. Decety J. (ed.). *Empathy: From Bench to Bedside.* MIT Press; 2011.
2. Hojat M. *Empathy in Patient Care: Antecedents, Development, Measurement, and Outcomes* (Vol. 77). New York: Springer; 2007.
3. Halpern J. *From Detached Concern to Empathy: Humanizing Medical Practice.* Oxford University Press; 2001.
4. Matsumoto DE, Hwang HC, Frank MG. *APA Handbook of Nonverbal Communication.* American Psychological Association; 2016; pp. xxiv–626.
5. Price R. *A Whole New Life: An Illness and a Healing.* 4th ed. Scribner; 2000.
6. Sweet V. *Slow Medicine: The Way to Healing.* Riverhead Books; 2017.

References

1. Parsons T. *The Social System.* Glencoe, IL: Free Press; 1951; pp. 428–479.
2. Parsons, T. Definitions of health and illness in the light of American values and social structure. In: Jaco EG, ed. *Patients, Physicians and Illness.* New York: Free Press; 1958; pp. 165–187.

3. DiMatteo MR, Prince LM, Taranta A. Patients' perceptions of physicians' behavior: Determinants of patient commitment to the therapeutic relationship. *J Community Health.* 1979; 4: pp. 280–290.
4. DiMatteo MR, DiNicola DD. *Achieving Patient Compliance.* Pergamon Press; 1982.
5. Rapport. *The American Heritage Dictionary of the English Language.* Accessed January 4, 2024. https://ahdictionary.com/word/search.html?q=rapport
6. Freidson E. *Profession of Medicine.* New York: Dodd, Mead; 1970.
7. Cassell EJ. *The Healer's Art: A New Approach to the Doctor-Patient Relationship.* New York: Penguin Books; 1976.
8. Lorber J. Good patients and problem patients: conformity and deviance in a general hospital. *J Health Soc Behav.* 1975; 16: pp. 213–225.
9. Eisenberg L. The search for care. *Daedalus.* 1977; 106: pp. 235–246.
10. DiMatteo MR, Taranta A, Friedman HS, Prince LM. Predicting patient satisfaction from physicians' nonverbal communication skills. *Med Care.* 1980; 18(4): pp. 376–387.
11. Haskard Zolnierek KB, DiMatteo MR. Physician communication and patient adherence to treatment: a meta-analysis. *Med Care.* 2009; 47(8): pp. 826–834.
12. DiMatteo MR, Giordani PJ, Lepper HS, Croghan TW. Patient adherence and medical treatment outcomes: a meta-analysis. *Med Care.* 2002; 40(9): pp. 794–811.
13. Janssen SM, Lagro-Janssen AL. Physician's gender, communication style, patient preferences and patient satisfaction in gynecology and obstetrics: a systematic review. *Patient Educ Couns.* 2012; 89(2): pp. 221–226.
14. Hurley EA, Harvey SA, Keita M, et al. Patient-provider communication styles in HIV treatment programs in Bamako, Mali: a mixed-methods study to define dimensions and measure patient preferences. *SSM Popul Health.* 2017; Dec; 3: pp. 539–548.
15. Perez Jolles M, Richmond J, Thomas KC. Minority patient preferences, barriers, and facilitators for shared decision-making with health care providers in the USA: a systematic review. *Patient Educ Couns.* 2019; 102(7): pp. 1251–1262.
16. Emanuel EJ, Emanuel LL. Four models of the physician-patient relationship. *JAMA.* 1992; 267(16): pp. 2221–2226.
17. Roter DL, Hall JA. *Doctors Talking with Patients/Patients Talking with Doctors: Improving Communication in Medical Visits.* 2nd ed. Westport, CT: Greenwood Publishing Group; 2006.
18. Beisecker AE, Beisecker TD. Using metaphors to characterize doctor-patient relationships: paternalism versus consumerism. *Health Commun.* 1993; 5: pp. 41–58.
19. Charles C, Gafni A, Whelan T. Decision-making in the physician-patient encounter: revisiting the shared treatment decision-making model. *Soc Sci Med.* 1999; 49(5): pp. 651–661.
20. Coulter A. Paternalism or partnership? Patients have grown up—and there's no going back. *BMJ.* 1999; 319(7212): pp. 719–720.
21. Beisecker AE. Aging and the desire for information and input in medical encounters: patient consumerism in medical encounters. *Gerontologist.* 1988; 28: pp. 330–335.
22. Benbassat J, Pilpel D, Tidhar M. Patients' preferences for participation in clinical decision making: a review of published surveys. *Behav Med.* 1998; 24(2): pp. 81–88.

23. Cornacchia HJ, Barrett S. *Consumer Health: A Guide to Intelligent Decisions.* St. Louis, MO: Mosby; 1980.
24. Roter DL, Stewart M, Putnam SM, Lipkin M, Jr., Stiles W, Inui TS. Communication patterns of primary care physicians. *JAMA.* 1997; 277(4): pp. 350–356.
25. Hardey M. "E-health": the internet and the transformation of patients into consumers and producers of health knowledge. *Information, Communication & Society.* 2001; 4(3): pp. 388–405.
26. Gusmano MK, Maschke KJ, Solomon MZ. Patient-centered care, yes; patients as consumers, no. *Health Aff (Millwood).* 2019; 38(3): pp. 368–373.
27. Beisecker AE, Beisecker TD. Patient information-seeking behaviors when communicating with doctors. *Med Care.* 1990; 28(1): pp. 19–28.
28. Keslar L. The evolution of the doctor-patient relationship. *Medical Economics Journal.* 2023; 100(10): pp. 84–103.
29. Hoffmann TC, Légaré F, Simmons MB, et al. Shared decision making: what do clinicians need to know and why should they bother? *Med J Aust.* 2014; 201(1): pp. 35–39
30. Stanier J, Purtell R, Thomas D, Murray W. Part of the team: effecting change and sharing power in healthcare settings. *Patient Experience Journal.* 2023; 10(1): pp. 164–172.
31. Quill TE, Brody H. Physician recommendations and patient autonomy: finding a balance between physician power and patient choice. *Ann Intern Med.* 1996; 125(9): pp. 763–769.
32. Stewart M, Brown JB, Donner A, et al. The impact of patient-centered care on outcomes. *J Fam Pract.* 2000; 49(9): pp. 796–804.
33. Lussier MT, Richard C. Because one shoe doesn't fit all: a repertoire of doctor-patient relationships. *Can Fam Physician.* 2008; 54(8): pp. 1089–1092, 1096–1099.
34. Trust. *The American Heritage Dictionary of the English Language.* Retrieved January 4, 2024. https://ahdictionary.com/word/search.html?q=trust
35. Caterinicchio RP. Testing plausible path models of interpersonal trust in patient-physician treatment relationships. *Soc Sci Med Med: Psychol Med Sociol.* 1979; 13A(1): pp. 81–99.
36. Haskard KB, Williams SL, DiMatteo MR, Rosenthal R, White MK, Goldstein MG. Physician and patient communication training in primary care: effects on participation and satisfaction. *Health Psychol.* 2008; 27(5): pp. 513–522.
37. Korsch BM, Gozzi EK, Francis V. Gaps in doctor-patient communication. 1. Doctor-patient interaction and patient satisfaction. *Pediatrics.* 1968; 42(5): pp. 855–871.
38. Francis V, Korsch BM, Morris MJ. Gaps in doctor-patient communication. Patients' response to medical advice. *N Engl J Med.* 1969; 280(10): pp. 535–540.
39. Jansen J, van Weert JC, de Groot J, van Dulmen S, Heeren TJ, Bensing JM. Emotional and informational patient cues: the impact of nurses' responses on recall. *Patient Educ Couns.* 2010; 79(2): pp. 218–224.
40. Doyle BJ, Ware JE Jr. Physician conduct and other factors that affect consumer satisfaction with medical care. *J Med Educ.* 1977; 52(10): pp. 793–801.
41. Kafetsios K, Anagnostopoulos F, Lempesis E, Valindra A. Doctors' emotion regulation and patient satisfaction: a social-functional perspective. *Health Commun.* 2014; 29(2): pp. 205–214.

42. Weng HC. Does the physician's emotional intelligence matter? Impacts of the physician's emotional intelligence on the trust, patient-physician relationship, and satisfaction. *Health Care Manage Rev.* 2008; 33(4): pp. 280–288.
43. Beck RS, Daughtridge R, Sloane PD. Physician-patient communication in the primary care office: a systematic review. *J Am Board Fam Pract.* 2002; 15(1): pp. 25–38.
44. Ong LM, de Haes JC, Hoos AM, Lammes FB. Doctor-patient communication: a review of the literature. *Soc Sci Med.* 1995; 40(7): pp. 903–918.
45. Stiles WB. Stability of the verbal exchange structure of medical consultations. *Psychology & Health.* 1996; 11(6): pp. 773–785.
46. Francis L, Monahan K, Berger C. A laughing matter: the use of humor in medical interactions. *Motivation and Emotion.* 1999; 23(2): pp. 155–174.
47. Pinna MÁC, Mahtani-Chugani V, Sánchez Correas MÁ, Sanz Rubiales A. The use of humor in palliative care: a systematic literature review. *Am J Hosp Palliat Care.* 2018; 35(10): pp. 1342–1354.
48. Wanzer MB, Sparks L, Frymier AB. Humorous communication within the lives of older adults: the relationships among humor, coping efficacy, age, and life satisfaction. *Health Commun.* 2009; 24(2): pp. 128–136.
49. Bitner MJ. Evaluating service encounters: the effects of physical surroundings and employee responses. *Journal of Marketing.* 1990; 54: pp. 69–82.
50. Kuller R, Ballal S, Laike T, Mikellides B, Tonello G. The impact of light and colour on psychological mood: a cross-cultural study of indoor work environments. *Ergonomics.* 2006; 49(14): pp. 1496–1507.
51. Rapoport A. *The Meaning of the Built Environment.* Beverly Hills, CA: Sage Publications; 1982.
52. Mehrinejad Khotbehsara E, Safari H, Askarizad R, Somasundaraswaran K. Investigating the role of spatial configuration on visitors' spatial cognition in health-care spaces: case studies in Gilan, Iran. *Facilities.* 2022; 40(9/10): pp. 617–637.
53. Gharipour M, Tyne IA, Afsary S, Hemme N, Trout AL. A community healthcare clinic in Baltimore: healing environment, design criteria, and assessment metrics. *Archnet-IJAR.* 2023; 17(4): pp. 609–627.
54. Dijkstra K, Pieterse M, Pruyn A. Physical environmental stimuli that turn healthcare facilities into healing environments through psychologically mediated effects: systematic review. *J Adv Nurs.* 2006; 56(2): pp. 166–181.
55. Ulrich RS. Effects of health facility interior design on wellness: theory and recent scientific research. *Journal of Health Care Design.* 1991; 3: pp. 97–109.
56. Martin DP, Hunt JR, Hughes-Stone M, Conrad DA. The Planetree Model Hospital Project: an example of the patient as partner. *Hosp Health Serv Adm.* 1990; 35(4): pp. 591–601.
57. Nesmith EL. *Health Care Architecture: Designs for the Future.* Washington, DC: American Institute of Architects Press; 1995.
58. Martin DP, Diehr P, Conrad DA, Davis JH, Leickly R, Perrin EB. Randomized trial of a patient-centered hospital unit. *Patient Educ Couns.* 1998; 34(2): pp. 125–133.
59. Miller KM. *Planning, Design, and Construction of Health Care Facilities.* Joint Commission Resources; 2006.
60. Ulrich RS. Natural versus urban scenes: Some psychophysiological effects. *Environment and Behavior.* 1981; 13: pp. 523–556.

61. Ulrich RS. How design impacts wellness. *Health Care Forum Journal.* 1992; pp. 20–25.
62. Heerwagen JH, Heerwagen DR. Lighting and psychological comfort. *Lighting Design Application.* 1986; 6: pp. 47–51.
63. White JM. Music therapy: an intervention to reduce anxiety in the myocardial infarction patient. *Clin Nurse Spec.* 1992; 6(2): pp. 58–63.
64. Allan EL, Suchanek-Hudmon KL, Berger BA, Eiland SA. Patient treatment adherence. Facility design and counseling skills. *J Pharm Technol.* 1992; 8(6): pp. 242–251.
65. Kwallek N, Woodson H, Lewis CM, Sales C. Impact of three interior color schemes on worker mood and performance relative to individual environmental sensitivity. *Color Research & Application.* 1998; 22(2): pp. 121–132.
66. Haider A, Tanco K, Epner M, et al. Physicians' compassion, communication skills, and professionalism with and without physicians' use of an examination room computer: a randomized clinical trial. *JAMA Oncol.* 2018; 4(6): pp. 879–881.
67. Houston TK, Ray MN, Crawford MA, Giddens T, Berner ES. Patient perceptions of physician use of handheld computers. *AMIA Annu Symp Proc.* 2003; pp. 299–303.
68. Rouf E, Whittle J, Lu N, Schwartz MD. Computers in the exam room: differences in physician-patient interaction may be due to physician experience. *J Gen Intern Med.* 2007; 22(1): pp. 43–48.
69. Devlin AS, Arneill AB. Health care environments and patient outcomes: a review of the literature. *Environment and Behavior.* 2003; 35(5): pp. 665–694.
70. Mead N, Bower P. Patient-centredness: a conceptual framework and review of the empirical literature. *Soc Sci Med.* 2000; 51(7): pp. 1087–1110.
71. Laine C, Davidoff F. Patient-centered medicine. A professional evolution. *JAMA.* 1996; 275(2): pp. 152–156.
72. Stewart MB, Brown JB, Weston WW, McWhinney IR, McWilliam CL, Freeman TR. *Patient-centered Medicine: Transforming the Clinical Method.* Thousand Oaks, CA: Sage Publications; 1995.
73. Probst JC, Greenhouse DL, Selassie AW. Patient and physician satisfaction with an outpatient care visit. *J Fam Pract.* 1997; 45(5): pp. 418–425.
74. Kleinman A. *The Illness Narratives: Suffering, Healing and the Human Condition.* New York: Basic Books; 1988.
75. Platt FW, Gaspar DL, Coulehan JL, et al. "Tell me about yourself": The patient-centered interview. *Ann Intern Med.* 2001; 134(11): pp. 1079–1085.
76. Smith RC, Hoppe RB. The patient's story: integrating the patient-and physician-centered approaches to interviewing. *Ann Intern Med.* 1991; 115(6): pp. 470–477.
77. Beckman HB, Frankel RM. The effect of physician behavior on the collection of data. *Ann Intern Med.* 1984; 101(5): pp. 692–696.
78. Barrier PA, Li JT, Jensen NM. Two words to improve physician-patient communication: what else? *Mayo Clin Proc.* 2003; 78(2): pp. 211–214.
79. Haidet P, Paterniti DA. "Building" a history rather than "taking" one: a perspective on information sharing during the medical interview. *Arch Intern Med.* 2003; 163(10): pp. 1134–1140.
80. Levinson W, Gorawara-Bhat R, Lamb J. A study of patient clues and physician responses in primary care and surgical settings. *JAMA.* 2000; 284(8): pp. 1021–1027.

81. Marvel MK, Epstein RM, Flowers K, Beckman HB. Soliciting the patient's agenda: have we improved? *JAMA*. 1999; 281(3): pp. 283–287.
82. Hall JA, Irish JT, Roter DL, Ehrlich CM, Miller LH. Satisfaction, gender, and communication in medical visits. *Med Care*. 1994; 32(12): pp. 1216–1231.
83. Jackson LD. Information complexity and medical communication: the effects of technical language and amount of information in a medical message. *Health Commun*. 1992; 4(3): pp. 197–210.
84. Street R. Information-giving in medical consultations: the influence of patients' communicative styles and personal characteristics. *Soc Sci Med*. 1991; 32(5): pp. 541–548.
85. Schillinger D, Piette J, Grumbach K, et al. Closing the loop: physician communication with diabetic patients who have low health literacy. *Arch Intern Med*. 2003; 163(1): pp. 83–90.
86. Betancourt JR, Carrillo JE, Green AR. Hypertension in multicultural and minority populations: linking communication to compliance. *Curr Hypertens Rep*. 1999; 1(6): pp. 482–488.
87. Kleinman A, Eisenberg L, Good B. Culture, illness, and care: clinical lessons from anthropologic and cross-cultural research. *Ann Intern Med*. 1978; 88(2): pp. 251–258.
88. Elderkin-Thompson V, Silver RC, Waitzkin H. Narratives of somatizing and nonsomatizing patients in a primary care setting. *J Health Psychol*. 1998; 3(3): pp. 407–428.
89. Robinson JW, Roter DL. Psychosocial problem disclosure by primary care patients. *Soc Sci Med*. 1999; 48(10): pp. 1353–1362.
90. Anfinson TJ, Bona JR. A health services perspective on delivery of psychiatric services in primary care including internal medicine. *Med Clin North Am*. 2001; 85(3): pp. 597–616.
91. Bertakis KD, Callahan EJ, Azari R, Robbins JA. Predictors of patient referrals by primary care residents to specialty care clinics. *Fam Med*. 2001; 33(3): pp. 203–209.
92. Patterson ML. *Nonverbal Behavior: A Functional Perspective*. New York: Springer-Verlag; 1983.
93. Craig KD, Prkachin KM, Grunau RVE. The facial expression of pain. In: Turk DC, Melzack R, eds. *Handbook of Pain Assessment*. New York: Guilford; 2001. pp. 153–169.
94. Feldt KS. The checklist of nonverbal pain indicators (CNPI). *Pain Manag Nurs*. 2000; 1(1): pp. 13–21.
95. Prkachin KM, Craig KD. The communication and interpretation of facial pain signals. *J Nonverbal Behav*. 1995; 19(4): pp. 191–205.
96. Ekman P, Friesen WV. Detecting deception from the body or face. *J Pers Soc Psychol*. 1974; 29(3): pp. 288–298.
97. Rinn WE. Neuropsychology of facial expression. In: Feldman RS, Rimer B, eds. *Fundamentals of Nonverbal Behavior*. Cambridge, UK: Cambridge University Press; 1991. pp. 3–30.
98. Rosenthal R, Hall JA, DiMatteo MR, Rogers PL, Archer D. *Sensitivity to Nonverbal Communication: The PONS Test*. Baltimore, MD: Johns Hopkins University Press; 1979.
99. Ekman P, Friesen WV, Hager JC. *The Facial Action Coding System*. 2nd ed. London: Weidenfeld & Nicolson; 2002.

100. Kurtz SM, Silverman J, Draper J. *Teaching and Learning Communication Skills in Medicine*. Abingdon, Oxon, UK: Radcliffe Medical Press; 2005.
101. Mast MS. On the importance of nonverbal communication in the physician-patient interaction. *Patient Educ Couns.* 2007; 67(3): pp. 315–318.
102. Kelly M, Nixon L, Broadfoot K, Hofmeister M, Dornan T. Drama to promote non-verbal communication skills. *Clinical Teacher.* 2019; 16(2): pp. 108–113.
103. Liu C, Lim RL, McCabe KL, Taylor S, Calvo RA. A web-based telehealth training platform incorporating automated nonverbal behavior feedback for teaching communication skills to medical students: a randomized crossover study. *J Med Internet Res.* 2016; 18(9): e246.
104. Roter DL, Hall JA, Kern DE, Barker LR, Cole KA, Roca RP. Improving physicians' interviewing skills and reducing patients' emotional distress. A randomized clinical trial. *Arch Intern Med.* 1995; 155(17): pp. 1877–1884.
105. Tumulty PA. What is a clinician and what does he do? *NEJM.* 1970; 283(20–24): p. 21.
106. Harrigan JA, Oxman TE, Rosenthal R. Rapport expressed through nonverbal behavior. *J Nonverb Behav.* 1985; 9(2): pp. 95–110.
107. Hall JA, Harrigan JA, Rosenthal R. Nonverbal behavior in clinician patient interaction. *Appl Prev Psychol.* 1995; 4(1): pp. 21–37.
108. Colliver J, Willis MS, Robbs RS, Cohen DS, Swartz MH. Applied research: assessment of empathy in a standardized-patient examination. *Teach Learn Med.* 1998; 10: pp. 8–11.
109. Blondis MN, Jackson BE. *Nonverbal Communication with Patients*. New York: Wiley & Sons; 1977.
110. Duncan S. On the structure of speaker-auditor interaction during speaker turns. *Language in Society.* 1974; 2: pp. 161–180.
111. Tickle-Degnen LG, Gavett E. Changes in nonverbal behavior during the development of therapeutic relationships. In: Philippot P, Feldman RS, Coats EJ, eds. *Nonverbal Behavior in Clinical Settings*. New York: Oxford; 2003. pp. 75–110.
112. Haskard KB, Williams SL, DiMatteo MR, Heritage J, Rosenthal R. The provider's voice: patient satisfaction and the content-filtered speech of nurses and physicians in primary medical care. *J Nonverb Behav.* 2008; 32: pp. 1–20.
113. Hall JA, Roter DL, Rand CS. Communication of affect between patient and physician. *J Health Soc Behav.* 1981; 22(1): pp. 18–30.
114. Milmoe S, Rosenthal R, Blane HT, Chafetz ME, Wolf I. The doctor's voice: postdictor of successful referral of alcoholic patients. *J Abnorm Psychol.* 1967; 72(1): pp. 78–84.
115. Ambady N, Laplante D, Nguyen T, Rosenthal R, Chaumeton N, Levinson W. Surgeons' tone of voice: a clue to malpractice history. *Surgery.* 2002; 132(1): pp. 5–9.
116. Morse DS, Edwardsen EA, Gordon HS. Missed opportunities for interval empathy in lung cancer communication. *Arch Intern Med.* 2008; 168(17): pp. 1853–1858.
117. Reynolds WJ, Scott B. Do nurses and other professional helpers normally display much empathy? *J Adv Nurs.* 2000; 31(1): pp. 226–234.
118. Bertman S, Krant MJ. To know of suffering and the teaching of empathy. *Soc Sci Med.* 1977; 11(11–13): pp. 639–644.
119. Feighny KM, Monaco M, Arnold L. Empathy training to improve physician-patient communication skills. *Acad Med.* 1995; 70(5): pp. 435–436.

120. Hojat M, Mangione S, Nasca TJ, Gonnella JS, Magee M. Empathy scores in medical schools and ratings of empathic behavior in residency training 3 years later. *J of Social Psychology*. 2005; 145(6): pp. 663–672.
121. Fine VK, Therrien ME. Empathy in the doctor-patient relationship: skill training for medical students. *J Med Educ*. 1977; 52(9): pp. 752–757.
122. Malle BF. The actor-observer asymmetry in attribution: a (surprising) meta-analysis. *Psychol Bull*. 2006; 132(6): pp. 895–919.
123. Ross L. The intuitive psychologist and his shortcomings: distortions in the attribution process. In: Berkowitz L, ed. *Advances in Experimental Social Psychology*. Vol. 10. New York: Academic Press; 1977. pp. 173–220.
124. Choi I, Nisbett RE. Situational salience and cultural differences in the correspondence bias and actor-observer bias. *Pers and Soc Psychol Bull*. 1998; 24(9): pp. 949–960.
125. DiMatteo MR. Variations in patients' adherence to medical recommendations: a quantitative review of 50 years of research. *Med Care*. 2004; 42(3): pp. 200–209.
126. Pedersen R. Empirical research on empathy in medicine—a critical review. *Patient Educ Couns*. 2009; 76(3): pp. 307–322.
127. Roter DL, Frankel RM, Hall JA, Sluyter D. The expression of emotion through nonverbal behavior in medical visits. Mechanisms and outcomes. *J Gen Intern Med*. 2006; 21(Suppl 1): pp. S28–S34.

Chapter 4
Communication and Decision-Making

Perhaps it goes without saying that people cannot follow health directives they do not understand and cannot remember. This is true, even if they like their health professional very much, or trust the source of a health message from a broader system like their public health department.

Unfortunately, there tend to be serious limitations in the communication that typically takes place during a medical visit. By the time they leave the medical office, patients on average have forgotten 40–80% of what they were told. Of the points they do recall hearing about, they remember about half incorrectly.[1] This is a poor start to behavior change and treatment adherence.

Certainly, many patients become anxious in the unfamiliar environment of their medical visits; they are sometimes confused by the information given to them, and their clinicians often use medical terms that patients have never heard before.[2,3] But even when health professionals are quite clear and supportive in their communications, many patients have limited comprehension; their *health literacy* is lacking and they have no framework for successfully engaging with the information they are told.

Health literacy

Health literacy involves an individual's ability to obtain, process, understand, and use health information in order to make decisions about their healthcare, modify their health behaviors, and follow through with medical recommendations for their treatment.[4-6] Although related to general literacy and numeracy (the ability to read, write, and understand numbers), health literacy and health numeracy are more specifically focused on the healthcare context.[4] Patients with low health literacy often do not understand verbal or written information from their clinicians.[7,8] Meta-analyses, reviews, and nationally representative large-scale studies conclude that only about 12% of U.S. adults are proficiently health literate.[9] The remainder (88%) have health literacy challenges: about half have intermediate proficiency, 22% have basic proficiency, and 14% have below basic proficiency, making it difficult to navigate the healthcare system, know the names of prescribed medications and take them correctly, and understand directions for over-the-counter medicines. Patients with limited health literacy, which is often unrecognized by their clinicians, are likely to miss follow-up appointments for tests and referrals and may not understand the costs and coverage of their health insurance. Health literacy is somewhat correlated with general education,[10] but high intelligence can coexist with a low level of medical knowledge and inaccurate beliefs about health.

In general, health professionals overestimate their patients' understanding of health information, and use medical terms that confuse patients.[11,12] Consequently, patients forget a large proportion of what they are told in their visit, particularly if the information is complicated.[13–15] Patients rarely ask questions or assert their need for clarification;[16] therefore, straightforward, jargon-free communication is essential.[17–18] One study found that patients correctly understood medical terms only 36% of the time.[17] Another, in which 71% of 224 participants were college-educated, found poor understanding of 50 common general medical terms. Only 10 participants correctly defined all the terms, and no term was defined correctly by everyone in the study.[19]

Assessment and notation in the medical record of a patient's level of health literacy, can be very helpful in appropriately targeting information to their level of comprehension.[20,21] Providers can use simpler language when necessary, and offer printed materials designed for lower–health literacy patients.[22] Those with higher health literacy might be offered more detailed and complex information.

Time is always at a premium, of course, and there may be little opportunity for such assessment in the medical visit. Best practice, then, would involve the use of "universal precautions" for health literacy; every patient would be assumed to have limited health literacy and simple communication would be initially offered. The U.S. Public Health Service's Agency for Healthcare Research and Quality (AHRQ) commissioned the development of a "toolkit" (available online[23]) that offers ways to communicate simply and clearly with patients, and verify their understanding.[24]

Use of the "teach-back" method can check patient comprehension. The healthcare professional asks their patient to repeat back, in their own words, what they understand about the essential information they need to know.[25]

This method verifies accurate comprehension, allows for corrections and clarifications, and helps the patient consolidate the information into memory.[20] The teach-back technique is effective across a broad range of settings, patient types, and outcomes.[26] This technique may also help health professionals to check that they themselves have been clear and complete in their directives to their patients; sometimes in their busy practices, health professionals fall short of ideal communication. In one study, for example, patients were not explicitly told instructions for the dosing and timing of their new medications *almost half of the time*. Only about a third of the time were patients told how long they would be taking the medication and any potential adverse effects.[27]

Information processing and recall

Effective communication in medical settings is not easy to achieve; it is more likely to occur if clinicians have tools to help their patients comprehend and recall essential information. Throughout this chapter, we focus on the first stage of the Information-Motivation-Strategy model (outlined in Chapter 2). We examine methods for checking on patients' understanding, and ways for the healthcare team to reinforce important health messages—particularly early in treatment when a new diagnosis is potentially confusing, and patients may be distressed. We also address communication issues in broader public health messages with an eye toward maximizing understanding and retention. This chapter reviews basic principles of information processing and remembering, as well as the factors essential to formulating decisions to adhere to medical treatment. We examine the most effective ways for patients, in conjunction with their providers, to weigh options, risks, and benefits as they decide what healthcare actions they will take and maintain. We will briefly introduce some technological aids that can facilitate understanding and follow-up (noting that Chapter 8 will present a detailed examination of these and other options).

Let's begin this section with a few basic, and necessarily simplified, facts about how memory works. The *memory process* can be divided into three essential components: encoding, storage, and retrieval. *Encoding* refers to the process of putting information into memory, and it requires attention and effort. *Storage* involves the maintenance of information in memory—which is a dynamic and constructive process, rather than a static entity. Studies show that memories can change over time, with some elements degrading and others integrated with old and new information. *Retrieval* refers to the process of recalling information that has been stored and integrated, bringing it back into conscious awareness.

Sometimes a stored memory is difficult to retrieve; it feels close to awareness but can't quite be accessed. This is called the "tip-of-the-tongue phenomenon."[28] When we successfully recall a stored memory, we experience the aspect of memory process that most people think of as "memory"; several steps have preceded this one, however. Let's examine these preliminary steps in more detail.

Focusing attention and encoding

Largely without even thinking about it, we all filter information and focus on, or "attend" to, some things, while ignoring others. If we didn't, we would be quickly overwhelmed by the sheer volume of incoming information. The first step in the memory process involves noticing and paying attention to something that we can integrate into our short-term or "working" memory; we generally attend to things that are important to us and notice things that are consistent with our preexisting ideas and expectations.

Our immediate, or short-term memory, is quite limited, however; most people are only able to store about seven things there at once. In computer terms, short-term memory is analogous to RAM (random access memory) which is used for active processing of information in real time and is constantly being "written over." This is in contrast with long-term memory, similar to a computer's ROM (read-only memory), which has a much larger capacity to store information permanently. Working memory contains items that are occurring right now as well as any previously stored information that we make conscious in order to help us solve a current problem.[29] Compared with younger people (ages 17–32), older adults (about ages 61–80) tend to have poorer understanding and memory for information in situations where demands on working memory are high.[30] Older age is a negative predictor of memory performance in situations such as medical visits, when complex information is presented in a fast-paced manner. Issues of working memory are particularly relevant to treatment adherence. An older person might, for example, remember that their medication dose is due soon, but fail to take the pill when distracted by a phone call. Intrusions to working memory can change a person's focus, leaving them wondering, "Now, why did I come into the kitchen?" With practice, rehearsal, and memory-enhancing strategies, information can be maintained at the forefront of attention until a task is completed or moved from short-term, working memory to long-term storage, where the capacity is believed to be limitless.

Memory storage

Studies have shown that memory is not stored in a single, particular *place* in the brain nor is ongoing electrical activity required for memories to be maintained.[31,32] Memory involves a process called long-term potentiation (LTP) in which certain neural pathways become strengthened through activity; the neurons in a sense develop "habits" in the ways they communicate with each other. Certain neurotransmitters influence the ease with which these "habits" are formed.

The brain also has "plasticity" meaning that different areas can take over tasks and memory storage that were once done by other parts (which might have been damaged by traumatic brain injury or stroke). These characteristics of memory are important to understanding adherence and health behavior change.

Emotion and memory

Some of our past experiences seem to be etched in our memories, and some of our memories are much more vivid than others. This may be due partly to the emotional content of the experiences. A "flashbulb memory" is one that is so emotionally intense and significant that it is remembered in great detail.[33] When experiences are emotionally charged, the brain's *amygdaloid complex* is more active;[34] this area of the brain interacts over the short term with stress hormones to increase the strength of stored memories that are emotionally potent.[35,36]

Receiving information about a health threat is likely to be an emotionally charged experience for many individuals, making the event quite salient and enhancing some aspects of memory. Most people are unlikely to forget the *experience* of receiving their diagnosis, although many do forget its technical name and what they must do to treat or manage it. When people receive a diagnosis, they are typically upset, and their heightened emotional state can be detrimental to the encoding of any treatment details they are subsequently given. While memory of the moment when problematic test results were first described might be quite clear, the distress that followed is likely to have interfered with focus and encoding of instructions for treatment and follow-up.[37]

One series of studies has demonstrated that when the content of a message is emotionally charged, a simple main point can be remembered well; memory for the surrounding information tends to be impaired by the emotional content, however.[38] Health professionals must keep this in mind in order to direct their patients' attention to the most crucial, actionable information that follows a distressing diagnosis. Both reassurance and effective communication strategies are essential; some basic principles for helping patients remember medical information are summarized in Table 4.1.

Although an emotionally charged diagnosis has the potential to make encoding, storage, and recall of follow-up medical information more difficult, clearly linking the diagnosis to the recommendations that follow can minimize this barrier. Health promotion advice is more likely to be recalled when it is directly related to a diagnosis.[39] It is likely that if health *risks* can

Table 4.1 What Health Professionals Can Do to Help Patients Remember Medical Information

1.	Speak slowly and do not rush through the information being provided to the patient.
2.	Refrain from using medical jargon.
3.	Check frequently to make sure the patient has understood.
4.	Know the patient's level of health literacy and convey information at an appropriate level. If the patient's health literacy cannot be determined, apply universal precautions and present information as if the individual is on the lower end of health literacy, adjusting when necessary (e.g., if the patient asks a question that indicates a more sophisticated understanding).
5.	Understand that patients receiving a diagnosis may be emotionally upset and their ability to remember treatment and follow-up information might be impeded.
6.	Provide comfort and reassurance to patients to alleviate their anxiety and increase their capacity to attend and remember.
7.	Pair information about behavior change with other meaningful information, such as support options available.
8.	Be aware of patients' health beliefs.
9.	Tailor and personalize information for each patient.
10.	Do not give too much information at once.
11.	Put the most important information first and last (see *primacy* and *recency* effects).
12.	Encourage patients to take notes.
13.	Suggest, or provide, memory aids (e.g., written materials, illustrations, mnemonics, etc.).

be made salient to patients, and those risks can be shown to be reduced by certain health behaviors, recommendations might be more accurately remembered.

If the emotional experience is *extremely* intense or traumatic, of course, the individual's memory encoding will likely be affected negatively. If anxiety is too high, the individual might simply "tune out" and conclude (often incorrectly) that nothing can be done.[40] Clearly, the time of diagnosis may represent a teachable moment for behavior change, but the patient's anxiety must be managed well so that this moment is not lost, and the patient can effectively understand and remember the steps necessary for self-management.

Chronic stress

Stress can interfere with attention and focus, as well as physiological functioning, in ways that negatively affect memory. Long-term stress, such as over the course of an illness or difficult life circumstance, can interfere with cognitive processing and memory, in part by causing atrophy of the part of the brain called the hippocampus.[35,41] Patients who struggle with the stresses of a serious disease over time may have increasing difficulty remembering essential elements of their treatment plan. Indeed, meta-analytic research shows that the adherence of patients with serious diseases tends to be worse when patients are more severely ill.[42] Such patients may need additional help to remember treatment details, especially when changes are made to an already-familiar regimen. In Chapter 7, we examine in more detail both trauma and stress in long-standing life circumstances; we consider the effects of chronic stress and trauma deriving from socioeconomic and environmental inequality on health behavior, adherence, healthspan, and longevity.

Self-enhancement bias

When the emotions associated with "bad news" are recalled, people's recollections often tend to err toward a self-enhancement bias; many come to believe that things are better than they actually are. In one study, the people who received the worst cholesterol test and cardiovascular risk results were most likely to recall, several months later, results that were better than they actually had been. Those with the worst health-risk profiles engaged in the most self-enhancing memory bias.[43] When information about health behavior is particularly disturbing (e.g., that a person is exercising far less, or that their diet is far worse, than ideal), research shows that instead of improving their behavior, individuals reduce their stress by changing their views of the situation.[44] According to the theory of cognitive dissonance (see Chapter 2), people are sometimes driven to seek consistency by changing their attitudes (e.g., about the importance of exercise or a good diet) to be in line with their behaviors.[45]

Cultural context

Several quite prominent and stable qualities of individual identity also tend to influence memory. These features include ethnicity, religion, family, and other cultural influences, and need to be understood and considered during the medical encounter. In Chapter 2, we examined the importance of beliefs to health behavior change; as we further explore memory, we can begin to understand the pervasive effects of these beliefs, through the mechanism of culture.

Briefly, we know that beliefs are maintained, in part, through the process of "cognitive filtering" in which individuals tend to notice and are more attentive to information that confirms what they already believe to be true; contradictory information is often ignored or discounted.[46] Individuals interpret ambiguous information so as to be consistent with what they think they already know.[47] And greater weight is placed on information that is important to them and consistent with their preconceptions.[48] This cognitive filtering process can create dramatic differences in understanding.

Cultural factors play an important role in this filtering process, and they affect an individual's willingness to engage with a health message and the ease with which they change their health behaviors. We examine culture and behavior change in more detail in Chapter 7, where we consider several issues and cases. Here, we note simply that a person whose family environment and sociocultural context encourage an active orientation toward health is likely to pay attention to risk factors and diagnoses; they may tackle the challenges of disease management head-on.[49] When dietary recommendations are dramatically different from an individual's cultural norms, however, resistance to dietary change is quite likely. If there are strong pressures on a patient to use "natural, herbal" family remedies in place of prescribed pills, adherence to a medication regimen may be much more difficult. In terms of the first component of the Information-Motivation-Strategy model, where understanding and remembering are essential, it is important to note that the sociocultural context can strongly influence attention to and initial encoding of health information, affecting whether the individual is willing and able to eventually take action.

Additional factors affecting understanding and recall

Some studies find gender differences, such that women's memories for personally experienced events may be better than men's; there are, however, no sex differences in memory for verbal information.[50,51] Despite individual variations, older age is a fairly reliable negative predictor for some kinds of memory.[52] Memory for contextual material,[53] as well as for rapidly presented information with high demands on working memory, are more problematic for older adults.[30] When working with older patients, it is important that their health professionals keep in mind issues of information processing and memory, and make efforts to accommodate their needs.

Consider the nurse practitioner, Kristina, who makes a conscious effort not to rush when she makes her weekly phone calls to 85-year-old Leroy. Her queries about his blood glucose, blood pressure, and sodium intake (all of which he manages for himself) are typically made in the same order. She consciously tries to offer a patterned familiarity to their conversations. She also encourages him to make notes for himself and to write down the date and hour each time he takes his medications. This helps him remember to take his prescriptions and prevents taking double doses.

Transient characteristics, such as sleep-deprivation, certain medications, and substance use can also play a crucial role in memory. Although direct links between sleep deprivation and the establishment of new memory traces are not entirely clear in research, sleep deprivation is consistently associated with a variety of cognitive ill-effects including difficulty concentrating.[54,55] Interference with attention is likely to affect memory, and for a variety of tasks and experiences, recall and task performance are better when followed by sleep.[56,57] New memory traces, which tend to be relatively fragile, are reactivated and strengthened during sleep and are better translated into long-term memories.[58,59] A sleep-deprived person may have difficulty concentrating, and will tend to forget health information provided during the medical visit. Inquiring about a patient's sleep is an important element of effective medical care.

Substances, including alcohol and even some prescription medications, can impair an individual's initial ability to focus on and appropriately attend to their medical visit, and can hinder memory consolidation.[36] The length of the medical visit can also influence memory and recall; in longer medical visits, patients have better recall[39] and visit duration is linked to higher quality of care.[60,61] How long is long enough? Researchers believe that at least 20 minutes may be essential to ensure enough time for true patient participation, information sharing, and fully answering patients' questions.[60] Making effective use of whatever time is available becomes even more crucial when 20 minutes cannot be achieved. In Chapter 8, we consider time constraints in medical care delivery, and examine how the medical team and new technologies can make the most of the time available.

Strategies for improving memory and recall

Let's examine some well-researched strategies for helping patients remember what they are told in the medical visit. These include: tailoring information to the unique characteristics and needs of the patient; offering various options to aid memory; taking care to present elements of information in the order that best facilitates their recall; and using techniques such as mnemonics and "chunking" of information.

Tailoring information

In various healthcare settings, it is common to find "one size fits all" informational pamphlets and website links. Although these can sometimes offer helpful strategies, they are often too general to be of much help to an individual managing a disease. Patients might also discount general communication, feeling it is not designed for them. Today's technologies, as we will see in Chapter 8, allow the management of individual behavioral plans for patients. Physical therapists and registered dieticians can create targeted exercise and eating plans based on patients' individual needs. Even with a low-tech approach, healthcare professionals should, as much as possible, individually tailor materials to supplement their verbal information and recommendations to their patients.[62] A theoretical model by Petty and

Cacioppo[63] called the Elaboration Likelihood Model (ELM) proposes that tailored messages prompt people to engage more thoughtfully with targeted material than they would with general messages, resulting in more effective behavior change; tailored messages are more likely to improve a variety of health-relevant behaviors, including nutrition, physical activity, disease screening, and smoking cessation.[64-66]

Tailored messages do interact with self-efficacy for behavior change such that for people with high self-efficacy, a tailored message is more effective than a generic message; those with low self-efficacy, however, respond more negatively to a tailored message, feeling threatened and generating counterarguments to the message.[67] Knowing a patient allows for more effective targeting of a message in order to be as non-threatening and encouraging as possible. When tailored messages are impractical, general information should still be given, but only *following* a discussion of the personalized issue or problem, helping a patient to feel that their health professional means it specifically for them.[68] A verbal health message accompanied by a written prescription (such as for exercise)[69] and an informational pamphlet can be most effective.

Patients are more likely to read information chosen specifically for them; because they attend to it better, they are also more likely to remember it. Of course, some patients have such low health literacy that written materials are not helpful, and accommodations may be necessary.[70,71]

Memory aids

Encouraging patients to take notes during the visit (if they have adequate levels of literacy) can be very helpful to their participation and recall. Note-taking can also be quite effective to supplement verbal information and instructions with illustrative materials. A review of the utility of visual aids, for example, has found that pairing pictures and illustrations with verbal content can improve comprehension, recall, and adherence.[72] These effects can be dramatic, and simple pictures that reinforce verbal information are particularly effective. Illustrations and visual aids cannot take the place of verbal instruction but should reinforce and further explain what is already part of the health literacy-appropriate medical communication, serving as a supplement, not a substitute. When a picture is used to integrate information that the patient doesn't understand in the first place, it is useless; worse, the patient might use the picture to try to guess (incorrectly) what they are supposed to do.[73]

As noted earlier, any materials (e.g., instructional videos) should be tailored to specifics of the patient's case to be most helpful. Patients tend to prefer and better comprehend material in illustrations depicting individuals who are similar to them (e.g., the same ethnicity)[74,75]

Ordering of information

A well-known finding from the learning and memory literature is that people are most likely to remember the first and the last things that a speaker presents. These tendencies are called *primacy effects* (remembering the first) and *recency effects* (remembering the last).[76] This quirk of memory can be used as a tool by the astute clinician who places the most crucial pieces of information at the beginning and the end of the visit. In addition to aiding recall, patients tend to view as most important the things they hear first.[13]

Mnemonics and chunking

Two more memory aids that can help patients with self-directed behavior change include: *mnemonics*, which are phrases or acronyms representing the elements of what must be remembered, and *chunking*, which is organizing information into more manageable groups. The utility of these is enhanced when health professionals advocate their use, such as with an eye-catching poster offering illustrations of health behaviors.[72]

Decision-making

Andi is 55 years old, and she has struggled with obesity for most of her adult life. She's tried many different diets, including one where she ate only pickles and lettuce for supper and another where she had nothing but high-energy milkshakes week after week. While on these diets, she did lose weight, but quickly regained it once she returned to "normal" eating. Andi exercises each day, although only for a few minutes, because she defines "exercise" generously to include walking from the parking lot and up one flight of stairs to her office. Andi is searching for an alternative weight-loss strategy, and decides to try a new over-the-counter weight-loss pill that offers dubious claims with no scientific evidence. Although the testimonials are glowing, and the ingredient list appears to Andi to contain only plant extracts, the US Food and Drug Administration (FDA) has fined the company repeatedly for making health claims without research. Andi doesn't care; she is tired of limiting her food intake and she is looking for a quick solution. This product seems to be it.

While it is tempting to hope that most people make health decisions based on carefully reasoned analyses of accurate and relevant data, this is rather far from the case. Studies suggest that few people conduct truly thoughtful and thorough comparisons of the evidence, strengths, weaknesses, benefits, and costs of health action before they try something they think will achieve their goals. Grocery shoppers are commonly lured by attractive packaging that claims a food product is "nutritious" instead of by its actual nutritional value. Andi has been lured by the prospect of an easy fix to her weight problem; and as far as she can tell, nothing harmful appears to be on the ingredient list.

Even when we do try to be logical, we are typically unaware of many factors that enter into our decision-making process. These include emotional state, social context, cultural background, and the salience of the stimuli encountered. These factors are considered throughout this book, and they pose challenges to reasoned decision-making. Therefore, structured decision-making processes can be helpful.

Evaluating risk in making medical decisions

How does one decide whether a particular health action is worth taking, relative to other options that include doing nothing at all? How does one decide if a treatment is worth the side effects or the cost in money, time, and trouble? How does one decide if the potential risk of a poor disease outcome makes it worthwhile to engage in a "health risk behavior" like smoking, alcohol consumption, or unsafe sex?

There are usually no simple answers. Over two million articles are published every year in the field of medicine, and when medical researchers do more than one study on a specific issue (as they ideally would), the results are bound to vary along with subjects, methods, measurements, and covarying factors. Summarizing a body of research and offering a simple, correct clinical recommendation can be challenging. Yet, people want exactly that from their doctors and their public health officials. This desire was quite clear during the COVID-19 pandemic in 2020, when a novel virus attacked an immunologically naïve world population. Over the months of 2020 and well into 2021, research data about how the virus behaved in the population and what people might do to protect themselves came in slowly. Individuals, health professionals, and public health leaders did their best to make decisions in the context of limited scientific information.

Fortunately, for most preventive and medical treatment decisions, there exists abundant empirical data; for some clinical topics, there is so much research information that sorting through it is a huge challenge. As we will see in this section, when there are no simple answers, there are some strategies for evaluating the risks and benefits of health action. One of these is meta-analysis, to which we have already been briefly introduced. The need for this approach is particularly acute in public health and medicine, where a great quantity of information must be managed in order to address a research or clinical question. Later in this chapter, we will address meta-analysis in greater detail, after we have laid some groundwork for understanding effect sizes and other components needed for the meta-analytic approach.

Medical decision analysis

Medical decision analysis is a formal process for assessing both the probabilities and the importance of various health outcomes;[77,78] it involves several steps including building and modeling a "decision tree" that maps out possibilities for and consequences of various courses of action. Medical decision analysis examines relevant probabilities, evaluates potential outcomes, and relies on sensitivity analyses.[79-81]

Individuals can be helped to make better choices by using some of the important elements of medical decision analysis including understanding probabilities and systematically evaluating possible actions and outcomes. Applying some of the concepts of structured decision analysis to personal decision-making (even without using the fully structured approach) can lead to more thoughtful and reasoned decisions.

A crash course in Bayesian methods

At first glance, the phrase *Bayesian statistics* seems a little intimidating. But, the concept of a Bayesian approach is simple, and each of us carries out many informal Bayesian analyses every day, from deciding how fast to drive on a slick road to deciding just how spicy a dish to order at a favorite Thai restaurant.

Let us first consider a strict "frequentist" approach that defines probability as the relative frequency of a particular event over a large number of trials or "opportunities" for the event to happen. This approach restricts our analysis to the specific issue under consideration and discourages any subjective decisions about which data to consider. Many decisions we make every day are based on frequentist probability estimates; the closer these estimates come to reality, the better our decisions based on them will tend to be. If a weather app lists an 80% chance of rain, one would do well to carry an umbrella; if that number is 20%, one might not bother. If a fetal genetic test reveals a one in 50 chance of a particular disorder, a prospective parent might decide on further testing; a one in 10,000 chance of the disorder might prompt a different decision.

Compared with a frequentist approach, a Bayesian approach reflects reality more accurately because it includes assumptions and additional available information.[82] When deciding whether to seek medical care for symptoms, a frequentist approach would involve simply paying attention to the symptoms. A Bayesian approach, however, would involve attending to the symptoms *and* drawing on a wider knowledge base, including recollections of past experience with the same symptoms. In a Bayesian approach, the individual might consider these questions: "When I felt this way before, did I get better or worse? What was my diagnosis? How did I resolve the problem?"

Although many studies in medicine, public health, and psychology have historically relied on traditional, frequentist approaches, Bayesian analyses are increasingly utilized.[83] Bayesian research methods rely on existing knowledge to set a priori (prior to experience) assumptions. Specific hypotheses are tested in the context of these assumptions; the results are used to update the knowledge base which then helps to set the next a priori assumptions. The emphasis is on constantly refining and strengthening understanding.

Our worldviews and belief systems constitute our "knowledge base," which we use to create and test hypotheses about many aspects of our lives—including actions we might take to improve our health. Let's recall Andi's decision to try a weight-loss supplement. Her "knowledge base" (which might be inaccurate) contains the following: *(1)* pills might help; *(2)* some pills can be harmful; *(3)* (according to advertisers) plant-based derivatives are not harmful because they are natural; and *(4)* (according to fashion influencers) life will be more fulfilling at a lower weight. Thus, Andi's working hypothesis is that buying and taking this new supplement will improve her life by helping her lose weight; she purchases the product and begins her own experiment to see if it produces the desired effect.

Within the first couple of days, Andi notices a difference—indeed, she's already lost three pounds. But she has also been experiencing lightheadedness, heart palpitations, and gastrointestinal distress. After one week on the pills, she quits taking them, convinced that they are making her sick. Her recent experience is added to her knowledge base, which now includes the idea that plant-based derivatives might not be so harmless after all, and any weight loss benefits might not outweigh the downside health risks.

The Bayesian approach is used in complex ways in research, relying on specific statistical methods for assessing a priori and a posteriori (based on past experience) probabilities. Even without these technical statistical tools, people can make good decisions by mapping out the differences between probabilities that are a priori and those that are a posteriori and deciding where the "truth" lies for them. (Note that we have put the word *truth* in quotes because implicit in this approach is the idea that our understanding will change over time as we obtain more and more data.) The Bayesian approach emphasizes the importance of effectively using preexisting information to enlighten interpretations of current information, and then making modifications in our assumptions as the data dictate.

Our preexisting knowledge base is typically derived from a variety of sources including our culture, past experiences, and empirical research (some of which is offered by those with a vested interest in the outcome).[84] That information might be distilled through health reporters who fail to mention potential sources of bias[85] or who sensationalize findings to gain and maintain an audience. The media sometimes exaggerate health risks to gain attention, and contribute to misunderstanding about various health threats.[86] As we will see further in Chapter 7, social media can complicate the situation, with influencers of all sorts (some with medical degrees) spouting information and misinformation at a fast pace. When individuals seek out their own health information, the chances are non-negligible that it is incorrect or that they will interpret it incorrectly. Studies of the types and quality of information available on the internet suggest that less than 10% of websites purporting to promote health behavior change were useful according to clinical practice guidelines set out by the U.S. Public Health Service.[87] On a variety of common health-related topics, even "credible" websites were only moderately accurate in the information they presented.[88]

Critical evaluation of health information and understanding of research results are crucial skills needed to engage in effective decision-making. Toward the goal of achieving these, let us turn now to an examination of the ways in which risks are presented, and what the numbers really mean.

Understanding risks and risk reduction

Researchers and practitioners in medicine and public health use a variety of specific statistical terms that allow them to communicate with each other about risk. Three terms that are often used are: *odds ratio*, *risk ratio* (or relative risk), and *hazard ratio* (or relative hazard). Each of these terms is a *relative* measure (as opposed to an absolute measure, which is a difference score rather than a ratio); each presents risks relative to one another in slightly different ways.

Odds ratios

An odds ratio (commonly abbreviated OR) represents the association between exposure to a particular risk factor and an outcome. It can be thought of as the ratio of two things: the odds of experiencing some outcome in a group that is exposed to a risk versus the odds in a group that has not been exposed to the risk. As an example, imagine a group of 100 smokers and a group of 100 nonsmokers. If 50 of the smokers develop lung cancer and 10 of the nonsmokers develop lung cancer, the odds of developing lung cancer for the two groups can be expressed as follows: smokers → 50/100 (1:1 odds) and nonsmokers → 10/100 (1:9 odds).

The *odds ratio* is expressed as: [odds of lung cancer for the exposed group (smokers)/odds of lung cancer for the unexposed group (nonsmokers)] or [(1/1)/(1/9)] → [1/.11] = 9.1. Thus, the odds of getting lung cancer are about nine times greater for a smoker compared to a nonsmoker.

Odds ratios are commonly used in many kinds of studies including clinical trials, case-control studies, meta-analyses, and various forms of survey research. When the outcome frequency is high in the population as a whole (e.g., if a certain kind of cancer were to occur naturally in 25% of the population), the odds ratio, when it is greater than one, will tend to overestimate the relative probability of the outcome in one group as compared to another. (This relative probability is known as the risk ratio, and it is discussed in the next section). When the odds ratio is less than one (and the outcome frequency in the population is high), the relative probability will be underestimated. Only when a particular outcome happens infrequently does the odds ratio closely approximate the risk ratio.

As an example, let's consider a real study of neonates using odds ratios.[89] This study looked at disease-related mortality predictors for low-birthweight infants in the neonatal units of two separate hospitals. After correcting mortality rates to account for the fact that disease severity was not the same at the two hospitals, the adjusted odds ratio of Hospital One to Hospital Two was 3.27. At first glance, this would suggest that low birthweight neonates in Hospital One had a three times greater risk of death than those in Hospital Two. But in cases like this, where the outcome variable (neonatal death) is common in the study population, the adjusted odds ratio is likely an overestimate of the true risk and it may need to be corrected in order to better represent the actual risk associated with one hospital versus the other.[90] This weakness of the OR approach should be kept in mind when evaluating studies that report their results in terms of ORs.

Risk ratios

Just like the odds ratio, the risk ratio (commonly abbreviated RR and also called the relative risk) compares the likelihood of a particular outcome for different groups. As illustrated in the prior section, when the incidence of an outcome in a study population is low, the results from ORs and RRs are almost the same. But the risk ratio contains a slight twist. Here, instead of odds, we are talking about the proportion (or percentage) of individuals experiencing a particular outcome in an exposed versus an unexposed group. So, using our lung cancer example from above, we see that the risk for those in the smoking group is 50%, whereas the risk for those in the nonsmoking group is only 10%. Our equation now uses these percentages instead of odds: [50%/10%] = 5. This means that an individual in the smoking group is five times as likely to develop lung cancer as is someone in the nonsmoking group.

This conceptualization is easier to interpret and makes better intuitive sense to most people than does the odds ratio, and so risk ratios are also quite commonly reported in the research literature.[91] It must be noted, however, that some study designs, such as the case-control study, and techniques such as the logistic regression, make it impossible to calculate the risk ratio directly from the data.

We should point out, also, that the interpretation of relative risks can be tricky for a couple of reasons. One is that the RR is dependent on whether we are framing our question in terms of an outcome happening or *failing* to happen (i.e., which group is placed in the numerator versus the denominator). Thus, when reading studies that use RRs, we must keep in mind that a small relative change on one side corresponds to a larger relative change on the reciprocal side. Let's use the simple example of gender as a risk factor for Pepper Syndrome (yes, we made that one up). If the male probability of developing Pepper Syndrome is 83% whereas the female probability is only 33%, the RRs are quite different depending on who is in the numerator. If we divide the male probability by the female probability (.83/.33) the RR is 2.5 but if we divide the female probability by the male probability (.33/.83) the RR is now 0.4. Keeping in mind the fact that 2/5 (0.4) and 5/2 (2.5) are reciprocal fractions will keep these numbers from becoming confusing.

Another reason that interpreting relative risks (or odds ratios, for that matter) may sometimes be perplexing is that the baseline likelihoods are sometimes not taken into account. Consider the challenge for Dr. Sanchez, who enters the examination room to find her usually calm patient, Tyler, agitated. Her queries reveal that he recently read an article that linked a medication he is currently taking with a doubled risk for a rare form of cancer. Although he doesn't have a history of cancer in his family, cancer is salient to him because he vividly recalls the death from cancer of the grandfather of a close friend. Tyler's current medication is serving him well, but after reading this article he doesn't want to take it anymore. He feels he would rather go back to one of the medications he tried before. He prefers dealing with some of their side effects rather than facing a twofold increase in his risk for this dreaded disease.

Dr. Sanchez is sympathetic to Tyler's concern; he is absolutely correct in his interpretation of what the study results show. But she points out one thing he has overlooked, which is that the likelihood of this rare cancer in someone with his constellation of characteristics is very low to start with—about one in a million. A doubling of this risk still leaves him with almost no chance of contracting the disease—only two chances in a million. When this additional information is taken into account, Tyler is relieved and glad that he can continue to take his current medications without worry, avoiding the side effects of other medication options.

Hazard ratios

The hazard ratio (often abbreviated HR or RH for "relative hazard") is a form of what is called "survival analysis." Practically, it can be thought of as a variation on the risk ratio or relative risk.[92] Cox's proportional hazards regression[93] is probably the most commonly used of the hazard ratios in the health-related literature,[94] and just as with risk ratios, it describes the degree of risk associated with being in one group versus another. One advantage of the hazard approach is that individuals who do not complete a study can still be included in its statistical analysis. These individuals are said to be "censored," but the data they provided before they dropped out are still valuable.

Survival analyses may, in fact, involve actual survival—that is, the likelihood of still being alive at a particular point in time. Such analyses might also represent something else entirely, like the "survival" or continuation of a behavior over time. For instance, a survival analysis can be used to estimate an individual's likelihood of continuing to exercise when enrolled in an exercise-support group versus the likelihood when working at exercise maintenance alone.

Whatever the event of interest, the relative hazard represents the probability that it will occur at any given point in time, based on group membership (e.g., a group exposed to a risk versus an unexposed group; a group that received a drug versus a group that received a placebo). This type of analysis involves a continuous time-hazard function (i.e., the likelihood of some event occurring during the next assessment period, if it has not happened already). Therefore, it describes the relative risk (or protection, if the numerator and denominator are reversed) associated with group membership *at any particular time point*. One common error when interpreting hazard ratios is to assume that they represent relative speed toward the outcome[95] such as looking at an RH for smoking of 1.3 and taking this to mean that smokers die at a 30% faster rate than nonsmokers. The correct interpretation is that at any given time point, someone from the smoking group has about a 30% greater chance of being dead compared with someone from the nonsmoking group. If the order of comparison groups is reversed, we see an RH of 0.70, indicating that nonsmokers experience only about 70% of the risk of death that smokers experience (at any given point in time).

Risk ratios and correlation

As we saw earlier, when an outcome is common in a population, the odds ratio tends to overestimate risks that are greater than one and to underestimate those that are less than one. When the base rate of a condition is very different in two groups, both odds ratios and risk ratios can be misleading. An illustration can be found in Table 4.2, which presents two scenarios, each with a relative risk of about two, but with different base rates.

Table 4.2 Illustration of the Influence of Base Rates on Risk Ratios and Correlations

Scenario 1: Poor outcomes are common because the disease is common.

		Health Outcome		
		Good	Poor	
Adherent to medications	Yes	34	16	50
	No	16	34	50
		50	50	100

Risk Ratio = 34/16 = 2.12
There is slightly more than twice the risk of a poor outcome if patients are nonadherent than if patients are adherent.
Phi Coefficient correlating adherence with health outcome = .36

Scenario 2: Poor outcomes are rare because the disease is very rare

		Health Outcome		
		Good	Poor	
Adherent to medications	Yes	49	1	50
	No	48	2	50
		97	3	100

Risk Ratio = 2/1 = 2
Here, there is also twice the risk of a poor outcome if patients are nonadherent versus if patients are adherent.
Phi Coefficient correlating adherence with health outcome = .06

In these two scenarios, the actual relationship (i.e., the correlation measured by the Phi Coefficient) between adherence and outcome is quite different (.36 versus .06) even though the risk ratio is almost exactly the same. This occurs because the distribution of good versus poor outcomes is different. In Scenario 1, the risk of a poor outcome is twice as high with nonadherence, and it is quite consequential because poor outcomes can occur frequently. In Scenario 2, where the disease is rare, twice the risk of nonadherence still makes a poor outcome a low probability event.

The landscape of study results and the value of meta-analysis

Each day, Hakim is bombarded with a great deal of health information and advice. Caffeine is harmful to your health ... coffee can improve your health. Chocolate isn't good for you ... wait, yes, it *is* good for you. Eggs are high in cholesterol and you should eat, at most, one or two per week; wait a minute, eggs contain 22% less cholesterol than previously thought and eating one per day may increase HDL ("good" cholesterol) levels. Not only are many health messages contradictory, their sheer number is daunting. While this might be exasperating for many of us, Hakim embraces each new recommendation enthusiastically. He cut eggs from his diet almost completely, then added them back in when a new study showed them to be healthy. He abstained from all alcohol until he read that a glass of wine each evening can lower the risk of cardiovascular disease. Margarine, marshmallows, multivitamins, mocha-lattes, and mackerel all appear and disappear from his diet with surprising regularity. By always following the latest health recommendations, Hakim feels assured that, barring an untoward event, he will live a long and healthy life.

In any given set of research studies, there are usually conflicting results. The odds ratios, risk ratios, and relative hazards described above are very useful for thinking about the likelihoods of various outcomes, but they typically vary from one study to another, usually because they use different methods and examine a variety of outcome measures. Each study has its own set of biases, as well, including the participants and how they are recruited, the study design, the measurement tools, and the statistical analyses of the data. It is also possible that even a very well-conducted study may miss something important or may produce a finding that is true in that sample but not relevant in the larger population.

Study results can be compared, of course, according to their "statistical significance," that is, if they meet a stated criterion for whether their results occurred by chance. A commonly used cut-off is that of $p < .05$, which means that the probability of being *wrong* when claiming a finding to be true, based on its evidence in a particular study, is less than 5%. Another way of saying this is that the likelihood of being right when making such a claim is at least 95%.

The statistical term *Type I error* refers to detecting a change (or difference) by chance in a sample when there is not actually one in the population from which the sample was drawn (i.e., a false positive). The statistical term *Type II error* involves failing to detect a change (or difference) when it actually does exist (i.e., a false negative). These two types of errors are tightly linked to one another; a higher p value decreases the likelihood of missing an effect that really exists but increases the likelihood of "finding" something that merely occurred by chance. Avoiding "false findings" by setting a more stringent p value (such as $p < .01$) also makes it more likely that a true finding will be missed. Increasing the size of a study sample gives the researcher more "power" to find effects that are real; as a sample gets larger, it more closely approximates the size of the actual population. If a sample contains only 10 people, and several are atypical in ways that are important to the study, results can be skewed. A sample of thousands would better reflect the population and allow inferences to be made about it.

The findings of various studies, such as whether coffee or eggs are good or bad for a person, might disagree because of biases inherent in the way research questions are framed, participants are recruited, and data are collected. Inconsistencies might occur because of between-study variations such as sample size and data analytic tools. One way to find out the "real answer" (so Hakim can know what to include in his diet) is to combine the results of several studies. This statistical approach is called "meta-analysis" and it allows researchers to find areas of consensus among a variety of studies and examine the factors that contribute to variation among them. We have already reviewed the results of several meta-analyses in previous chapters and have noted the strength of the evidence that they produce.

A meta-analysis can be thought of as an analysis of research studies that serve as the "participants." Instead of gathering information from individuals, a meta-analysis pools information from many empirical investigations that all examine the same research question, and it computes summary statistics to represent the overall results from all studies combined. For example, suppose a meta-analysis examines the question of whether walking reduces the risk of cardiovascular disease (CVD). Indeed, such a meta-analysis was done, combining the results from 18 different studies and reporting a hazard ratio for CVD of 0.69 for those who walked the most versus those who walked the least.[96] With a *p* value of less than .001, we can feel confident that walking actually does decrease one's chances of developing cardiovascular disease. The likelihood that the reported findings are merely due to chance and not generally true is less than one in a thousand.

Studies that remain unpublished, usually because their findings did not reach statistical significance, are unlikely to be included in meta-analyses. To address this problem, researchers calculate a number called the "fail-safe *N*," which represents the number of new, unpublished, or not retrieved studies with "no effect" that would need to be included in the meta-analysis in order to make its results nonsignificant.[97] If this number is small, it indicates that just a few contradictory study results could nullify the conclusions of the meta-analysis. A large number indicates a robust conclusion; many studies would need to contradict the findings before they would be rendered nonsignificant.

When we review research evidence, we hope to find well-done meta-analyses because their results carry greater weight than any single study, and they increase our confidence in choosing various treatment options and behavioral modifications.

Cumulative and interactive effects

Hakim was confused about the many, and often contradictory, health-relevant findings that turned up in his study of best dietary choices. His strategy was to respond to the most recent findings because he believed that research results are cumulative. That is, Hakim believed that if four different studies found four different behaviors that reduced heart disease risk each by 8%, combining those behaviors should reduce risk by 32%. Unfortunately, these behaviors co-occur and "share variance" with one another; their intercorrelations need to be statistically controlled. When behaviors are intercorrelated, adopting them all does not yield an additive outcome.

Even if the effects were additive, Hakim's baseline heart attack risk would still need to be taken into account. If his disease risk is high, a 32-percent decrease (or any decrease at all) could be quite important. But Hakim's chance of a heart attack is only about three in 10,000; he is very young, has low blood pressure, low cholesterol, and no family history of heart disease. A percentage decrease in risk would not be very meaningful because his a priori risk is very low.

When evaluating study results, it is also crucial to keep in mind the ways in which an individual is similar to, or different from, the people who participated in the research. Gender differences may be important in determining similarity of disease risk. The health behaviors (e.g., diet, exercise, smoking, and alcohol use) of research participants can make various studies relevant to someone like Hakim, or unlikely to apply to him. Careful reading of research and discussion with one's health professional are necessary to keep findings on health risk behaviors in perspective.

Patient involvement in decision-making

Health professionals and their patients typically go through the decision process on their own, as they consider the best course of action to promote the patient's health. Doctors evaluate evidence, arrive at diagnoses, and tell their patients what they think should be done. Patients consult the internet, and then either agree or disagree with their doctors; sometimes they just ignore what their doctors have to say. It should not be like this. A medical decision should be a course of action that has been evaluated and agreed upon together, by the provider who has specialized knowledge to evaluate the evidence, *and* the patient who ultimately must carry out the plan. Collaboration, teamwork, and shared decision-making are essential.

A considerable body of research shows that patients who collaborate in making medical decisions are more adherent to their jointly-decided-upon treatment regimens and more satisfied with the care they receive; they often experience more positive health outcomes than those who are not involved in treatment decisions.[98,99] Meta-analytic findings indicate that excellent communication (including shared decision-making) is related to better outcomes such as patients' emotional health, control of their symptoms, engagement in health behaviors (e.g., vaccinations), and lower decisional conflict.[100-102] In addition, meta-analyses show that provider-patient partnerships and greater patient involvement and participation in their care are associated with greater patient satisfaction and treatment adherence.[103,104]

While some don't want to be involved at all, most people wish to have a voice in decisions that affect their health; they are not, however, equally equipped to participate in those decisions. And, while many healthcare practitioners want to make decisions with their patients, some are singularly unenthusiastic about doing so.[105] Thus, the degree to which participation occurs is quite variable;[106] across more than 3,500 clinical decisions made in outpatient facilities, one study found that only 9% involved informed, joint decision-making.[107]

Asking patients, up front, how much involvement they desire, and offering them opportunities to be involved in their care, can be helpful.[105] Some simple tools for evaluating patients' preferences might aid this process, and allow exploration of how much information and discussion a patient would like to have.[108] Clinicians' preferences for involving patients can also be assessed.[105] Knowing these predispositions ahead of time can smooth the process of collaboration. Some aspects of the Transtheoretical Model of Change (outlined in Chapter 2) might be used to aid healthcare practitioners in working with patients who are just getting accustomed to the idea of being actively involved in decisions and are at different levels of "readiness" to participate in their care.[109]

There are many informal ways in which providers can invite patients to be involved in their healthcare decisions. These include actively listening to the patient's story, nonverbally communicating sensitivity to and interest in patient preferences, and asking the patient about their concerns and opinions. More formal methods of patient engagement exist as well, and these are the focus here.

Tools for participatory decision-making

There are always uncertainties attached to proposed treatments, and (perhaps with the exception of emergency treatment) patient preferences are always relevant. Medical decision-making requires an individual to choose the level of risk (such as of treatment related side effects) that they may be willing to tolerate for a particular benefit or disease management outcome.[78,110] A patient might prefer to initially try dietary management and wait to start medications to manage hypertension, for example. Another might be willing to accept a very high risk of medication side effects in treatment for cancer, in order to have a chance to attain a very good outcome such as cure. Likewise, people vary in what they are willing to do to avoid a highly undesirable condition. Some people are willing to restrict their diet and alcohol use, exercise nearly every day, and take medications in order to manage their diabetes; others might refuse to change one bit of their lifestyle to accommodate their condition. *Decision trees*, part of clinical decision analysis mentioned earlier in this chapter, can help patients and members of their healthcare team weigh the costs and benefits associated with various treatment options for all kinds of conditions.[80] In a decision tree, a set of options is generated, and the probabilities of particular outcomes are listed, with their relative importance or "utility values" assigned for each. Case Study 4.1 and Figure 4.1 present a sample decision tree that might help a patient named Peter decide how to proceed.

Case Study 4.1 Sample Decision Tree and a Simplified (hypothetical) Medical Decision Analysis

Peter could use some help choosing among multiple treatment options for tankurvi syndrome (an imaginary disease we created for this illustration). Partly because of his family history, and partly because of his own habits, Peter has developed tankurvi, although thankfully he is in the very early stages of the disease. Right now, he has two basic courses of action to prevent the worsening of his condition: *(1)* strict dietary modifications that may be very difficult for Peter to adhere to, or *(2)* moderate changes to his diet coupled with a medication that usually has no bothersome side effects.

The decision tree in Figure 4.1 shows the two possible results (events) associated with each decision option, and the probabilities for each. The utility (or "value") for Peter that is associated with each outcome is also included. Based on these, it is not surprising that Peter prefers to take a moderate dietary approach along with medication (Option 2).

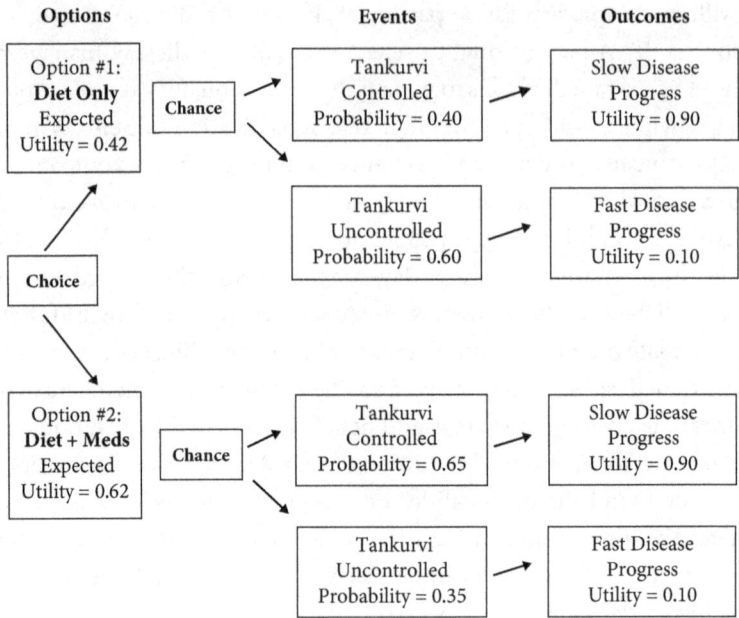

Figure 4.1 Sample Decision Tree

As we see in Case Study 4.1, Peter's input is crucial, because only he knows his personal preference for eating whatever he wants with a few modifications versus practicing strict self-control. The decision that must be made is *preference sensitive*; it is one in which the ratios of cost to benefit depend, to some degree, upon the individual's personal preferences and values. In this case, it is especially important that Peter's healthcare provider help him evaluate his options in terms of the scientific evidence.[111] A collaborative decision-making process, using appropriate aids as illustrated in the case study box and Figure 4.1, can result in better understanding of the issues, more realistic expectations about outcomes, less decisional conflict, and a final decision that best reflects the patient's values.[111]

There exist a number of methods for engaging patients in decision-making, including interactive computer programs, videos, or apps that present patients with information about risks, side-effects, and likely outcomes associated with different treatment approaches.[112,113]

Sometimes, these approaches include input from the point of view of patients who have struggled with the same health issues; others remind patients of questions they should ask. For the clinician, web resources provide tools that can be used to guide patients. One particularly useful website is that maintained by the Beckwith Center for Shared Decision Making at the University of Pittsburgh Medical Center, which offers numerous decision aids for both clinicians and patients. The URL for accessing these tools is: https://www.upmc.com/healthcare-professionals/shared-decision-making. Ideally, decision aids can be used at home by patients, so that they can discuss options with their loved ones before a final decision is reached.[114,115] When used properly, decision aids are beneficial in increasing patients' knowledge and collaboration, which are essential for health behavior change and treatment adherence.[115]

Joint decision-making and maximizing quality-adjusted life years

When they consider how to proceed with various options for treatment or health behavior change, patients typically do not explicitly mention their desire to maximize their "quality-adjusted life years." This is often, however, exactly their implicit goal. People generally want to live as well as possible for as long as possible; but while some treatments might increase length of life, they might also reduce its quality by virtue of their difficulty, side effects, and/or ultimate health outcomes. It is fairly easy to quantify survival (length of life); certain medical interventions might make additional years of life more likely (although all predictions can only be made in probabilistic terms). Attaching an assessment of *quality of life* is more complex. Values that individuals place on various "states of being" may be quite unique to them. For some, taking daily medication injections, experiencing increased but tolerable pain, or having significant dietary restrictions might be considered unbearable. For others, these might be considered manageable, requiring adjustment but still allowing a life worth living. It is the balance between length of life and its quality that patients, ideally with the help of their physicians, try to achieve.

In the study of population-based health outcomes in the field of health economics, the quality-adjusted life year (QALY) is a statistical measure based on the value of a health outcome to a population of people who experience it combined with the length of life (based on attendant probabilities) afforded by the treatment.[116] The QALY thus combines two different potential benefits of treatment—length of life and quality of life—into a single number that can allow comparison across different types of treatments in a particular period of time.

The statistical measurements are less important in our discussion here than the concept itself. One can imagine that considerable value could be added to physician-patient discussions and joint decision-making by simply keeping in mind various potential costs and benefits in terms of both life expectancy and effects on quality of life.

Joining the perspectives of providers and patients

Health professionals and their patients sometimes have different perspectives on disease and treatment, and their cognitive and personal constructs might not be aligned. Their differences can make shared decision-making a significant challenge. In the context of a chronic disease like rheumatoid arthritis, for example, the physician considers disease markers in blood tests and on imaging scans, and the results of a physical examination, to measure disease progression and treatment success. The physician recognizes that the patient's disease is chronic, and the goal is long-term management. The patient focuses on the subjective experience of pain and stiffness, and might expect that when a treatment does help to relieve these symptoms, the condition is cured. Such a conclusion might be tempting, especially if the treatment is burdensome, like self-injected medication or an intravenous infusion. When the condition is serious and asymptomatic (such as hypertension), a misalignment of perspectives might be especially problematic and lead to nonadherence and poor health outcomes.

In this chapter, we have focused much attention on the importance of provider-patient communication including analysis and assessment of health risk. We have also examined provider-patient joint decision-making about courses of action to achieve the best possible outcomes for the patient. We have emphasized that medical decisions can be complex and that patients need their clinicians' guidance in evaluating health risks and potential healthcare choices. As we have examined in the health behavior models guiding us in Chapter 2, patients make decisions about what they will, or will not, do based on their understanding of the regimen, their beliefs about the disease and treatment, their commitment and social context, and the resources available to them. Patients do strive for autonomy in their choices, but they need guidance and support from their health professionals, who play a pivotal role in their healthcare choices. Decisions about prevention and management of serious and chronic illnesses are often complex and difficult, and some conditions may not even be "fixable." While patients ultimately decide what health behaviors they will enact as well as how much, and what kind of, medical care they will receive, they *are* affected (as we saw in Chapter 3) by their interpersonal connections with their health professionals. The "power of the physician" lies not in the ability to control or compel the patient, but (as we will see in Chapter 5), in the ability to persuade, motivate, and fully inform the patient, who is ultimately free to choose.

Summary

A basic premise of this chapter is that patients cannot follow treatments or health directives they do not understand and cannot remember. Anxiety, limited health literacy, and limited comprehension can conspire to challenge an individual's ability to obtain, process, understand, and use health information in order to make healthcare decisions, modify health behaviors, and adhere to medical treatment. When messages from health professionals or public health authorities are inconsistent, unclear, or incomplete, nonadherence is likely to result. In Chapter 4, we examine the best ways that patients can be helped to understand and remember information; we consider ways to improve attention, focus, recall, the storage of memories, the management of emotions and stress, the tailoring of information, and the effects of cultural contexts. And we review the most effective ways for patients to weigh options, risks, and benefits in deciding, in conjunction with their providers, what healthcare actions they will take and maintain. We consider decision analysis issues including Bayesian methods, meta-analysis, decision-making strategies, and odds, risk, and hazard ratios. We examine shared decision-making, in which provider and patient work together to consider options and discuss and incorporate patient values, preferences, abilities, and self-efficacy to carry out the regimen. We consider patients' needs for information, guidance, and support in the context of patient autonomy. We examine quality-adjusted life years as a concept to aid in physician-patient discussions and joint decision-making while focusing choices on both life expectancy and the patient's assessments of quality of life.

Tools for instruction and self-study

Learning objectives

By the end of this chapter, readers should be able to

1. Describe the challenges faced by those with low health literacy.
2. Summarize the methods that clinicians can use to more effectively communicate with their patients who have varying health literacy levels.
3. Explain how emotion and stress affect memory.
4. Identify different types of memory aids that may be helpful to patients in a medical visit.
5. Explain how a Bayesian approach might be used in medical decision-making.
6. Justify the use of meta-analysis in combining the results of several studies examining the same research question.
7. Describe the benefits of patients being actively involved in medical decision-making.

Review questions

1. How is health literacy different from standard literacy?
2. What are the three components of memory? Include a brief description of each.
3. Name four specific things a clinician can do to help patients remember medical information.
4. Briefly outline what we know about individually-tailored medical information.
5. What is the primacy effect and what is the recency effect? How can clinicians use these concepts to guide the order in which they present information to patients?
6. What is the purpose of a decision tree, how is it structured, and how does it work?
7. How is a Bayesian analytical approach different from a frequentist approach?
8. What is the difference between an odds ratio (OR) and a risk ratio (RR)?

9. What are meta-analyses? Why are they so important?
10. What are Type I and Type II errors? What is their relationship to one another?
11. Overall, what does research show regarding outcomes of shared decision-making?
12. What are quality-adjusted life years?

Prompts for discussion and further study

1. Describe the value of universal precautions for health literacy, and suggest some cautions for using this approach.
2. What are the pros and cons associated with bringing family members into the medical decision-making process? Under what circumstances might they facilitate good decisions and under what conditions might they hinder them?
3. In terms of policy, what types of things can be done to improve health literacy? Think broadly—not just in medicine but in other fields as well (e.g., education).

Suggested reading

1. Roter DL, Hall JA. *Doctors Talking with Patients/Patients Talking with Doctors: Improving Communication in Medical Visits.* 2nd ed. Praeger; 2006.
2. Sox HC, Higgins MC, Owens DK, Schmidler GS. *Medical Decision Making.* 3rd ed. Blackwell; 2024.
3. Douthat R. *The Deep Places: A Memoir of Illness and Discovery.* Convergent Books; 2021.
4. Bowler K. *Everything Happens for a Reason: And Other Lies I've Loved.* Random House; 2018.

References

1. Kessels RP. Patients' memory for medical information. *J R Soc Med.* 2003; 96(5): pp. 219–222. doi: 10.1177/014107680309600504
2. DiMatteo MR, Haskard-Zolnierek KB, Martin LR. Improving patient adherence: a three-factor model to guide practice. *Health Psychol Rev.* 2011; 6(1): pp. 74–91.

3. Zolnierek KB, DiMatteo MR. Physician communication and patient adherence to treatment: a meta-analysis. *Med Care.* 2009; 47(8): pp. 826–834. doi: 10.1097/MLR.0b013e31819a5acc
4. Institute of Medicine (US) Committee on Health Literacy. *Health Literacy: A Prescription to End Confusion.* Nielsen-Bohlman L, Panzer AM, Kindig DA, eds. Washington (DC): National Academies Press (US); 2004.
5. Office of Disease Prevention and Health Promotion, U.S. Department of Health and Human Services. *Healthy People 2030.* Retrieved December 21, 2023 from https://health.gov/healthypeople. Washington, DC: U.S. Government Printing Office, August 2020.
6. Kalichman SC, Ramachandran B, Catz S. Adherence to combination antiretroviral therapies in HIV patients of low health literacy. *J Gen Intern Med.* 1999; 14(5): pp. 267–273.
7. Scott TL, Gazmararian JA, Williams MV, Baker DW. Health literacy and preventive health care use among Medicare enrollees in a managed care organization. *Med Care.* 2002; 40(5): pp. 395–404. doi: 10.1097/00005650-200205000-00005
8. Schillinger D, Bindman A, Wang F, Stewart A, Piette J. Functional health literacy and the quality of physician-patient communication among diabetes patients. *Patient Educ Couns.* 2004; 52(3): pp. 315–323. doi: 10.1016/S0738-3991(03)00107-1
9. Lopez C, Kim B, Sacks K. Health literacy in the United States: enhancing assessments and reducing disparities. Milken Institute (creative commons license); 2022. https://milkeninstitute.org/report/health-literacy-us-assessments-disparities
10. Paasche-Orlow MK, Parker RM, Gazmararian JA, Nielsen-Bohlman LT, Rudd RR. The prevalence of limited health literacy. *J Gen Intern Med.* 2005; 20(2): pp. 175–184.
11. Voigt-Barbarowicz M, Brütt AL. The agreement between patients' and healthcare professionals' assessment of patients' health literacy-a systematic review. *Int J Environ Res Public Health.* 2020; 17(7): p. 2372. doi: 10.3390/ijerph17072372
12. Seligman HK, Wang FF, Palacios JL, et al. Physician notification of their diabetes patients' limited health literacy: a randomized, controlled trial. *J Gen Intern Med.* 2005; 20(11): pp. 1001–1007. doi: 10.1111/j.1525-1497.2005.00189.x
13. Ley P. Memory for medical information. *Br J Soc Clin Psychol.* 1979; 18(2): pp. 245–255.
14. Ley P. Satisfaction, compliance and communication. *Br J Clin Psychol.* 1982; 21 (Pt 4): pp. 241–254.
15. Jansen J, Butow PN, van Weert JC, et al. Does age really matter? recall of information presented to newly referred patients with cancer. *J Clin Oncol.* 2008; 26(33): pp. 5450–5457.
16. Mathews JJ. The communication process in clinical settings. *Soc Sci Med.* 1983; 17(18): pp. 1371–1378.
17. Hadlow J, Pitts M. The understanding of common health terms by doctors, nurses and patients. *Soc Sci Med.* 1991; 32(2): pp. 193–196.
18. Jackson LD. Information complexity and medical communication: the effects of technical language and amount of information in a medical message. *Health Comm.* 1992; 4: pp. 197–210.

19. Thompson CL, Pledger LM. Doctor-patient communication: is patient knowledge of medical terminology improving? *Health Comm.* 1993; 5: pp. 89–97.
20. Schillinger D, Piette J, Grumbach K et al. Closing the loop: physician communication with diabetic patients who have low health literacy. *Arch Intern Med.* 2003; 163(1): pp. 83–90.
21. Wetta RE, Severin RD, Gruhler H, Lewis N. Capturing health literacy assessment in the electronic health record through evidence-based concept creation: a review of the literature and recommendations for action. *Health Informatics Journal.* 2019; 25(3): pp. 1025–1037. doi: 10.1177/1460458217739341
22. Schwartzberg JG, Cowett A, VanGeest J, Wolf MS. Communication techniques for patients with low health literacy: a survey of physicians, nurses, and pharmacists. *Am J Health Behav.* 2007; 31 Suppl 1: S96–104.
23. AHRQ Health Literacy Universal Precautions Toolkit, 2nd ed. Prepared by Colorado Health Outcomes Program, University of Colorado Anschutz Medical Campus. Rockville, MD: Agency for Healthcare Research and Quality. https://www.ahrq.gov/health-literacy/improve/precautions/toolkit.html
24. DeWalt DA, Broucksou KA, Hawk V, et al. Developing and testing the health literacy universal precautions toolkit. *Nurs Outlook.* 2011; 59(2): pp. 85–94. doi: 10.1016/j.outlook.2010.12.002
25. Villaire M, Mayer G. Chronic illness management and health literacy: an overview. *J Med Pract Manage.* 2007; 23(3): pp. 177–181.
26. Talevski J, Wong Shee A, Rasmussen B, Kemp G, Beauchamp A. Teach-back: a systematic review of implementation and impacts. *PLoS ONE.* 2020; 15(4): e0231350. doi: 10.1371/journal.pone.0231350
27. Tarn DM, Heritage J, Paterniti DA, Hays RD, Kravitz RL, Wenger NS. Physician communication when prescribing new medications. *Arch Intern Med.* 2006; 166(17): pp. 1855–1862. doi: 10.1001/archinte.166.17.1855
28. Schwartz BL. Tip-of-the-tongue states: phenomenology, mechanism, and lexical retrieval. *Metacognition and Learning.* 2002; 1(2): pp. 149–158.
29. Engle RW. Working memory capacity as executive attention. *Current Directions in Psychological Science.* 2002; 11: pp. 19–23.
30. Stine EL, Wingfield A, Poon LW. How much and how fast: rapid processing of spoken language in later adulthood. *Psychol Aging.* 1986; 1(4): pp. 303–311.
31. Lashley KS. In search of the engram. *Symposium of the Society for Experimental Biology.* New York: Cambridge University Press; 1950.
32. Gerard RW. *What Is Memory?* New York: Freeman; 1953.
33. Brown R, Kulik J. Flashbulb memory. *Cognition.* 1977; 5: pp. 73–99.
34. Cahill L, Haier RJ, Fallon J, et al. Amygdala activity at encoding correlated with long-term, free recall of emotional information. *Proc Natl Acad Sci USA.* 1996; 93(15): pp. 8016–8021.
35. McEwen BS, Sapolsky RM. Stress and cognitive function. *Curr Opin Neurobiol* 1995; 5(2): pp. 205–216.
36. McGaugh JL. Memory consolidation and the amygdala: a systems perspective. *Trends Neurosci.* 2002; 25(9): p. 456.

37. Kessels RP. Patients' memory for medical information. *J R Soc Med.* 2003; 96(5): pp. 219–222.
38. Christianson SA, Loftus EF. Remembering emotional events: the fate of detailed information. *Cogn Emot.* 1991; 5(2): pp. 81–108.
39. Flocke SA, Stange KC. Direct observation and patient recall of health behavior advice. *Prev Med.* 2004; 38(3): pp. 343–349.
40. Beck KH, Frankel A. A conceptualization of threat communications and protective health behavior. *Soc Psychol Q.* 1981; 44(3): pp. 204–217.
41. Kim EJ, Pellman B, Kim JJ. Stress effects on the hippocampus: a critical review. *Learn Mem.* 2015; 22(9): pp. 411–416. doi: 10.1101/lm.037291.114
42. DiMatteo MR, Haskard KB, Williams SL. Health beliefs, disease severity, and patient adherence: a meta-analysis. *Med Care.* 2007; 45(6): pp. 521–528.
43. Croyle RT, Loftus EF, Barger SD, Sun YC, Hart M, Gettig J. How well do people recall risk factor test results? Accuracy and bias among cholesterol screening participants. *Health Psychol.* 2006; 25(3): pp. 425–432.
44. Gerrard M, Gibbons FX, Benthin AC, Hessling RM. A longitudinal study of the reciprocal nature of risk behaviors and cognitions in adolescents: what you do shapes what you think, and vice versa. *Health Psychol.* 1996; 15(5): pp. 344–354.
45. Festinger L. *A Theory of Cognitive Dissonance.* Stanford, CA: Stanford University Press; 1957.
46. Nisbett RE, Ross L. *Human Inference.* Englewood Cliffs, NJ: Prentice Hall; 1980.
47. Taylor SE, Crocker J. Schematic bases of social information processing. In: Higgins ET, Herman CP, Zanna MP, eds. Hillsdale, NJ: Lawrence Erlbaum; 1981. pp. 89–134.
48. Fiske SE, Taylor SE. *Social Cognition.* 2nd ed. New York: McGraw Hill; 1991.
49. Umberson D. Gender, marital status and the social control of health behavior. *Soc Sci Med.* 1992; 34(8): pp. 907–917.
50. Herlitz A, Nilsson LG, Backman L. Gender differences in episodic memory. *Mem Cognit.* 1997; 25(6): pp. 801–811.
51. Kimura D, Clarke PG. Women's advantage on verbal memory is not restricted to concrete words. *Psychol Rep.* 2002; 91(3 Pt 2): pp. 1137–1142.
52. Verhaeghen P, Marcoen A, Goossens L. Facts and fiction about memory aging: a quantitative integration of research findings. *Journals of Gerontology: Psychological Sciences.* 1993; 48: pp. 157–171.
53. Spencer WD, Raz N. Differential effects of aging on memory for content and context: a meta-analysis. *Psychol Aging.* 1995; 10(4): pp. 527–539.
54. Harrison Y, Horne JA. Sleep loss and temporal memory. *Q J Exp Psychol A.* 2000; 53(1): pp. 271–279.
55. Maquet P. The role of sleep in learning and memory. *Science.* 2001; 294: pp. 1048–1052.
56. Fenn KM, Nusbaum HC, Margoliash D. Consolidation during sleep of perceptual learning of spoken language. *Nature.* 2003; 425(6958): pp. 614–616.
57. Peigneux P, Laureys S, Fuchs S et al. Are spatial memories strengthened in the human hippocampus during slow wave sleep? *Neuron.* 2004; 44(3): pp. 535–545.
58. Sutherland GR, McNaughton B. Memory trace reactivation in hippocampal and neocortical neuronal ensembles. *Curr Opin Neurobiol.* 2000; 10(2): pp. 180–186.

59. Fishbein W, McGaugh JL, Swarz JR. Retrograde amnesia: electroconvulsive shock effects after termination of rapid eye movement sleep deprivation. *Science.* 1971; 172(978): pp. 80–82.
60. Chen LM, Farwell WR, Jha AK. Primary care visit duration and quality: does good care take longer? *Arch Intern Med.* 2009; 169(20): pp. 1866–1872. doi:10.1001/archinternmed.2009.341
61. Neprash HT, Mulcahy JF, Cross DA, Gaugler JE, Golberstein E, Ganguli I. Association of primary care visit length with potentially inappropriate prescribing. *JAMA Health Forum.* 2023; 4(3): e230052. doi: 10.1001/jamahealthforum.2023.0052
62. Skinner CS, Strecher VJ, Hospers H. Physicians' recommendations for mammography: do tailored messages make a difference? *Am J Public Health.* 1994; 84(1): pp. 43–49.
63. Petty RE, Cacioppo JT. *Attitudes and Persuasion: Classic and Contemporary Approaches.* Dubuque, IA: William A. Brown; 1981.
64. Krebs P, Prochaska JO, Rossi JS. A meta-analysis of computer-tailored interventions for health behavior change. *Prev Med.* 2010; 51(3–4): pp. 214–221. doi: 10.1016/j.ypmed.2010.06.004
65. Hao L, Goetze S, Alessa T, Hawley MS. Effectiveness of computer-tailored health communication in increasing physical activity in people with or at risk of long-term conditions: systematic review and meta-analysis. *J Med Internet Res.* 2023; 25: e46622. doi: 10.2196/46622
66. Noar SM, Benac CN, Harris MS. Does tailoring matter? Meta-analytic review of tailored print health behavior change interventions. *Psychol Bull.* 2007; 133(4): pp. 673–693. doi: 10.1037/0033-2909.133.4.673
67. Holt CL, Clark EM, Kreuter MW, Scharff DP. Does locus of control moderate the effects of tailored health education materials? *Health Educ Res.* 2000; 15(4): pp. 393–403.
68. Kreuter MW, Chheda SG, Bull FC. How does physician advice influence patient behavior? Evidence for a priming effect. *Arch Fam Med.* 2000; 9(5): pp. 426–433.
69. Swinburn BA, Walter LG, Arroll B, Tilyard MW, Russell DG. The green prescription study: a randomized controlled trial of written exercise advice provided by general practitioners. *Am J Public Health.* 1998; 88(2): pp. 288–291.
70. Gazmararian JA, Baker DW, Williams MV et al. Health literacy among Medicare enrollees in a managed care organization. *JAMA.* 1999; 281(6): pp. 545–551.
71. Hochhauser M. Plain language needed. *Appl Clin Trials.* 2003: pp. 14–15.
72. Lee K, Nathan-Roberts D. Using visual aids to supplement medical instructions, health education, and medical device instructions. *Proceedings of the International Symposium on Human Factors and Ergonomics in Health Care.* 2021; 10(1): pp. 257–262.
73. Fillippatou D, Pumfrey PD. Pictures, titles, reading accuracy and reading comprehension: a research review. *Educ Res.* 1996; 38: pp. 259–291.
74. Dowse R, Ehlers MS. The evaluation of pharmaceutical pictograms in a low-literate South African population. *Patient Educ Couns.* 2001; 45(2): pp. 87–99.
75. Hosey GM, Freeman WL, Stracqualursi F, Gohdes D. Designing and evaluating diabetes education material for American Indians. *Diabetes Educ.* 1990; 16(5): pp. 407–414.

76. Castro CA. Primacy and recency effects. In: Craighead WE Nemeroff CB, eds. *The Corsini Encyclopedia of Psychology and Behavioral Science*. 3rd ed. Vol. 3. New York: Wiley. pp. 1241–1243.
77. Keeney RL. Decision analysis: an overview. *Oper Res*. 1982; 30(5): pp. 803–838.
78. Weinstein MC, Fineberg HV. *Clinical Decision Analysis*. Philadelphia, PA: W.B. Saunders Company; 1980.
79. Detsky AS, Naglie G, Krahn MD, Naimark D, Redelmeier DA. Primer on medical decision analysis: part 1—Getting started. *Med Decis Making*. 1997; 17(2): pp. 123–125.
80. Richardson WS, Detsky AS. Users' guides to the medical literature. VII. How to use a clinical decision analysis. B. What are the results and will they help me in caring for my patients? Evidence Based Medicine Working Group. *JAMA*. 1995; 273: pp. 1610–1613.
81. Richardson WS, Detsky AS. Users' guides to the medical literature. VII. How to use a clinical decision analysis. A. Are the results of the study valid? Evidence-Based Medicine Working Group. *JAMA*. 1995; 273: pp. 1292–1295.
82. Etzioni RD, Kadane JB. Bayesian statistical methods in public health and medicine. *Annu Rev Public Health*. 1995; 16: pp. 23–41.
83. Jaynes ET. *Probability Theory: The Logic of Science*. Cambridge: Cambridge University Press; 2003.
84. Baker CB, Johnsrud MT, Crismon ML, Rosenheck RA, Woods SW. Quantitative analysis of sponsorship bias in economic studies of antidepressants. *Br J Psychiatry*. 2003; 183: pp. 498–506.
85. Hochman M, Hochman S, Bor D, McCormick D. News media coverage of medication research: reporting pharmaceutical company funding and use of generic medication names. *JAMA*. 2008; 300(13): pp. 1544–1550.
86. Frost K, Frank E, Maibach E. Relative risk in the news media: a quantification of misrepresentation. *Am J Public Health*. 1997; 87(5): pp. 842–845.
87. Neuhauser L, Kreps G. Rethinking communication in the e-health era. *J Health Psychol*. 2003; 8(1): pp. 7–23.
88. Kunst H GD, Latthe PM, Latthe M, Khan KS. Accuracy of information on apparently credible websites: survey of five common health topics. *Br Med J*. 2002; 324: pp. 581–582.
89. Tarnow-Mordi W, Ogston S et al. R. Predicting death from initial disease severity in very low birthweight infants: a method for comparing the performance of neonatal units. *BMJ*. 1990; 300(6740): pp. 1611–1614.
90. Zhang J, Yu KF. What's the relative risk? A method of correcting the odds ratio in cohort studies of common outcomes. *JAMA*. 1998; 280(19): pp. 1690–1691.
91. Schechtman E. Odds ratio, relative risk, absolute risk reduction, and the number needed to treat—which of these should we use? *Value Health*. 2002; 5(5): pp. 431–436.
92. Cantor A. *Survival Analysis Techniques for Medical Research*. Cary, NC: SAS Publishing; 2003.
93. Cox DR. Regression models and life tables (with discussion). *Journal of the Royal Statistical Society Series B*. 1972; 34: pp. 187–220.
94. Cox DR, Oakes D. *Analysis of Survival Data*. London: Chapman and Hall; 2001.
95. Tyring SK, Douglas JM Jr., Corey L, Spruance SL, Esmann J. A randomized, placebo-controlled comparison of oral valacyclovir and acyclovir in

immunocompetent patients with recurrent genital herpes infections. The Valaciclovir International Study Group. *Arch Dermatol.* 1998; 134(2): pp. 185–191.
96. Hamer M, Chida Y. Active commuting and cardiovascular risk: a meta-analytic review. *Prev Med.* 2008; 46(1): pp. 9–13.
97. Rosenthal R, Rosnow RL. *Essentials of Behavioral Research: Methods and Data Analysis.* New York: McGraw-Hill; 1991.
98. DiMatteo MR. Evidence-based strategies to foster adherence and improve patient outcomes. *JAAPA.* 2004; 17(11): pp. 18–21.
99. Golin CE, DiMatteo MR, Gelberg L. The role of patient participation in the doctor visit. Implications for adherence to diabetes care. *Diabetes Care.* 1996; 19(10): pp. 1153–1164.
100. Stewart MA. Effective physician-patient communication and health outcomes: a review. *CMAJ.* 1995; 152(9): pp. 1423–1433.
101. Scalia P, Durand MA, Elwyn G. Shared decision-making interventions: an overview and a meta-analysis of their impact on vaccine uptake. *J Intern Med.* 2022; 291(4): pp. 408–425. doi: 10.1111/joim.13405
102. Wyatt KD, List B, Brinkman WB et al. Shared decision making in pediatrics: a systematic review and meta-analysis. *Acad Pediatr.* 2015; 15(6): pp. 573–583. doi: 10.1016/j.acap.2015.03.011
103. Hall JA, Roter DL, Katz NR. Meta-analysis of correlates of provider behavior in medical encounters. *Med Care.* 1988; 26(7): pp. 657–675.
104. Harrington J, Noble LM, Newman SP. Improving patients' communication with doctors: a systematic review of intervention studies. *Patient Educ Couns.* 2004; 52(1): pp. 7–16.
105. Jahng KH, Martin LR, Golin CE, DiMatteo MR. Preferences for medical collaboration: patient-physician congruence and patient outcomes. *Patient Educ Couns.* 2005; 57(3): pp. 308–314.
106. Street RL, Jr., Krupat E, Bell RA, Kravitz RL, Haidet P. Beliefs about control in the physician-patient relationship: effect on communication in medical encounters. *J Gen Intern Med.* 2003; 18(8): pp. 609–616.
107. Braddock CH, 3rd, Edwards KA, Hasenberg NM, Laidley TL, Levinson W. Informed decision making in outpatient practice: time to get back to basics. *JAMA.* 1999; 282(24): pp. 2313–2320.
108. Golin CE, DiMatteo MR, Leake B, Duan N, Gelberg L. A diabetes-specific measure of patient desire to participate in medical decision making. *Diabetes Educ.* 2001; 27(6): pp. 875–886.
109. Guadagnoli E, Ward P. Patient participation in decision-making. *Soc Sci Med.* 1998; 47(3): pp. 329–339.
110. Barry MJ, Mulley AG, Jr., Fowler FJ, Wennberg JW. Watchful waiting vs immediate transurethral resection for symptomatic prostatism. The importance of patients' preferences. *JAMA.* 1988; 259(20): p. 3010.
111. O'Connor AM, Legare F, Stacey D. Risk communication in practice: the contribution of decision aids. *BMJ.* 2003; 327(7417): pp. 736–740.
112. Kasper JF, Mulley AG, Jr., Wennberg JE. Developing shared decision-making programs to improve the quality of health care. *QRB Qual Rev Bull.* 1992; 18(6): pp. 183–190.
113. Levine MN, Gafni A, Markham B, MacFarlane D. A bedside decision instrument to elicit a patient's preference concerning adjuvant chemotherapy for breast cancer. *Ann Intern Med.* 1992; 117(1): pp. 53–58.

114. Barry MJ. Health decision aids to facilitate shared decision making in office practice. *Ann Intern Med.* 2002; 136(2): pp. 127–135.
115. O'Connor AM, Rostom A, Fiset V, et al. Decision aids for patients facing health treatment or screening decisions: systematic review. *BMJ.* 1999; 319(7212): pp. 731–734.
116. Weinstein MC, Torrance G, McGuire A. QALYs: the basics. *Value in Health.* 2009; 12: pp. S5–S9.

Chapter 5
Persuasion and Motivation

Every day, we are bombarded with persuasive messages about products, services, and political candidates. These messages come to us on TV and radio, in social media posts, on highway billboards, and on the sides of buses. Sometimes they succeed in changing our beliefs, attitudes, and behaviors. Advertisers tend to be particularly successful at persuading and motivating, partly because the products, services, and entertainment they offer generally represent enjoyable additions to our lives.

Perhaps because of their entreaties to *give up* some of life's pleasures in the service of health behavior change, however, clinical and public health professionals face more challenges in their efforts to persuade. Health professionals ask reluctant patients to take their medications regularly, eat whole food diets with less salt and fat, and limit their intake of sweets. They try to influence people to take a walk, or enroll in an exercise class, or accept a vaccination. If the abysmal adherence statistics we examined earlier are any guide, it is clear that patients need plenty of persuasion to overcome their natural tendencies to live in the moment, take health risks, and jeopardize their future well-being.

Persuasion

Throughout this book, we offer numerous strategies to support health professionals' efforts to improve their patients' health behaviors, and we examine the major determinants of behavior change in the context of medical care (broadly defined to include public health). One of these determinants is *persuasion*. The act of *persuading* is an attempt, let's say by a health professional, to move or change a person's beliefs, attitudes, or course of action by means of argument or entreaty. A patient might be firmly against getting a flu vaccination, but after their physician explains the dangers of serious illness from the flu, the patient accepts the shot. Sometimes the simple endorsement by a trusted health professional (e.g., with a poster at the clinic) is enough to change behavior. Indeed, one meta-analysis found that primary care practitioners' promotion of physical activity to sedentary adults significantly increased their physical activity levels 12 months later.[1]

Persuasion can be simple and focused on a specific belief, as compared with conversion, which involves completely changing a broad set of behaviors and beliefs. Conversion isn't necessary; our patients don't need to become "exercise fanatics" or Instagram fitness stars. We would be happy with them simply viewing a specific action, such as going for a walk, somewhat more positively than they did before; their attitude change can set them on a healthier course and get them actually walking.

In Chapter 2, we reviewed several theoretical models that have guided thinking and research on health behavior change, providing an historical perspective on major developments in the field. These models offer guidance in understanding individuals' thought processes when they "decide" how to behave regarding their health and healthcare. We put "decide" in quotes here because, as we will see in Chapter 6, many health behaviors are automatic; their enactment is cued by conditions in the environment or by the behavior of other people, not by conscious, individual decisions.

Further, as we examine persuasion and motivation here, we should keep in mind a basic concept—that people generally will not do what they are *told* to do. People will do what they *want* to do, typically based on what matters to them. Case Study 5.1 presents an example.

Case Study 5.1 What Persuaded and Motivated People to Get the COVID-19 Vaccination?

Accepting a health policy directive to be vaccinated for a communicable disease such as COVID-19 will usually depend on the outcomes an individual expects and desires. Any potential benefits offered by a health action need to satisfy personal expectations about one's physical, psychological, and social well-being. Many people believe a vaccination that prevents severe illness or death is worth getting, both for their own long-term well-being and to spare their family pain and loss. Others value personal liberty so highly that they are willing to take a greater risk. In the case of the COVID-19 vaccination, global rates of acceptance and uptake were only about 68% and 42%,[2] respectively. This occurred for a wide variety of reasons. For some, proof of vaccination was required for work or to attend a valued activity like a concert. Others fully believed in "the scientific endeavor" and in vaccine safety and effectiveness. Some got the shot only in response to pressure from their spouses. Many skipped it, believing that they were personally not susceptible to illness; "I never get sick" was a common argument. Some cited a social media post about someone who believed the vaccine made them sick.

During the COVID-19 pandemic, persuasion by public health officials did work somewhat to change behavior, at least in the short term. Many of the recommended, and sometimes required, public health measures (such as masking and social distancing) were initially adopted by many, and there is a lot of evidence that people generally acted in rational ways to keep themselves and their families safe during the worst waves of the COVID-19 pandemic.[3,4] One large-scale study conducted in the United States, however, found that even when people had accepted the initial two-shot vaccination series, by the time a booster shot became available, less than half elected to receive it.[5]

Resistance to persuasion

Resistance involves the exertion of force in opposition to pressure being exerted.[6] We can easily envision a variety of reasons for cognitive and behavioral resistance to health recommendations. For some, historical atrocities like the Tuskegee Syphilis Study[7] have led to distrust of the medical establishment. Based on a report by the Kaiser Family Foundation, resistance to vaccinations may derive less from distrust of the vaccine itself and more from not wanting to be *told what to do*.[8] Resistance may arise as a push-back to perceived limits on personal freedom. This study also found that since the COVID-19 pandemic started, there has been a reduction in the percentage of school-age children who are fully vaccinated against all childhood diseases.[8] Attitudes regarding personal freedom appear to drive resistance more than do concerns about vaccine safety or even distrust of science. Other studies have similar findings, across a variety of vaccination types from COVID-19 to HPV.[9,10] This concept of pushing back when one senses that personal freedoms are being threatened is known in psychology as "reactance,"[11] and it represents a genuine threat to the success of persuasive health-related messages (see Case Study 5.2).[12]

> ### Case Study 5.2 The Sturgis Motorcycle Rally, July 2020
>
> A classic example of reactance is the Sturgis, South Dakota, motorcycle rally, which took place at the height of the COVID-19 pandemic,[13,14] when the country was reeling from fears of this unknown but deadly virus. In July of 2020, roughly 460,000 people attended an annual rally in a small rural town and created what infectious disease experts called "a superspreading event." While outdoor motorcycle rides were generally considered safe, much of the rally activity took place indoors at eating establishments, bars, concerts, and tattoo parlors. People gathered in large crowds in poorly ventilated venues; few followed public health recommendations to wear masks or maintain distance from others. While difficult to track precisely, the rally was believed to be responsible for multiple COVID-19 outbreaks in other states across the Midwest. During the pandemic, the South Dakota governor did not put into place any public health mandates, noting that people should simply be given information to protect their health and then should be free to make their own choices about personal risk and enjoy their chosen way of life.

The upshot of our discussion so far has been that sometimes persuasion works, sometimes people resist it, and sometimes they pay attention—but only to the parts they want to hear. Let's examine persuasion in more detail and unpack some of the complexity that has driven a major field of psychological research for decades.

Persuasive messages

The field of social psychology has taught us much about persuasion. Several decades ago, the idea of subliminal persuasion was a hot topic, especially in the United States. People speculated about the ways in which advertisers might hide subliminal messages on billboards or flash images onto movie screens for a microsecond, influencing the public to buy the products (e.g., new cars, popcorn) that were being promoted. Although subliminal perception does exist (and has been studied for well over 100 years), it tends to be weak and transient. Persuasion through conscious processing tends to be more powerful and, as we will see, can occur through multiple pathways.

Social psychologists have studied the types of messages and messengers most likely to persuade us (these are summarized in Table 5.1). The characteristics of the persuasive messenger include the individual's expertise and our liking for the person. Let us look at each of these issues in a bit more detail.

Table 5.1 Summary of Elements of Persuasive Messages in Healthcare

Messenger Expertise	This is the perception that the messenger, a respected health professional, has special knowledge and experience and their message is worthy of attention.
Liking for the Messenger	People who are liked are better able to persuade others; attractive individuals, those who are familiar, and those who are seen as similar to oneself tend to be best liked. Building familiarity and trust, and pointing out parallels between provider and patient, can increase the persuasiveness of a message.
Perceptions of Scarcity	When opportunities are limited, they tend to be more highly valued; emphasizing the importance of timely action may reduce patients' procrastination.
Norm of Reciprocity	The natural desire to reciprocate can encourage patients' attention to and cooperation with health messages.
Desire to be Consistent	People generally want to maintain consistency between their beliefs and actions; awareness and reconciliation of inconsistencies can support steps toward health behavior change.
Fear Induction	Fear of the negative consequences of poor health behaviors can be persuasive and motivate change, but only if fear is not overwhelming and manageable steps to avoid the frightening outcome are offered.
Teachable Moments	People's own experiences, and those of others to whom they are close, can make the need for change more salient. A health professional who is aware of these experiences can create opportunities to teach and motivate more effectively.
Message Framing	Persuasive messages can be framed in terms of what might be gained if a health behavior is adopted, or what might be lost if it is not. Which type of framing is most effective depends on the type of health behavior being targeted.
Expectations	People's expectations for what will happen if they perform (or don't perform) a certain behavior can influence whether or not they attempt it. Their expectations of the responses of others to the behavior are also important influences on behavioral adoption.

Expertise and other forms of power

Information offered by an expert such as a health professional carries more weight than the same information conveyed by someone without expertise;[15] *expert power* is authority by virtue of one's knowledge and experience.[16,17] Healthcare providers can also use *informational power* (based on the content of the expert's communication), *reward power* (the capacity to give rewards), *coercive power* (the capacity to control or withhold), and *referent power* (the capacity to provide an appropriate reference point for the patient). Examples of each of these can be found in Table 5.2. These various forms of social power can be quite effective. Health professionals already have the appropriate expertise, information, reward resources, and anecdotal examples to encourage adherence and health behavior change. They are in a perfect position to persuade their patients to pursue effective health behaviors.[18]

Liking

Many studies demonstrate that a well-liked messenger has greater persuasive power.[16] This issue was particularly salient in Chapter 3, where we examined

Table 5.2 Examples of Persuasive Power in Use

Expert Power	"In my experience, Katrina, people with blood pressure levels as high as yours usually can't control their hypertension with diet and exercise alone. I've seen a lot of cases like this and, trust me, medication really will help."
Informational Power	"Mona, despite the fact that you feel healthy, your hemoglobin A1c has been consistently over 8%. I also see some small changes occurring in your retinas. The damage isn't severe enough to qualify as diabetic retinopathy yet, but regulating your blood glucose is now more crucial than ever."
Reward Power	"We've got a new incentive program for those in our 'walk fit' group, Curtis. Those who walk an extra 5,000 steps per week over the next month will get two free tickets to the County Health Expo! Do you want to sign on for that?"
Coercive Power	"I'm sorry Mr. Balcom, but I can't make that referral for you until we can get your weight within the target range. I know that you're in a lot of pain, but it simply makes no sense, and could be dangerous, to undergo knee replacement surgery when you're this heavy."
Referent Power	"Victor, I struggle to eat right, too—believe me, I enjoy burgers and fries as much as the next person. But I made a commitment to follow this eating plan almost ten years ago now. It took me nearly a year of small steps and changes to get it right, but I'm now at the point where I can resist the temptation to snack between meals and I honestly feel that I enjoy my occasional 'splurges' more than I used to."

trust in the practitioner-patient relationship. We tend to like people who we think are attractive[19] and similar to us,[20] and with whom we are more familiar.[21,22] Although attractiveness is subjective and may not be changeable, the latter two characteristics are easier to target. Healthcare providers can increase perceptions of similarity and familiarity by briefly sharing some of their own experiences (e.g., describing their own exercise challenges). Building a therapeutic alliance increases familiarity and a sense of comfort within the provider-patient relationship.

Scarcity, reciprocity, and consistency
Messages are also most persuasive when they involve some of the following: *(1)* perceptions of scarcity (such as of time, when someone believes that an opportunity is "now or never"); *(2)* norms of reciprocity (the desire to return, in kind, what one receives); and *(3)* the desire to be consistent in one's behaviors. Each of these principles can be used in formulating and delivering persuasive messages to patients, as we see in the following examples.

Suppose that a nurse educator believes their patient would benefit from a two-hour free seminar offered by the medical practice on the self-management of diabetes. They might encourage the patient to register by pointing out (if it is true) that there are only a few open spaces left for the upcoming session and that it will be several weeks before another session will be scheduled. The fact of scarcity may increase the seminar's appeal to the patient.

The norm of reciprocity might involve a token gift from the medical office, such as a refrigerator magnet picture frame with a dry erase area to record the next appointment. This small gift might encourage the patient to reciprocate and keep their appointment or call early if needing to reschedule. When offering a specialty referral to their patient, a physician might emphasize the talent and expertise of the specialist, encouraging the patient's reciprocity in promptly making and keeping the appointment.

Finally, particular behaviors can be highlighted by the healthcare provider to encourage consistency in healthy behavior patterns. For example, a nutritionist might remind the patient that they have already decreased dietary sodium and remind the patient of their own statements about wanting to cut down on salt. This can illustrate how reasonable the next dietary steps might be and can reinforce the patient's consistency and perseverance.

As we will examine in detail in Chapter 6, the desire of many people to remain consistent and fulfill their commitments can contribute to the success of a *behavioral contract* created with the patient to support their treatment plan. A behavioral contract outlines the action steps to which the patient is committing, and it is signed by provider and patient. The patient's desire to maintain consistency and fulfill the agreement can create subtle pressure to adhere and even to adopt additional health behaviors within the aims of the signed contract.

Fear induction

Fear induction is a persuasive technique, but one that can be misused. Fear inducing messages can be complex, and although they are potentially powerful motivators, using them can sometimes backfire. A meta-analysis of the literature on "fear appeals" found that fear-provoking messages are the most emotionally powerful, but to be effective, they should be paired with equally powerful information about how one might avoid the feared outcome.[23] This information must be framed to maximize the individual's sense of self-efficacy; the individual must be confident that they are *able* to take the necessary action to minimize the threat.

When people are simply frightened, they are not likely to engage in preventive health behaviors. Instead, their fear activates defensive responses such as avoidance or reactance.[23] A large body of research on this topic suggests that trying to simply scare a person into health behavior change (e.g., telling them they will die if they keep smoking) is unlikely to be successful without the provision of clear steps to take that can change the outcome.

Teachable moments

As with so many things in life, timing is important, and there are times when people are especially receptive to change. These are called "teachable moments" and in the health domain they tend to have two things in common: *(1)* an emotionally motivating component, such as a "close call" or a friend's diagnosis; and *(2)* a reasoned realization that change is necessary, such as when an emotionally charged event leads to a closer examination of one's health risks and ways to minimize them.[24,25] One person might be motivated to eat a healthier diet and exercise regularly after their best friend is diagnosed with diabetes. Another might finally quit smoking after a sibling is diagnosed with emphysema.

Naturally occurring, emotionally motivating, events are not always available; imagery or role-playing might be used in their place to facilitate a teachable moment. For example, a clinician might encourage a patient who is a smoker to close their eyes and imagine their family's thoughts, feelings, and behaviors on the day of their funeral. Or, the clinician might ask them to play the role of a patient receiving a diagnosis of terminal cancer caused by smoking. If the patient actively engages in this role-play experience, it might motivate real change in their life. Studies just like this have shown that smokers who role-play someone with lung cancer are more likely to change their attitudes and their smoking behaviors, and to maintain these changes over time compared with smokers who simply received information about the dangers of smoking.[26,27]

Moments of opportunity, if recognized and timed to fit with a persuasive message, can vastly increase its salience and strength, and ultimately contribute to enhancing behavior change.[28] Toward this end, it makes sense for a health professional to keep track of psychosocial information that might help create or amplify teachable moments.

Dr. Claude is a family practice physician who sees Marisol regularly for her cardiovascular disease. Marisol is moderately successful at managing her condition, but Dr. Claude's efforts to engage her in additional preventive actions, including mammogram screening for breast cancer, have been largely unsuccessful. In his last meeting with her, Marisol attributed her failure to make and keep mammogram appointments to the stress and extra work she has taken on since her sister began treatment for breast cancer. Dr. Claude noted this attribution and asked about her sister, and how their family was coping. After a brief discussion, Dr. Claude revisited Marisol's own mammography screening, emphasizing her family history of breast cancer and the importance of early detection for the most effective treatment and cure. Because of her sister's situation, this information was now more salient and compelling to Marisol; two days later she scheduled a mammogram, and she kept the appointment. This example illustrates the importance of keeping track of health-relevant details in patients' lives, even if they are not the patients' own health issues, because they might help motivate them to take health action.

Message framing
Another aspect of persuasive communication relevant to health behavior change is *message framing*, which refers to the way in which a message is presented. A *gain-framed* message is presented in terms of its positive value (or the gain) that might come from listening to it, taking it seriously, and acting upon it. A *loss-framed* message is presented in terms of what will be lost if the message is ignored or minimized.

Both gain-framed and loss-framed messages can help to convince people to change their health behavior,[29] but responses often depend upon the context in which the message is delivered. If a health behavior is designed to prevent or screen for an illness such as cancer, a loss-framed message might be more effective in convincing a person to adopt the behavior. For example, it is important for women to have regular cervical cancer screening, but the procedure itself is not pleasant; after several repetitions of negative test results, a woman might decide to put off the next recommended but uncomfortable procedure. Reminders that regular cervical cancer screening is important in preventive care and encouragement to care for one's body are likely to be less effective than reminders framed in terms of loss—what might happen if the screening is put off and precancerous cells are, in fact, present. On the other hand, if a behavior (e.g., exercise) is focused primarily on improving overall health, a gain-framed message may be most beneficial because it emphasizes potential positive outcomes, such as being able to walk farther, feel better, and have more energy.

Expectations

The last element of persuasion involves *expectations*. Expectations can be social (which we will examine in detail in Chapter 7) or outcome-related. Outcome expectations refer to beliefs that certain behaviors will result in specific outcomes, such as the conviction that brushing and flossing one's teeth regularly will result in healthy gums, sweet-smelling breath, and fewer cavities. Outcome expectations are important in the goal-adoption process; indeed, meta-analytic studies show that expectations about health outcomes have significant modest- to medium-sized effects on fostering positive health behaviors.[30,31]

Goal setting

In Chapter 2, we outlined several important theoretical models that underpin our knowledge of behavioral change toward the goal of health. These models lead us to some practical questions about what factors persuade an individual to adopt particular health-related goals and what factors keep the individual motivated to pursue them.

Sometimes people target certain health objectives because of their emotions and feelings; at other times they are driven by social comparisons, logical reasoning, or even some kinds of direct pressure. An individual might suddenly *feel* compelled to undertake a challenge, such as training to run a 10K race, after spending the afternoon watching the track and field events of the summer Olympics. Inspiration from watching the athletes may propel the individual to plan a workout schedule in order to achieve the cardiovascular fitness and stamina required by a 10K race. Sometimes, though, people adopt goals that are rooted in social comparisons, such as when a parent observes other parents swimming with their children and then decides to join in for both exercise and fun.

Sometimes health goals are established after a well-reasoned decision-making process, such as when one elects to change several behaviors at the same time to achieve better cardiovascular health. The available information and data support the goal behaviors, and any arguments against their adoption are clearly outweighed by evidence. Take the example of Ja'Marr who has recently been diagnosed with hypertension and worryingly high LDL (low density lipoprotein or "bad") cholesterol. Together, these conditions place him at high risk for cardiovascular disease. He needs to make some sweeping dietary changes and increase his level of daily exercise. In addition, his physician has recommended that he begin taking medications to lower his cholesterol and control his high blood pressure. Ja'Marr has accepted this advice and has set several health-related goals for himself. He has the long-term goals of lowering blood pressure and cholesterol, and the short-term goals of consistently taking his medications, walking each evening after work, and replacing many of the processed foods in his diet with more lean meats, and fresh fruits and vegetables. Ja'Marr believes that each of these goals is achievable, despite the possibility of unpleasant side effects associated with one of his prescribed medications. In weighing the potential risks and benefits, Ja'Marr judges the arguments in favor of taking medication to be stronger than the arguments against it.

Health goals are often adopted directly in response to some form of persuasion. It is common for people to be influenced by media campaigns or by press pieces that report research findings from scientific studies. For example, a journalist might write about the extensive research supporting sleep as crucial for health and longevity. More than a decade ago, *New York Times* journalist Eric Nagourney reviewed the compelling research evidence[32] showing that disrupted sleep patterns are associated with problems regulating blood sugar and might be linked to diabetes. He cited empirical data published in the *Proceedings of the National Academy of Sciences* and was convincing enough to motivate many people to change their behavior and pursue the goal of healthy sleep. Many of our own students, after reading the *New York Times* article, were convinced of the importance of sleep and said that they would make a concerted effort to get enough of it. They didn't wait for meta-analytic findings published in 2016[33] showing that the magnitude of health risk from inadequate sleep is comparable to that of traditional risk factors such as sedentary lifestyle and unhealthy eating. They were already believers.

It is important to have high quality health information available to help people set reasonable health goals;[34] studies show that accurate information about the risks and benefits of health behaviors can indeed influence people's choices.[35] Information is the crucial *first step* in goal-setting because people need to *know what to do* in order to move in the right direction, and they must be persuaded that putting knowledge into action makes sense for them. Goal-setting depends upon a combination of reason and emotion, and a person needs to feel confident that it is *possible* for them to achieve the identified goal.

Goal pursuit

Once a goal has been chosen, what motivates someone to pursue that goal despite obstacles and failures, and beyond initial successes? Several of the factors that prompt initial investment in a goal also predict ongoing motivation and goal pursuit: the desires of others, the expectations of outcome success, and an individual's self-efficacy. Those who set their health goals partly on the basis of what they think others (e.g., parents, spouses, or friends) expect of them are likely to be motivated to continue pursuing their goals because of these same expectations. These socially-derived motivations are discussed in greater detail in Chapter 7. It is important to keep in mind, though, that not everyone is equally motivated by the expectations of others; some people really don't care much about any opinions but their own. Further, different people derive different degrees of satisfaction from goal attainment and different degrees of distress or negative emotion when they experience failure.[36-38] What people believe about the likely outcomes of their behavior can also play an important role in determining whether they continue to persevere over time with their newly minted habits.

Optimism

Optimism is a trait or characteristic that appears to be a major determinant of goal-directed behavior and tenacity. Some people are optimistic; they have a natural tendency to expect positive outcomes.[39] Optimistic people persevere and keep trying, despite difficulties.[40]

Particularly in the realm of health, however, optimism functions in some apparently contradictory ways. Individuals who are optimistic expect positive outcomes if they try to change, but sometimes they do not recognize the need to modify their own behaviors in order to attain those outcomes. In other words, optimists predict good health outcomes for themselves even when they do little or nothing to work toward those outcomes. (Says an optimist: "This super-sized banana split is a good choice for meeting my daily fruit needs.") Optimists can feel so good about their situation that they have little motivation to change even though they actually see themselves as capable of making changes once they decide to make them. Optimists feel good about their abilities, and they are more likely than non-optimists to attempt behavioral modifications once they decide to do so.[41]

Optimistic self-beliefs do not operate equally across all types and phases of behavior change. Some individuals may feel quite optimistic about initiating change in some areas but not others; some feel competent to start a new behavior but frustrated and pessimistic when facing the inevitable difficulties and barriers in its long-term maintenance. Optimistic beliefs may also be inconsistent in their value across different types of health-relevant behaviors. These beliefs might help a person face a health crisis or meet primary prevention goals like exercise, but prove to be less helpful in maintaining ongoing treatment for chronic illness or when assessing potential health risks.[42,43]

The coping strategy called *constructive thinking* has emerged as a more adaptive "cousin" to optimism, capturing much of what seems useful about optimism while avoiding the naïve aspects of that construct. Constructive thinking involves the ability to solve problems (delaying gratification as necessary) under stressful circumstances while maintaining a positive outlook.[44,45] The problem-solving aspects of constructive thinking seem especially useful in predicting a range of health behaviors, from managing substance use, to making behavioral adjustments during pregnancy, to strictly adhering to medical treatments.[45-47]

Self-efficacy

Optimistic self-beliefs are similar in many ways to self-efficacy, which involves the sense that one is capable of performing the behaviors necessary to achieve a particular outcome.[48] Psychologist Albert Bandura proposed four specific sources for an individual's self-efficacy (in order of effectiveness): *(1)* past experience in performing specific behaviors (i.e., recognizing that one has been able to achieve past similar goals); *(2)* vicarious experiences (i.e., watching those similar to oneself successfully perform behaviors); *(3)* verbal persuasion (i.e., being told that one is capable); and *(4)* the experience of physiological arousal (i.e., an adrenaline surge interpreted as excitement). A strong sense of self-efficacy makes it more likely that an individual will initiate a behavior and expend sustained effort over time to maintain it. Sustained effort is likely to lead to greater achievement, which then further increases self-efficacy for a given task or behavior, and a cycle of success is created.[48] Some researchers have suggested that if a particular behavior (such as exercise) is possible for a person, self-efficacy might be more simply viewed as their *willingness* to perform it.[49,50]

Whether self-efficacy is just a willingness to try, or something more complicated, a rich body of literature shows that self-efficacy leads to better health behaviors including commitment to exercise, weight management, consistent contraception, and decreased cigarette and alcohol use.[51] Studies also show that it is possible to change a person's sense of self-efficacy (at least over the short term) so as to enhance their positive behavioral outcomes.[52,53] Some techniques for doing this are summarized in Table 5.3. It is important to recognize, however, that while verbal persuasion is the most frequently used method for increasing self-efficacy, it is also one of the least effective. While it is certainly acceptable for health professionals to verbally encourage their patients, it is more effective when they also use other approaches, such as helping patients identify role models (people just like them who are facing challenges and succeeding) and supporting patients in creating situations in which they can succeed. Small successes (made more likely by breaking larger goals into smaller, manageable components) can be powerful motivators as they strengthen an individual's sense of self-efficacy. Starting with short bouts of physical activity and gradually working up to longer exercise sessions, for example, can be more effective than immediately jumping into a full exercise regimen.[54] Talking with patients to identify past success can also help to make future goal-attainment more likely.[55]

Table 5.3 Strategies for Increasing Patients' Self-Efficacy

Enactive Attainments	Personal experiences of success	1. Set small steps toward behavior change so that success can be experienced early. 2. Discuss with patients their past successes so that these are salient.
Vicarious Experiences	Seeing the successes of similar others	1. Share with patients the success stories of others who are like them. 2. Engage patients in groups of similar others where they can view successful change. 3. Provide motivational videos that combine helpful tips along with "real life" stories of success in implementing them.
Verbal Persuasion	Being told that one is capable	1. Assure the patient of their own abilities; be a cheerleader. 2. Provide rationale for your beliefs about the patient's capability to be successful.
Physiological Arousal	Understand, manage, and use arousal	1. Help patients recognize and learn to channel the "rush of adrenaline" or "butterflies in the stomach" to motivate their successful behaviors (e.g., learn to channel nervous energy about an upcoming 5K race into one's performance in training runs). 2. Work with patients to manage physiological arousal that might impede their goals (e.g., remind the patient to deep-breathe when embarking on participation in a support group).

Perceptions of benefits and costs

Analysis of the potential benefits and costs of various health-related actions is an important next step in the behavior change process. As we saw in several of the Chapter 2 models, behavior change and maintenance depend partly upon perceptions of the behavior's costs (e.g., cancer risks from smoking) versus benefits (e.g., social gains from "smoking breaks" with the boss). In Chapter 7, we discuss expectations and perceptions of social costs and benefits in detail; we begin to examine them here, in the next example.

Suppose an individual believes that their close family member expects and wants them to adopt a particular health behavior. There is an inherent cost associated with failing to do so: the family member will be disappointed or upset. Conversely, the expected approval and happiness of that person if the behavior is achieved promises a significant benefit or reward. Expected rewards can range from personal and intangible (e.g., feeling good about oneself for achieving an exercise goal) to very concrete (e.g., a reduction in one's health insurance premium after quitting smoking).

Several important elements of behavior change are necessary in order to build habits through behavioral conditioning, as we will see in detail in Chapter 6. Here we are focusing on perceptions of, and expectations for, the costs and benefits of potential health actions and noting that the first step in a behavior change process involves the individual's *desire* to obtain the benefits, and/or to avoid the costs of action, or inaction. Of course, perceived consequences, desirable or undesirable, will matter only if they are tightly linked to the behavior under consideration. For example, if one is planning to do an exercise program with a friend, perceptions of the benefits of *exercise itself* are necessary to sustain motivation. If the friend quits exercising and just wants to walk a block together to the bakery, the individual's plans for a dedicated exercise program will be in jeopardy. In addition, when expected outcomes for behavior are tightly linked to external (or extrinsic) rewards, a focus on internal (or intrinsic) rewards can be reduced or eliminated entirely.[56] Unless intrinsic rewards are also in operation, a behavioral goal might be abandoned when hopes for the external reward are thwarted. Research links intrinsic rewards to persistence in the pursuit of goals.[57] People are more likely to achieve their goal behaviors and experience greater well-being when they strive for intrinsically meaningful goals.[58] Care should be taken to strengthen expectations for intrinsic rewards if an individual's behavior is to be maintained over time; meta-analytic findings suggest that coupling extrinsic incentives with intrinsic goals can lead to the best chance for behavior change.[59]

Goal framing

As we saw earlier, the manner in which a message about behavior change is framed (i.e., presented) can influence the likelihood of its adoption. Framing can influence whether a person stays actively engaged in the pursuit of their goal, or simply gives it up. We have previously noted that when individuals compare themselves favorably to others, and perceive that they are increasing in task mastery, they experience higher levels of self-efficacy than if they feel inferior to others and are not improving in their skills. (This is *social comparison*, examined more in Chapter 7.) Similarly, research has shown that when people think about their goals as steps toward learning (as opposed to performance), they remain engaged in trying to achieve those goals, even after they have experienced failure.[60] If people frame their goals in terms of increasing their skills, they strive more earnestly and perceive their own abilities more positively than if they focus only on the potential outcomes of their efforts. Thus, the common tendency to focus attention on what we are trying to attain, rather than on the process of attaining it, can be a self-defeating strategy. This is especially true when we must maintain our efforts over time.[61]

Targeting goals

In this chapter, we have considered the reasons that individuals might take on and continue to pursue health goals. But, how do they choose their goals in the first place? Which goals should they choose, and how should they make that choice?

It is probably not surprising that setting ambitious goals can produce better outcomes than if goals are too easy.[62] Ambitious goals, of course, should be things the individual is *capable of achieving*.[63,64] Too often, people set unrealistic health goals (e.g., losing 10 pounds in two weeks), often spurred on by ads for weight-loss programs and fitness clubs. Empirical evidence suggests that a person should set and work toward clear, specific, and modest *subgoals* that are aimed at achieving the ultimate goal.[65] These lower order (or stepping-stone) subgoals help build self-efficacy with modest yet measurable achievements that increase ongoing mastery and skill refinement.

There likely exist several routes, through various subgoals, toward any desired health outcome. For example, achieving a healthy weight can involve multiple methods of balancing eating patterns and exercise. Plans that are individually tailored and allow for more personal choice are more likely to be maintained over time than rigid one-size-fits-all programs.[66] The likelihood of success is increased when subgoals are defined precisely for the individual, with specific techniques for implementing goal-directed behaviors and the chance for modification and adjustment at various points in time.[67]

It can be tricky to guide a person toward smaller, achievable goals when they are feeling motivated to take on a bigger and more ambitious task. Telling a patient, "I don't think you'll be able to do that" harms their sense of self-efficacy and is not likely to be productive. Yet, the medical professional may anticipate that the goal as it is currently framed is *not* likely to be something the patient can accomplish. By focusing discussion with the patient on the importance of gaining mastery over the process, and by tailoring stepping-stones with the patient's needs and expectations in mind, a plan can be established that maximizes the likelihood of success. Case Study 5.3 illustrates this for Maisie.

Case Study 5.3 Modifying but Not Discouraging Maisie's Goals

At her appointment with Lisa, her behavioral health specialist, Maisie was more upbeat than she'd been in a long time; she was encouraged by attending her weight-loss support group. She was now motivated to change! Maisie explained to Lisa that she planned to lose 70 pounds, and maybe even more, before her college class reunion (which was only seven months away). She enthusiastically described her plans for going to the gym four times per week, walking every day, and cutting her calorie consumption to about 1,200 per day. Lisa was glad to see Maisie's change in mood and motivation, but she could also see that Maisie was setting goals that would be very difficult to achieve. Her challenge now was to direct Maisie's goals appropriately without undermining her sense of self-efficacy.

LISA: "Maisie, that's wonderful! I'm so glad you found the group to be a helpful resource! I haven't seen you this motivated in a long time, so let's get right down to the specifics. Tell me more about what you'd like to accomplish."

MAISIE: "I'd like to really work hard and lose those 70 pounds that we've been talking about for so long."

LISA: "Class reunion, huh? That would motivate me, too! So, what have you thought about in terms of specific strategies?"

MAISIE: "Well, there's a gym not far from my house and I think I'll buy a membership there. I will be dedicated about it—I'm going to go four times per week, plus I'm going to walk *every* day, and I'm just going to have to cut down on my eating. I was thinking of restricting myself to 1,200 calories per day."

LISA: "You're an ambitious woman, Maisie. I've found with many of my other patients, though, that a step-up plan works best. This is one that eases you into the larger plan a little more slowly and almost always results in better long-term outcomes. I can tell that you're committed to really doing this, so I think an accelerated step-up plan that involves a focus on whole foods and healthy eating is something you could certainly handle. Shall we go ahead and map out some concrete goals?"

MAISIE: "Okay, let's see what that would look like."

* * * * * * * * *

LISA: "So, let's review what we've got. Until we see each other again in two weeks, you're going to keep a very detailed record of everything you eat. Don't try to restrict yourself, just make a note of everything. This will give us a good idea of your food preferences and choices and how we might modify them to limit processed foods and enhance your consumption of whole foods. Then we can work together to develop a food plan that you can work with."

MAISIE: "I don't want to go slowly; I want to just start cutting back so I can start losing weight."

LISA: "Well, keep in mind that your body will also be using more calories than it does now, because you're going to be moving more. So, you need an eating plan that will work to maintain your energy for your exercise."

MAISIE: "Right, so I'm going to wear my activity tracker all the time and my goal will be 10,000 steps per day for the first two weeks. Doesn't seem hard."

LISA: "Yes, you'll be surprised at how easy it is to fit in extra steps here and there. You might also be surprised, though, at how few steps you take now. I remember when I first started wearing an activity tracker and my estimates were way off. I thought I probably walked close to 10,000 steps in a day anyway but that first day I only logged 2,700!"

MAISIE: "And rather than spending all that money on a gym membership that I might not even use, I'm going to schedule two training sessions with that personal trainer you recommended. She can probably suggest a couple of things for me to buy..."

LISA: "Yes, elastic bands and dumbbells or maybe one of those exercise balls..."

MAISIE: "...and I will do whatever workout she recommends twice per week to start. I think you'll be surprised at just how hard I can push myself."

LISA: "I think you've got an excellent plan here. You're going to be practicing some good self-monitoring skills, as well as learning state-of-the-art fitness techniques from your trainer. And in two weeks we'll evaluate things. At that point we'll be able to make a plan for healthy eating as well. I know you are excited to get started!"

Motivation

In psychology, *motivation* typically refers to forces acting either on or within a person to initiate behavior.[68] We use the term casually when we talk about our willingness to follow a plan or work toward a goal that we have set for ourselves, as in, "I'm not very motivated to exercise today!" Our motivation gives us the impetus to begin taking action, and the drive to continue it. Sometimes we say we are motivated by those who inspire us; indeed, inspiration is everywhere. Our neighborhoods are filled with walkers and runners; our parks have seniors doing chair yoga and tai chi; friends and acquaintances offer their own stories of getting in shape and feeling better. Sometimes circumstances push us to go in a new health-related direction, to attempt something we had thought impossible, or to change our lives in ways we never imagined (see Case Study 5.4 for an example).

Case Study 5.4 A Father's Motivation to Help His Daughter

A simple, poignant, and classic story of motivation and a New Year's resolution appeared in the *Los Angeles Times* newspaper on January 1, 1998.

A 32-year-old father, who weighed 297 pounds, found out in December 1996 that his kidney was a perfect match for his 5-year-old daughter who needed a transplant. He was not approved for surgery, however,

> because his weight made the procedure of donating his kidney too dangerous.
>
> There was not much time. The little girl was undergoing dialysis for her kidney disease that was leading to kidney failure, and so her father went on a very strict, medically approved diet. He ate only one meal a day, cut out sweets and fats, and exercised. Within a year, he lost 103 pounds, and in December of 1997, the transplant surgery was performed successfully at the Cleveland Clinic.[69]

Unless one is very strongly motivated by unusual and compelling circumstances, motivation for behavior change is typically not so clear-cut or focused. Psychologists have long studied motivation and agree that helping someone, or ourselves, to be motivated is a complex process. People tend to have vague notions of wanting to be "better, stronger, healthier," and they imagine quantum change happening quickly (such as running a 10K comfortably, having lost 25 pounds, rather soon after being sedentary and vastly overweight). Behavior change typically does not occur in a quantum shift and change is usually not linear. Instead, it occurs gradually, as people move through a process of identifiable motivational stages (such as we have seen in our Chapter 2 discussion of the Transtheoretical Model).[70] As James Prochaska and colleagues noted in their extensive research on this model and in their book, *Changing to Thrive*,[70] change is not easy, and most people do not know how to do it.

Health behavior change tends to occur in steps, with some forward progress and some backsliding. Complicating the picture is the consistent research finding that most health behaviors tend to be *inter-correlated*; individuals tend to engage in *multiple health risk behaviors*, not just one.[71] For example, cigarette smoking tends to co-occur with poor diet and inactivity, as well as with excessive alcohol use. There are advantages to considering these behaviors together. Quitting smoking, for example, can support increased movement and efforts to eat a healthier diet. Or, improved diabetes management might increase the individual's energy, making regular exercise more likely. In multiple risk behavior change, the individual (and even the clinician) might feel overwhelmed, with too much change being required and too many opportunities for failure presenting themselves. Studies do show, however, that with high-risk populations, programs for change should be targeted to each individual, and health behavior change is most likely to be successful if behaviors are linked together.[71]

Motivational interviewing, motivational communication

The Transtheoretical Model forms the theoretical basis for a method of working with people to help develop and strengthen their motivation to change. Motivational Interviewing (and the related Motivational Communication) is not so much a set of techniques as it is a *style of interacting* that is meant to allow the examination of ambivalence and facilitate progress toward a goal or decision.[72]

Clinical psychologists William Miller and Stephen Rollnick wrote the classic book about this approach[73] and they offer strategies for healthcare providers to facilitate health behavior change and treatment adherence in their patients.[74] They make it clear that while persuasion and inspiration can kick-start motivation and offer the force necessary for a person to initiate behavior change, sustaining it requires clearly articulated goals and step-by-step plans for altering day-to-day actions.

A person needs to understand what they really feel about a behavior change in order to make that change every day over time. With the use of motivational interviewing and motivational communication, a health professional can help a patient understand both their willingness to change and their resistance to it. Making clear the individual's true desire *not* to change is an essential first step in the process. One's motivation to exercise, for example, can derive from expectations of its likely benefit, such as having more energy, getting in shape, and being healthier. Many people, however, are also resistant to exercise because they really dislike the "vibe" at their gym or they believe that exercise takes too much time. The desire for the behavior is not there.

There is no simple path to behavior change, and it typically occurs in stages and requires concrete goals for specific target behaviors (e.g., walking for 30 minutes, four evenings a week). Being specific is essential to tracking whether and how the behavior has been accomplished; vague goals like "getting more exercise" are difficult to pin down. Anyone beginning a new walking habit, will likely go through the stages as they work toward the change; Miller and Rollnick offer ideas for communicating to encourage patients through their steps to behavioral change. See Case Study 5.5 for an application of the Stages of Change and Motivational Interviewing.

> **Case Study 5.5 The Stages of Change and Motivational Interviewing Applied to Mercedes' Exercise Regimen**
>
> Physician's Assistant Elisa Hernandez talks with her patient about exercise. Mercedes is managing type 2 diabetes, and together they will set a goal for Mercedes to walk for 30 minutes, four evenings a week, after work or after dinner.
>
> Elisa knows that her patient is beginning this process in Stage 1, the stage of *Pre-contemplation.* Mercedes can easily list all the reasons *not* to walk ("I'm tired after work; I prefer to watch the news; I am busy after dinner helping my children with homework; I don't have the right shoes."). If she is encouraged to do so, Mercedes can probably come up with one reason to walk ("Walking my dog would make him happy"), but it's not easy. Mercedes is well aware of, and not reluctant to express, her resistance to the behavior change. The goal behavior itself seems far off.
>
> The next time they talk, Elisa asks Mercedes for her thoughts about walking, and she really listens to her patient's responses. Mercedes seems to be entering Stage 2, *Contemplation.* She says that she *intends* to start walking someday, maybe sometime in the summer, and she is becoming more aware of the potential positive effects of walking regularly (e.g., getting stronger, having more energy, managing her blood sugar). But Mercedes remains ambivalent because her resistance to walking is still strong ("I have too many things to do in the evening, like laundry and cleaning up from supper"). At this stage, though, she is open to being inspired by others who walk, such as several neighbors who walk their dogs in the evening. She still thinks about the negatives and feels resistance, but she is moving slightly closer to taking evening walks.
>
> Stage 3, *Preparation,* is just what it sounds like. Mercedes tells P.A. Elisa that she bought a pair of walking shoes and discovered that there is a later evening TV news show she can watch while folding laundry and doing chores after an evening walk. Mercedes has not yet started to exercise, but she is getting closer. Elisa's task is to support Mercedes' thinking

about the ways to overcome her resistance. Note that Elisa does not disagree with Mercedes' statements of resistance; she does not think that Mercedes is "making excuses." Elisa makes herself available as a sounding board and someone to guide the conversation as Mercedes solves the practical problems that she feels are standing in the way of her taking action.

Stage 4 is *Action*. It took a while to get here, but Mercedes' first evening of walking after dinner arrives. Elisa has reminded her that it is important to pay attention to the natural rewards of the action she has taken—the crisp, coolness of the evening, or the friendliness of the neighbors, or her dog's happiness, or how much better she feels after a walk. It is important to have a sense of pride in having taken action, and it will be easier for Mercedes if her family members are supportive of her health behavior. Elisa is also available through email to acknowledge Mercedes' success.

Stage 5 is *Maintenance*. When Elisa next sees Mercedes, a few weeks have passed; Elisa continues to offer encouragement and reinforcement. She also encourages Mercedes to keep track of her progress on her phone notes app, or on a chart, and to feel comfortable enjoying a small reward to herself for maintaining her health habit. As we will see in more detail in Chapter 6, the maintenance of health habits requires reinforcement. Adhering to plans for walking four evenings a week deserves a reward, perhaps a movie night after a month of success.

Elisa was not surprised when Mercedes told her that she had a *Relapse*, that is, a lapse in behavior and return to the previous state; it is very common and was bound to occur at some point. A week of rainy days and a head cold left Mercedes at home in the evenings, and then it became difficult for her to start walking again. Elisa explained that how one deals with relapse is crucial; Mercedes needs to remember the strategies she once used to start her evening walks. Elisa encouraged her to look into finding a place indoors to walk in bad weather, such as the local mall, or perhaps to purchase an inexpensive used treadmill or stationary bicycle to use at home. Mercedes will benefit greatly from Elisa's support and encouragement at this stage, as well as her reminders of what Mercedes has accomplished already and can accomplish again.

An important concept in Motivational Interviewing is the individual's "readiness to change." This is an overall feeling of one's current willingness to take action. At any point in their discussions leading up to

Mercedes' behavior change, Elisa can ask her a simple question: "On a scale from 0 to 10, where 0 means you are not at all ready to start walking for 30 minutes after work or after dinner, and 10 means you are ready to start right now ... where are you at this time?" When Mercedes indicates a low number on the scale, Elisa encourages her to express the reasons for her resistance: "Oh, you say 2. Can you talk about your choice? What would it take for you to be at 5 or 6?" Weeks later, when Mercedes says she is at 7, Elisa helps her to solidify her choice by expressing the reasons for her readiness to change: "Great, you say 7! So can you elaborate on your choice of a 7?"

There are four very important principles of Motivational Interviewing that Elisa can use in helping Mercedes toward her goal of behavior change. The first principle is *empathy*, which, as we saw in Chapter 3, involves understanding another person's perspective. Elisa can work with Mercedes' situational constraints (such as time limitations, family pressures, fears of evaluation by others, soreness, aches and pains) to help her find solutions to problems that stand in the way of her walking goals.

The second principle is *rolling with resistance*. Generally, this means not pushing back on the patient's resistance and not arguing for the person to change their perspective and their actions. Rather, it involves being more patient with their challenges and limitations. Elisa can use the principles of persuasion examined earlier in this chapter to maintain a more effective dialogue with Mercedes during times when she is feeling resistant to change.

Behavior change should never be viewed in terms of "success versus failure." Instead, by employing the third principle of *developing discrepancy*, Elisa reminds Mercedes: "Being able to do activities as a family is one of your key values as a parent. Let's talk about what's keeping you from getting back on track with your plan to be able to take your kids hiking on their spring break." In examining the discrepancy between the current behavior (being sedentary) and personal values (being active with family), cognitive dissonance is created, and this can provide motivation to shift one or the other—most likely the behavior.

Finally, there is *self-efficacy*. Elisa reminds Mercedes that it has been her own choice to develop a habit of walking and moving more. Together they review Mercedes' own desire to develop a habit of moving, and her own ideas about the best time and place to accomplish her goal of walking

> for 30 minutes four times a week. Elisa emphasizes Mercedes' agency in this entire process. This approach is far from simply giving a *prescription* for exercise, or offering a persuasive message based on fear. Mercedes is doing the work, with Elisa's help, to come to her *own* prescription for incorporating movement into her life, and she has developed the tools to solve problems and overcome her resistance.

From persuasion and motivation to behavior change

In this chapter, we have examined the many factors that affect acceptance of, versus resistance to, health messages. Whether these messages come from the family doctor who is known and trusted, or from public health authorities who seem remote and disconnected from everyday life, persuasion and motivation depend upon a variety of well-researched elements which, when achieved, position the individual to make and maintain behavioral change.

The steps to change require an understanding of how habits are developed and maintained. Fortunately, well established psychological principles and some recent developments in the "science of habits" can transform the desire and willingness to change into sustained action.[75] In Chapter 6, we will examine the evidence base for understanding, developing, and then sustaining lifelong habits and long-term behavioral change. In his valuable book *The Power of Habit*,[76] Charles Duhigg tells us that by understanding and enacting certain habit principles, we can recognize the cues in the environment that trigger our actions and the environmental elements that reinforce them. We can build or change any habit we put our minds to, and as health professionals, we can teach our patients to transform their day-to-day routines and improve their health.

Summary

In this chapter, we explore the factors that influence people to initially adopt, and then pursue, a health-related goal. We consider the role of persuasion, which is an attempt to move or change by means of argument a person's belief or position, and ultimately their action. We refer back to theoretical models in Chapter 2 and consider resistance to vaccinations and mitigation strategies against COVID-19 and other diseases. We examine the characteristics of persuasive messages and messengers, and suggest ways that healthcare providers can offer more compelling communications to their patients. We discuss the characteristics of messengers, their expertise, and how well they are liked, and we examine the role in persuasion of both fear and inspiration. We consider message framing, logical reasoning, expectations, and self-efficacy, as well as the importance of a sense of competence and self-esteem in goal-setting. We show how recognizing teachable moments is important, as is knowing the unique characteristics of the patient in order to target persuasive messages most effectively. Factors that influence goal pursuit, such as expectations, optimism, and perceptions of benefits and costs are also evaluated. We examine motivation to change both individual and multiple-health-risk behaviors, and we consider a practical case application of the Transtheoretical Model through the process of Motivational Interviewing/Motivational Communication. The importance of empathy, rolling with resistance, developing discrepancy, and self-efficacy are discussed.

Tools for instruction and self-study

Learning objectives

By the end of this chapter, readers should be able to

1. Relate the concept of resistance to health behavior choices during a pandemic.
2. Describe the elements of persuasive messages and messengers.
3. Articulate how fear induction plays a role in persuasion, as well as caveats for its use.
4. Demonstrate how teachable moments can inspire behavior change.
5. Explain how reason, emotion, and self-efficacy are involved in goal-setting.
6. Recognize how expectations, optimism, and cost-benefit analysis are related to goal pursuit.
7. Explain motivation in the context of individual and multiple health risk behavior change.
8. Apply the techniques of motivational interviewing and the stages of the transtheoretical model to a person working to change a health behavior.

Review questions

1. Why is simply having information about good health behaviors not sufficient?
2. Provide a brief definition of persuasion.
3. What is the key theoretical model for understanding motivation, as discussed in this chapter? Name and provide an example for each of its steps or stages.
4. Define "resistance" and "reactance."
5. Describe what is meant by the term "self-efficacy" and the role that it plays in the decision to change health behavior.
6. List three elements that increase the persuasiveness of a message. Provide an example for how each element might be used in a medical or health-related context.
7. What is constructive thinking and how is it different from optimism? Give an example of its application to treatment adherence.
8. What do you know about fear induction as a persuasive technique? In what contexts might it work as well as, or better than, other approaches?
9. Which is better for persuading people to change their health behaviors—subliminal persuasion or a direct, conscious route? Why?

Prompts for discussion and further study

1. This chapter discusses resistance and reactance, and how they might encourage people to make poor decisions regarding their health. What are your thoughts on individual freedoms when it comes to health behaviors? Is a decision that primarily affects only the individual (e.g., refusing to take a medication for diabetes or hypertension) different from a decision that affects others (e.g., smoking in the vicinity of others or refusing to be vaccinated against a communicable disease)?
2. What are some of the ethical issues involved in persuasion? What are some examples of persuasive communication in medicine, and what are the specific elements that make a messages persuasive? Are similar persuasive elements used in direct-to-consumer advertising of drugs and other health products?

3. We learned about fear-based messages in this chapter. When people are simply frightened, they are not likely to engage in preventive health behaviors. Instead, their fear activates defensive responses such as avoidance or reactance. Do you think this happened during the COVID-19 pandemic?

Suggested reading

1. Cialdini RB. *Influence: Science and Practice*, 4th ed. Pearson Education; 2009.
2. Rollnick S, Miller WR, Butler CC. *Motivational Interviewing in Health Care: Helping Patients Change Behavior (Applications of Motivational Interviewing)*, 2nd ed. Guilford Press; 2022.
3. Prochaska JO, Prochaska JM. *Changing to Thrive: Using the Stages of Change to Overcome the Top Threats to Your Health and Happiness.* Hazelden Publishing; 2016.

References

1. Orrow G, Kinmonth AL, Sanderson S, Sutton S. Republished research: effectiveness of physical activity promotion based in primary care: systematic review and meta-analysis of randomised controlled trials. *Br J Sports Med.* 2013; 47(1): p. 27. doi: 10.1136/bjsports-2012-e1389rep
2. Wang Q, Hu S, Du F, et al. Mapping global acceptance and uptake of COVID-19 vaccination: a systematic review and meta-analysis. *Commun Med (Lond).* 2022; 2: p. 113. doi: 10.1038/s43856-022-00177-6
3. Badillo-Goicoechea E, Chang TH, Kim E, et al. Global trends and predictors of face mask usage during the COVID-19 pandemic. *BMC Public Health.* 2021; 21: pp. 1–2.
4. Ciancio A, Kämpfen F, Kohler IV, et al. Know your epidemic, know your response: early perceptions of COVID-19 and self-reported social distancing in the United States. *PLoS One.* 2020; 15(9): e0238341. doi: 10.1371/journal.pone.0238341
5. Agaku IT, Adeoye C, Long TG. Geographic, occupational, and sociodemographic variations in uptake of COVID-19 booster doses among fully vaccinated US adults, December 1, 2021, to January 10, 2022. *JAMA Netw Open.* 2022; 5(8): e2227680. doi: 10.1001/jamanetworkopen.2022.27680
6. American Psychological Association. Persuasion. APA Dictionary of Psychology. April 19, 2018. https://dictionary.apa.org/persuasion
7. Scharff DP, Mathews KJ, Jackson P, Hoffsuemmer J, Martin E, Edwards D. More than Tuskegee: understanding mistrust about research participation. *J Health Care Poor Underserved.* 2010; 21(3): pp. 879–897. doi: 10.1353/hpu.0.0323

8. Sparks G, Kirzinger A, Brodie M. KFF-COVID-19 vaccine monitor: profile of the unvaccinated. Kaiser Family Foundation. June 11, 2021. https://www.kff.org/coronavirus-covid-19/poll-finding/kff-covid-19-vaccine-monitor-profile-of-the-unvaccinated/
9. Capurro G, Maier R, Tustin J, Jardine CG, Driedger SM. "They're trying to bribe you and taking away your freedoms": COVID-19 vaccine hesitancy in communities with traditionally low vaccination rates. *Vaccine.* 2022; 40(50): pp. 7280–7287. doi: 10.1016/j.vaccine.2022.10.058
10. Rosen BL, Thompson EL, Wilson KL, Smith ML. Do political and religious affiliations impact HPV vaccine mandate support? *Health Behavior and Policy Review.* 2017; 4(5): pp. 472–483. doi: https://doi.org/10.14485/HBPR.4.5.7
11. Brehm JW, Brehm SS. *Psychological Reactance: A Theory of Freedom and Control.* San Diego, CA: Academic Press; 1981.
12. Reynolds-Tylus, T. Psychological reactance and persuasive health communication: a review of the literature. *Frontiers in Communication.* 2019; 4: p. 56.
13. Sanchez R. South Dakota's Sturgis Motorcycle Rally: a "cautionary tale" in the age of COVID-19. CNN. August 8, 2021. https://www.cnn.com/2021/08/06/us/sturgis-motorcycle-rally-covid/index.html
14. Firestone MJ, Wienkes H, Garfin J, et al. COVID-19 outbreak associated with a 10-day motorcycle rally in a neighboring state—Minnesota, August–September 2020. *MMWR Morb Mortal Wkly Rep.* 2020; 69: pp. 1771–1776. doi: 10.15585/mmwr.mm6947e1
15. Cialdini RB. *Influence: Science and Practice.* Boston, MA: Allyn and Bacon; 2001.
16. French J, Raven BH. The basis of social power. In: Cartright D, ed. *Studies in Social Power.* Ann Arbor, MI: Institute for Social Research; 1959.
17. Rodin J, Janis IL. The social power of health-care practitioners as agents of change. *J Soc Issues.* 1979; 35(1): pp. 60–81.
18. Buchmann WF. Adherence: a matter of self-efficacy and power. *J Adv Nurs.* 1997; 26(1): pp. 132–137.
19. Eagly AH, Ashmore RD, Makhijani MG, Longo LC. What is beautiful is good, but…: a meta–analytic review of research on the physical attractiveness stereotype. *Psychol Bull.* 1991; 110(1): pp. 109–128.
20. Montoya RM, Horton RS, Kirchner J. Is actual similarity necessary for attraction? A meta-analysis of actual and perceived similarity. *J Soc Pers Relationships.* 2008; 25(6), pp. 889–922.
21. Zajonc RB. Attitudinal effects of mere exposure. *J Pers Soc Psychol.* 1968; 35: pp. 151–175.
22. Bornstein RF. Exposure and affect: overview and meta-analysis of research, 1968-1987. *Psychol Bull.* 1989; 106(2): pp. 265–289. doi: 10.1037/0033-2909.106.2.265
23. Tannenbaum MB, Hepler J, Zimmerman RS, et al. Appealing to fear: a meta-analysis of fear appeal effectiveness and theories. *Psychol Bull.* 2015; 141(6): pp. 1178–1204. doi: 10.1037/a0039729
24. Lawson PJ, Flocke SA. Teachable moments for health behavior change: a concept analysis. *Patient Educ Couns.* 2009; 76(1): pp. 25–30. doi: 10.1016/j.pec.2008.11.002
25. McBride CM, Clipp E, Peterson BL, Lipkus IM, Demark-Wahnefried W. Psychological impact of diagnosis and risk reduction among cancer survivors. *Psycho-oncology.* 2000; 9(5): pp. 418–427.

26. Janis IL, Mann L. Effectiveness of emotional role-playing in modifying smoking habits and attitudes. *J Exp Res Pers*. 1965; 1: pp. 84–90.
27. Mann L, Janis IL. A follow-up study on the long-term effects of emotional role playing. *J Pers Soc Psychol*. 1968; 8(4): pp. 339–342.
28. McBride CM, Emmons KM, Lipkus IM. Understanding the potential of teachable moments: the case of smoking cessation. *Health Educ Res*. 2003; 18(2): pp. 156–170.
29. Rothman AJ, Salovey P. Shaping perceptions to motivate healthy behavior: the role of message framing. *Psychol Bull*. 1997; 121(1): pp. 3–19.
30. Zhang CQ, Zhang R, Schwarzer R, Hagger MS. A meta-analysis of the health action process approach. *Health Psychol*. 2019; 38(7): pp. 623–637. doi: 10.1037/hea0000728
31. Casey B, Coote S, Shirazipour C, et al. Modifiable psychosocial constructs associated with physical activity participation in people with multiple sclerosis: a systematic review and meta-analysis. *Arch Phys Med Rehabil*. 2017; 98(7): pp. 1453–1475. doi: 10.1016/j.apmr.2017.01.027
32. Nagourney E. Insights: possible link between sleep and risk for diabetes. *New York Times*. 2008; January 15. Retrieved May 29, 2024 from http://www.nytimes.com/2008/01/15/health/15insi.html?_r=1
33. Anothaisintawee T, Reutrakul S, Van Cauter E, Thakkinstian A. Sleep disturbances compared to traditional risk factors for diabetes development: systematic review and meta-analysis. *Sleep Med Rev*. 2016; 30: pp. 11–24. doi: 10.1016/j.smrv.2015.10.002
34. Eng TR, Maxfield A, Patrick K, Deering MJ, Ratzan SC, Gustafson DH. Access to health information and support: a public highway or a private road? *JAMA*. 1998; 280(15): pp. 1371–1375.
35. DiMatteo MR, Haskard-Zolnierek KB, Martin LR. Improving patient adherence: a three-factor model to guide practice. *Health Psychol Rev*. 2012; 6(1): pp. 74–91, doi: 10.1080/17437199.2010.537592
36. Besser A, Flett GL, Hewlett PL. Perfectionism, cognition, and affect in response to performance failure vs success. *Journal of Rational-Emotive & Cognitive Behavior Therapy*. 2004; 22: pp. 301–28.
37. Oishi S, Diener E. Re-examining the general positivity model of subjective well-being: the discrepancy between specific and global domain satisfaction. *J Pers*. 2001; 69(4): pp. 641–666.
38. Sheldon KM, Kasser T. Pursuing personal goals: skills enable progress but not all progress is beneficial. *Pers Soc Psychol Bull*. 1998; 24: pp. 546–557.
39. Scheier MF, Carver CS. Optimism, coping, and health: assessment and implications of generalized outcome expectancies. *Health Psychol*. 1985; 4(3): pp. 219–247.
40. Boehm JK, Chen Y, Koga H, Mathur MB, Vie LL, Kubzansky LD. Is optimism associated with healthier cardiovascular-related behavior? Meta-analyses of 3 health behaviors. *Circ Res*. 2018; 122(8): pp. 1119–1134. doi: 10.1161/CIRCRESAHA.117.310828
41. Schwarzer R. Self-regulatory processes in the adoption and maintenance of health behaviors: the role of optimism, goals, and threats. *J Health Psychol*. 1999; 4(2): pp. 115–127.
42. Martin LR, Friedman HS, Tucker JS, Tomlinson-Keasey C, Criqui MH, Schwartz JF. A life course perspective on childhood cheerfulness and its relation to mortality risk. *Pers Soc Psychol Bull*. 2002; 28(9): pp. 1155–1165.

43. Epstein S. Coping ability, negative self-evaluation, and overgeneralization: experiment and theory. *J Pers Soc Psychol.* 1992; 62(5): pp. 826–836.
44. Epstein S, Meier P. Constructive thinking: a broad coping variable with specific components. *J Pers Soc Psychol.* 1989; 57(2): pp. 332–350.
45. Ammerman RT, Lynch KG, Donovan JE, Martin CS, Maisto SA. Constructive thinking in adolescents with substance use disorders. *Psychol Addict Behav.* 2001; 15(2): pp. 89–96.
46. Park CL, Moore PJ, Turner RA, Adler NE. The roles of constructive thinking and optimism in psychological and behavioral adjustment during pregnancy. *J Pers Soc Psychol.* 1997; 73(3): pp. 584–592.
47. Spernak SM, Moore PJ, Hamm LF. Depression, constructive thinking and patient satisfaction in cardiac treatment adherence. *Psychol Health Med.* 2007; 12(2): pp. 172–189.
48. Bandura A. Self-efficacy: toward a unifying theory of behavioral change. *Psychol Rev.* 1977; 84(2): pp. 191–215.
49. Kirsch I. Efficacy expectations or response predictions: the meaning of efficacy ratings as a function of task characteristics. *J Pers Soc Psychol.* 1982; 42: pp. 132–136.
50. Kirsch I. Response expectancy as a determinant of experience and behavior. *Amer Psychol.* 1985; 4: pp. 1189–1202.
51. Sheeran P, Maki A, Montanaro E et al. The impact of changing attitudes, norms, and self-efficacy on health-related intentions and behavior: a meta-analysis. *Health Psychol.* 2016; 35(11): pp. 1178–1188. doi: 10.1037/hea0000387
52. Allison MJ, Keller C. Self-efficacy intervention effect on physical activity in older adults. *West J Nurs Res.* 2004; 26(1): pp. 31–46.
53. Luszczynska A, Tryburcy M, Schwarzer R. Improving fruit and vegetable consumption: a self-efficacy intervention compared with a combined self-efficacy and planning intervention. *Health Educ Res.* 2007; 22(5): pp. 630–638.
54. Serdula MK, Khan LK, Dietz WH. Weight loss counseling revisited. *JAMA.* 2003; 289(14): pp. 1747–1750.
55. Elder JP, Ayala GX, Harris S. Theories and intervention approaches to health-behavior change in primary care. *Am J Prev Med.* 1999; 17(4): pp. 275–284.
56. Deci EL, Koestner R, Ryan RM. A meta-analytic review of experiments examining the effects of extrinsic rewards on intrinsic motivation. *Psychol Bull.* 1999; 125(6): pp. 627–668.
57. Rawsthorne LJ, Elliot AJ. Achievement goals and intrinsic motivation: a meta-analytic review. *Pers Soc Psychol Rev.* 1999; 3(4): pp. 326–344.
58. Williams GC, Grow VM, Freedman ZR, Ryan RM, Deci EL. Motivational predictors of weight loss and weight-loss maintenance. *J Pers Soc Psychol.* 1996; 70(1): pp. 115–126.
59. Cerasoli CP, Nicklin JM, Ford MT. Intrinsic motivation and extrinsic incentives jointly predict performance: a 40-year meta-analysis. *Psychol Bull.* 2014; 140(4): pp. 980–1008. doi: 10.1037/a0035661
60. Elliott ES, Dweck CS. Goals: an approach to motivation and achievement. *J Pers Soc Psychol.* 1988; 54(1): pp. 5–12.
61. Laitakari J, Vuori I, Oja P. Is long-term maintenance of health-related physical activity possible? An analysis of concepts and evidence. *Health Educ Res.* 1996; 11(4): pp. 463–477.

62. Locke EA, Latham GP. *Theory of Goal Setting and Task Performance.* Englewood Cliffs, NJ: Prentice Hall; 1990.
63. Cervone D, Jiwani N, Wood R. Goal setting and the differential influence of self-regulatory processes on complex decision-making performance. *J Pers Soc Psychol.* 1991; 61(2): pp. 257–266.
64. Locke EA, Frederick E, Lee C, Bobko P. Effect of self-efficacy, goals, and task strategies on task performance. *J Appl Psychol.* 1984; 69: pp. 241–251.
65. Strecher VJ, Seijts GH, Kok GJ, et al. Goal setting as a strategy for health behavior change. *Health Educ Q.* 1995; 22(2): pp. 190–200.
66. Dishman RK, Motl RW, Saunders R, et al. Enjoyment mediates effects of a school-based physical-activity intervention. *Med Sci Sports Exerc.* 2005; 37(3): pp. 478–487.
67. Gollwitzer PM, Brandstatter V. Implementation intentions and effective goal pursuit. *J Pers Soc Psychol.* 1997; 73(1): pp. 186–199.
68. Fuchs A. Motivation. In: Kirch W, ed. *Encyclopedia of Public Health.* Dordrecht: Springer; 2008. doi: 10.1007/978-1-4020-5614-7_2238
69. Father loses 103 pounds to donate kidney to his daughter. *Los Angeles Times.* January 1, 1998. https://www.latimes.com/archives/la-xpm-1998-jan-01-mn-4054-story.html
70. Prochaska JO, Prochaska JM. *Changing to Thrive: Using the Stages of Change to Overcome the Top Threats to Your Health and Happiness.* Hazelden Publishing; 2016.
71. Prochaska JJ, Prochaska JM, Prochaska JO. Building a science for multiple-risk behavior change. In: Hilliard ME, Riekert KA, Ockene JK, Pbert L, eds. *The Handbook of Health Behavior Change.* 5th ed. Springer; 2018; doi: 10.1891/9780826180148.0012
72. Rollnick S, Miller WR. What is motivational interviewing? *Behavioural and Cognitive Psychotherapy.* 1995; 23(4): pp. 325–334.
73. Miller WR, Rollnick S. *Motivational Interviewing: Helping People Change.* Guilford Press; 2012.
74. Rollnick S, Miller WR, Butler CC, Aloia MS. Motivational interviewing in health care: helping patients change behavior. *COPD: J Chronic Obstr Pulm Dis.* 2009; doi: 10.1080/15412550802093108
75. Weinschenk S. The science of habits. *Psychology Today.* April 19, 2019. https://www.psychologytoday.com/us/blog/brain-wise/201904/the-science-habits
76. Duhigg C. *The Power of Habit: Why We Do What We Do in Life and Business.* Random House; 2014.

Chapter 6
Habits

Many of us dream of quantum change, a sudden and most welcome improvement in our capabilities, functioning, and emotional resources. Inspirational podcasts, books, and weekend retreats can promise us life-changing insight and motivation. We have a strong desire to achieve our goals, and we envision ourselves much improved over the current versions that we are today.

A desire to change, however, is not the same thing as changing. As we saw in Chapter 5, change requires a kind of "spark" of insight or meaning to ignite one's hope for a better future self. Persuasion and motivation push along the process of knowledge and awareness, and it is helpful to have a sense that change is absolutely necessary. But lasting change requires *sustained, incremental effort*. The process is often slow and sometimes seems boring in contrast with the promise of a miracle. Quantum changes do exist, of course; a person's social media posts go viral or what was believed to be a chronic disease is suddenly eradicated and "cured." But miraculous changes, such as quick and significant weight loss or the rapid building of impressive muscle mass and strength, are the exception. Going in search of them can sometimes create problems such as the side effects of drugs and supplements. Furthermore, in passing up the opportunity to enact incremental change, people can miss the chance to gain control of their habitual behaviors for both the present and the future.

As we will see in this chapter, sustainable change can happen in small and gradual ways. Simple daily habits, strung together, can become larger, more complex patterns. Nowhere is this more important than in the management of health behavior and chronic illnesses. As we saw in Chapter 1, the incidence and prevalence of chronic diseases, even in relatively young persons, are growing; and the long-term dangers of poor health habits are increasing. Case Study 6.1 illustrates this in Gabriel's struggle to manage his multiple chronic conditions.

Case Study 6.1 Gabriel

Gabriel works as the parts manager in a car dealership. Much of his job is sedentary, working with customers at the parts department counter, or ordering parts on the computer. At the age of 29, after several years without consistent medical care, he finally has a job that offers him health insurance. Visits to his recently-assigned primary care physician have resulted in a new and significant diagnosis—high blood pressure—and a recognition that his type 2 diabetes (which was diagnosed when he was 14) is not well controlled.

Gabriel does not want to *manage* these chronic conditions for the rest of his life by taking medication, exercising every day, and changing his diet. Taken together, the new health directives from his physician comprise a formidable list: take several daily medications as prescribed; test his blood sugar several times a day; adjust his eating habits to keep his blood sugar in the acceptable range; and eat a heart-healthy diet of whole foods with much less salt and fat than he has grown accustomed to. Gabriel was also told to get regular physical exercise and maintain a healthier weight because he has borderline obesity. In addition, Gabriel's doctor recommends that he significantly limit his alcohol intake to a maximum of one drink a day, not smoke or vape, and get seven to eight hours of uninterrupted sleep every night in order to most effectively manage his chronic conditions.

Unfortunately, like many young adults with childhood-onset type 2 diabetes and hypertension, Gabriel has difficulty carrying out the simplest of these recommendations—to take his medications as prescribed. In some recent research among young people like Gabriel, medication nonadherence was as high as 80%.[1]

Managing all of these health requirements is difficult, and Gabriel understandably wishes that these conditions would simply go away. Sometimes he searches the web for simpler answers, or a cure; it is hard for him to accept that managing his diabetes and hypertension will require significantly altering and managing his day-to-day *habits* for the rest of his life.

Habits defined

The American Heritage Dictionary defines a habit as "a recurrent, often unconscious pattern of behavior that is acquired through frequent repetition."[2] Merriam-Webster defines a habit as "a settled tendency or usual manner of behavior; an acquired mode of behavior that has become nearly or completely involuntary" and as "a behavior pattern acquired by frequent repetition or physiologic exposure that shows itself in regularity or increased facility of performance."[3]

These definitions can be applied to health-promoting actions, such as a habit of taking vitamins or getting enough sleep. But, as we will see, *problematic behaviors* can also become habits. These might come in the form of addictions (smoking, drinking too much alcohol) or as regular avoidance of important health behaviors.

The "new" habit science

The past decade has produced many developments in the science of habit formation and maintenance. Indeed, many new assistive technologies such as reminder systems and online coaching and psychological support (from a human or artificial intelligence [AI]) are commonplace and in Chapter 8, we will review some of these valuable developments. Cognitive behavior modification (addressed later in this chapter) can help modify unwanted habits and help to establish desirable ones. Troubleshooting for "temptations" and "problem behaviors" and suggestions for alternate actions are available on the internet at a moment's notice. The good news is that now no one needs to struggle alone.

The basic principles of habit formation and maintenance, upon which new habit science and technologies are based, are not new at all, however. They comprise an entire field of psychology, begun in the early 1900s and formalized in the 1930s by the famous psychologist B.F. Skinner. This field is "behaviorism" or "applied behavior analysis," and it is built upon the principles of classical and operant conditioning. The interface of these principles with modern life in the 21st century *is* new; the "old habit science" has become more accessible and usable. Recent popular books about habit formation and maintenance can help individuals who know little about how to change; they make valuable suggestions and teach readers generalizable principles about habits, agency, efficacy, daily actions, tiny shifts, and nudges. These books help develop awareness of how our fast-paced environments can trigger and reinforce patterned behavior, for good or ill. They show how with many creatures—dogs, dolphins, and humans, alike—complex behaviors can be built upon the acquisition of individual simpler behaviors, each of which is reinforced. And, for some individuals, the new technological advancements in behavioral management (as we address in Chapter 8) can be lifesaving.

The basics of behavioral analysis and change

In the remainder of this chapter, we will examine basic issues in applied behavior analysis as they relate to health behavior change and treatment adherence. These principles apply whether an individual directs and keeps track of their own behavior (self-management with a notebook), is assisted by a human coach (in-person or online), or works with an app (including a very polite avatar).

Forming habits

Habit formation is complex and involves cognitive (thought-based) and neural (biological) processing, environmental prompting, and behavioral repetition. Repetition allows encoding of behavioral patterns in procedural memory, so that behavioral steps are carried on without conscious thought.[4] As described in Chapter 4, the encoding process involves strengthening of neural connections; this strengthening enables neurons to communicate with one another efficiently. When Gabriel first began his new job, for example, he relied on the real-time mapping app on his phone to find his way to the dealership and then to retrace his path back home. After a few days, however, the pattern of right and left turns had become part of his procedural memory. Now he pays little attention to his route, sometimes finding himself almost inexplicably at home after listening to a podcast or two. Gabriel's "going home" behavior has become so habitual that one day he drove several miles before he remembered that he had a dental appointment, even though he'd seen it on his calendar just moments before he left work. The combination of getting into his car in the familiar parking lot, and the late afternoon sun, cued him to drive home even though going home was not next on his schedule.

Behaviors and their contexts can become habitually associated through a process called "classical conditioning"; environmental triggers can exert influence over neural and physiological reactions which, in turn, prompt behaviors. It is important to keep in mind that some habits develop effortlessly whereas others require effort; the latter often characterizes health behavior change.

Classical conditioning
Classical conditioning was first described by Ivan Pavlov in 1927 and involves learning to associate unrelated stimuli to produce the same outcome. Pavlov labeled things that naturally evoke a particular reaction "unconditioned stimuli." In response to a potato chip in the mouth, salivation is a natural reaction. "Neutral stimuli" are those that do not initially evoke a reaction (e.g., the TV screen won't make a person's mouth water). But, with repeated pairing the unconditioned stimulus can impart some of its power to the neutral stimulus, turning it into a "conditioned stimulus." So, consistently snacking on potato chips when watching TV can eventually cause salivation and a desire for potato chips, even when one is watching TV with no snacks in sight.

This process explains one of the facets of habit formation and maintenance. A conscious effort can be made to create conditioned responses to environmental cues; these associations can foster habit strength and preservation over time. Once a habit has been formed, the original stimulus need not be present for the habitual response to be triggered; contextual factors can also initiate the behavioral response.[4] For example, Diego has created a playlist of 20 favorite songs and he always listens to them when he runs or power-walks. He's started to notice that simply hearing one of the songs prompts him to quicken his steps, and when he hears a coworker humming one of "his tunes" he suddenly feels motivated to take the stairs.

Operant conditioning
Another way in which habits can be created is through their association with reward.[5] Although reward has a physiological component (chemical releases in the pleasure-centers of the brain), the learning process in operant conditioning is more cognitive than in classical conditioning because it emphasizes *expectations* for what will follow a behavior. Associating good

things (rewards) with performing certain behaviors encourages their repetition because the memory of past rewards can be prompted by environmental cues.[5] In cases where the desired behavior is difficult to achieve, *shaping* can be used to move the person in small steps toward the larger goal. Shaping relies on the process of operant conditioning in which successive approximations of the goal behavior are rewarded; when the first step has been mastered, it is no longer rewarded and instead the next step must be achieved to gain the reward.

Rewards for behaviors
As we noted in Chapter 5, the adoption of new behaviors can be motivated by clear expectations of reinforcement; rewards can help build behavioral habits.[6,7] For example, a person might be able to motivate themselves to walk regularly by indulging in a hot bath after (and only after) a walk. Reinforcement techniques are most useful when they have certain characteristics. First, to create a sustainable habit, the reinforcements must truly be desirable and rewarding to the person. If a person much prefers showers to baths, a hot bath would not serve as an effective reward and might even be a deterrent. Second, the reward should not be counterproductive to the person's health. Rewarding each walk with a pint of ice cream might be great for reinforcing walking behavior but may ultimately do more harm than good.

Maintaining habits and reinforcement schedules
It is possible to imagine a perfect reward system in which an individual has a well-thought-out and consistent system of highly desired rewards for every health-related action. But perfect reward systems aren't very practical. A better goal is to create habits that can be sustained over long periods without constant reinforcement.

Research is very clear that for *initially* establishing new patterns of behavior, a continuous schedule of reinforcement is most effective; the target behavior should be rewarded every time it is carried out.[8] But, after a while, partial schedules of reinforcement (in which the desired behavior is rewarded only part of the time) should be instituted; the behavior will then persist for a longer time, even in the absence of reward.[9]

Partial reinforcement schedules may be fixed or variable and may be ratio- or interval-based. *Fixed* schedules reward a behavior in a consistent fashion—for example, every fifth time the behavior is done. The "ratio" indicates that it is the number of repetitions that is "fixed." Olivia might keep track of her gym workouts and treat herself to a movie each time she has completed five workouts. Or, she may wear an activity tracker and allocate herself an hour of television for every 10,000 steps she takes.

A fixed interval schedule is based on a time period. A behavior might be rewarded only after engaging in the behavior for five minutes. Walking on a treadmill for a fixed time is an example; regardless of how fast or slow Xavier walks (and how many steps he takes), he gives himself a point for every five minutes walked. If Xavier sets up a system in which he rewards himself with points, he might be quite motivated to walk an additional five minutes... and then five more. Depending on what is reinforcing to Xavier, he might use his points to allow himself rewards like clothing, tickets to music or sporting events, or even desserts.

Variable schedules are just like the fixed-ratio and fixed-interval schedules in terms of the elements of reinforcement except that instead of being "fixed" on a particular number (e.g., five repetitions or five minutes) they vary around that number. For example, the reward comes sometimes after four minutes (or 400 steps), sometimes after ten minutes (or 1,000 steps), and so on. Variable schedules are less predictable and so represent a way of keeping the system of rewards fresh and interesting. Higher numbers required for a reward might be seen as challenges while lower numbers are unexpected treats.

Implementing these types of schedules by oneself can be difficult; it is helpful to have someone else to help monitor and regulate the rewards, especially if one is inclined to "cheat" even a little. These behavior modification techniques can be fun and rewarding in themselves, increasing the sustainability of the process. Case Study 6.2 summarizes several creative reinforcement schedules and their implementation.

Case Study 6.2 Examples of Reinforcement Schedules for Health Behavior Change in Action

Olivia: Olivia wants to increase her walking. She has set up an interesting game, a contingency plan, whereby she "earns" television-watching time in five-minute increments. Each morning she rolls dice to determine the "price" of that day's television and has set up an equivalency for the number of steps to five minutes of TV. She keeps track of her daily steps with her smartwatch. Not only has this strategy increased her activity, it has made her more careful about what she watches on TV.

Anthony: Anthony is trying to stick to a healthy eating plan, but his office is very near to a donut shop. Simply bringing healthy snacks to work with him wasn't enough; he was still succumbing to temptation far too frequently. So, he controls his donut purchases by paying himself double the price of a donut every time he skips one. He keeps a box labeled "anti-donut" in his desk drawer to collect what he saves. Although he loves donuts, he also loves "gourmet" healthy food (but he hates spending the money!). Now he uses the "anti-donut" money to have a fancy but healthy meal at a restaurant with no guilt because he earned it by skipping donuts, and this process is keeping him on track with his healthy eating.

The Moreno Family: David and Julia Moreno want their children, Isla and Carmen, to learn a variety of good health habits. The entire family saves healthy-behavior points to "purchase" a variety of activities and other treats. In the kitchen, the family has a chart that lists "point values" for different health-behaviors and a grid on which each member can check off behaviors they have accomplished. For example, putting on sunscreen, tooth-brushing, and eating a serving of fruit or vegetables each net five points; drinking a glass of water nets two points; putting on a helmet for bicycling without being reminded nets 10 points. Parents participate too, and each week the family comes together to total the points. With their points, the children can purchase screen time, trips with friends, and so on. These rewards encourage them to engage in a broad range of positive health behaviors, with very little nagging from their parents.

Behavioral contracts and contingency plans

In Chapter 5, we introduced the behavioral contract as a way to motivate health behavior change. By committing in written form to a course of action, individuals can become more motivated to pursue that action and maintain consistency between their thoughts and behaviors. Behavioral contracts can do much more than motivate goal-engagement; they often contain formal schedules for administering rewards or negative consequences and can engage people to carry out their action plans. Behavioral contracts apply subtle social pressure by reminding people of their commitments. Contracts are effective across a variety of domains, from encouraging weight gain in individuals with anorexia[10] to motivating weight loss in overweight patients.[11]

Contingency contracts (also called contingency management techniques) utilize the same principles, typically setting up a system so that target behaviors are clear, providing reinforcements for those behaviors, and withholding incentives when they are not carried out.[12] Contingency management procedures are effective across a wide variety of clinical settings[13] ranging from self-care for transplant populations[14] to dietary interventions.[15]

Some "contracts" may be less formal than standard behavioral or contingency management contracts but still incorporate similar elements. Some may take the form of a worksheet rather than an agreement; by completing it with their health educator or with a support group, individuals can solidify their plans for implementing change. Such worksheets not only help patients identify specific actions they can take, and encourage them to commit to these actions, but may also strengthen their self-efficacy by prompting recollection of how they themselves, or people they know, have been successful at behavior change. These recollections of past successes encourage them to generalize from prior experience to future efforts, enhancing their sense of mastery and competence. Reflecting on the successes of similar others allows them to vicariously experience positive outcomes and proactively envision these for themselves.

Intrinsic motivation

Despite their utility, behavior-modification techniques require caution. Associating one's behavior with external rewards might diminish intrinsic motivation, which is essential for persistent goal-directed behavior, as shown in a meta-analysis of 128 different studies.[16] Behaviors supported by internal motivation and intrinsic rewards are better maintained than those enacted to gain external rewards which tend not to remain reinforcing for long. A target behavior will decrease unless a reward's value can be maintained indefinitely. A combination of extrinsic incentives and intrinsic rewards might be best, as these meta-analytic findings suggest.[16,17]

The reward of positive verbal feedback is easy to maintain and enhances intrinsic motivation rather than decreasing it. Supportive examples include: "You did that really well," and "I'm impressed at how you never gave up." The effectiveness of verbal feedback is an exception to the general finding that rewards diminish intrinsic motivation; meta-analysis shows that positive verbal feedback from members of a social network can provide effective and economical support for behavior change. As we will see in more detail in Chapter 7, other people can strongly influence one's willingness and ability to pursue and maintain behavior change. The reactions of an individual's social network to their attitudes and health behaviors can offer a potent source of reward and motivation.

Breaking bad habits

We have seen that some habits are easy to maintain over time; they tend to reinforce themselves. For some people, going for a run after work or taking a yoga class can be reinforcing; their tight, tense muscles finally relax, and they are rewarded with less stress and better sleep. For others, eating ice cream after work while lying on the couch watching television can feel good and be very rewarding. Behavioral patterns that are reinforced tend to continue.

Unfortunately, there are some habits we would prefer to extinguish, yet they persist. Smoking, eating high fat fast-food for dinner, and staying up late binge-watching TV instead of sleeping are good examples. The self-reinforcing aspects of many habits (e.g., drinking beer or eating chocolate every day) make them difficult to quit. The chocolate tastes very good; the beer facilitates relaxation and interactions with new people.

Most behaviors are, in fact, not associated with a single reward. Many of our favorite so-called "comfort foods" taste good and satisfy our hunger; they may also arouse feelings and memories (perhaps from childhood) of being well cared-for, safe, and secure. We may seek out these foods not only when we are hungry or want something delicious, but also when we are feeling anxious, sad, or lonely; these foods satisfy both physical and emotional needs. When multiple associations have been established, new "rewards" become possible and habitual behaviors, for good or for bad, are quite likely to be reinforced.

Can habits, even those established decades ago, be changed? Is it possible to replace habitual unhealthy actions with fresh, new ways of behaving? Yes, but (no surprise here) it isn't quick or easy. First, to change behavior we need to change what reinforces it. The reinforcement systems for unhealthy behaviors will need to be eliminated or at least weakened, and new, competing behaviors must be instituted in place of the old patterns. The process of replacing current rewards with more appropriate ones will take time and many repetitions.

There does not exist a set number of times that one must repeat a behavior to make it habitual, and experts suggest that if there were such a number, it would not be small. Persistence at repeating a behavioral pattern over time is required in order to create a habit. For example, exercising every day for a week will not create a strong habit of exercise. In addition, everyone has particular strengths and weaknesses, making certain behavioral changes easier than others.

Clearly the "demotivation" and elimination of problematic behaviors can be a complex undertaking. Certain habits, such as in the case of addictions, continue because the rewards are strongly linked to brain functioning (and may even require medical and pharmacological interventions to change). Recent research in the area of obesity conceptualizes overeating as strongly physiologically linked, with changes in body and brain chemistry driving behavioral patterns. In this book, we address addictions only briefly and in non-medical terms; we also refer the reader to some excellent sources on the topic (see the Suggested Reading list at the end of this chapter). Whether an addiction is strongly reinforced by changes in brain chemistry or a simple pattern of day-to-day actions, behaviors continue because of many environmental cues, triggers, and reinforcements. Changing behavior requires attention to and awareness of how cues, triggers, routines, and reinforcements drive action, as well as the development of methods to interrupt these patterns.

One simple process for demotivating, or breaking, a bad habit is to *substitute an incompatible behavior and reinforce* it until the new behavior becomes a strong habit. For example, instead of sitting on the couch eating snack foods, one might get outside and go for a walk (not toting a bag of chips). Instead of going out to a bar with friends, one might go bowling with them at a bowling alley that does not serve alcohol. When the environment changes, the former associations that once triggered and reinforced behavioral patterns are missing and there is a better chance to modify one's actions.

Many behaviors are complex and have multiple elements; sometimes whole sequences of actions must be established and reestablished again. These steps might be implemented most effectively with the help of a coach or provider who has the knowledge and awareness to help the individual with a psychological approach to behavior change.

The habit of not doing

"Not doing" can be a habit; it can involve not exercising, not taking medication, not eating fruits and vegetables. Earlier in this chapter we met Gabriel, and in Case Study 6.3, we see how his habit of "not doing" is problematic for managing his chronic disease.

> ### Case Study 6.3 Gabriel and His Habit of "Not Doing"
>
> As we saw in Case Study 6.1, Gabriel would rather not think about all the things his doctor advised to manage his two serious chronic conditions. The many adjustments he needs to make include eating whole foods, testing his blood sugar, taking medications, being physically active, limiting alcohol, and getting seven or more hours of sleep each night. Right now, nearly every day, Gabriel essentially reinforces himself for avoiding all or most of these behaviors.
>
> Gabriel knows he needs to take medications regularly, but he sees the pill bottles on the counter and walks past them to do something more interesting, deciding that he will think about the pills later. As thoughts of pills drift from his mind, his anxiety about them decreases and this is reinforcing; not taking medication eventually becomes a habit. The pill bottles have served as a cue to action; he sees them on the counter and experiences anxiety and stress as he is reminded of his diagnoses. He then enacts a behavioral routine in which he thinks "I'll deal with this later," and turns his attention to something else—an activity he chooses because it is rewarding in some way. In addition, his stress is reduced when he stops thinking about his diagnosis (this is "negative" reinforcement—the unpleasant anxiety is essentially "subtracted" from his experience). His habit of not taking medication is thus reinforced and becomes stronger.
>
> The same is true for food. When Gabriel arrives home from work, he grabs a bag of chips and a beer, which are reinforcing because they

require no effort to prepare and taste good. He sits down on the couch and consumes them while watching TV, and then falls into a fitful sleep. This is all understandable because he is so tired after work, but each time his behavior is reinforced by the immediate feel-good elements (taste, drifting off to sleep) he develops a stronger and stronger habit of not doing what he needs to do.

Are there reasons other than habit for not taking his medications? Of course. Gabriel might worry about their side effects and (perhaps because he has read about them online) believe that the medicines do more harm than good. They might be expensive, and he might feel that he is a person who "does not take medication." It is therefore relatively easy for Gabriel to "forget" to take his pills, and to become "distracted" by other things.

This example of Gabriel's habit of avoiding his medication is a simple one; many behaviors are more complex and require considerable analysis. All complex behaviors can be broken down into their constituent parts, however, so that they can be understood and changed.

Very small behavior changes

Two basic requirements of any habit change or formation are: *(1)* to be very specific about the behavior to be adopted, and *(2)* to scale the goal behavior down to very small behavioral components, appropriately called "tiny habits" (see Fogg, 2020, on the Suggested Reading list). We return to Gabriel in Case Study 6.4 to see how this "tiny habit" concept applies to chronic disease management.

Case Study 6.4 Gabriel and Small Habits

Imagine that Gabriel comes home and does not grab a bag of chips and flop down on the couch; instead, he drops his backpack and puts on his walking shoes. He walks to the mailbox and back (further, if he is so inclined). His goal is to interrupt his usual pattern. The next day, he can add to that routine by walking to the end of the block and then coming home, washing his hands, cutting up an apple or other piece of fruit, and perhaps taking it to the backyard to enjoy in the late afternoon sunshine. Or, better still, he might walk several blocks and talk with his neighbors. Each day, or week, he might add a simple behavior until he strings many of them together. He might test his blood sugar, steam some vegetables, and take his medications. By the time he has cleaned up from dinner, he might begin to wind down and watch the news or a favorite TV program while doing a few simple stretching exercises on the floor, and get to bed early. One goal is to figure out how each small behavior can build on others and fit into a naturally occurring behavioral routine. By enacting each small behavior and pairing it with an existing routine, Gabriel can add more small changes each day and reinforce them in a number of ways—by checking off a list on his phone app and saying to himself that he has done well or by using various methods of self-monitoring and self-reward (such as we will examine in Chapter 8). In Gabriel's case, his dual chronic medical conditions of diabetes and hypertension necessitate managing many large behavioral changes, which can be tackled with attention to many small behavioral components.

Self-knowledge and personality

It's often been said (first by Socrates) that "the unexamined life is not worth living." We might expand this to read, "the unexamined individual is not likely to change." Without understanding one's own strengths, weaknesses, preferences, and tendencies, one is not likely to choose effective strategies for implementing change.

Personality refers to a relatively stable set of personal characteristics that are rooted in biological and temperamental factors but have been shaped and molded by the interaction of those factors with the environment. Although it is not the case that personality *determines* people's behavior, it is true that personality influences how we interpret and respond to our environments. (Given the focus of this book, it is especially important to point out that myths about the "nonadherent personality" have not been supported by research.) The five fundamental personality traits considered very important by personality psychologists are summarized in Table 6.1.

Table 6.1 Brief Descriptions of the "Big Five" Personality Traits

Trait	Description
Openness to Experience	Individuals high on this trait tend to be open-minded, creative, and often artistic. They are imaginative and easily in tune with their emotions and feelings, and enjoy exploring different ideas.
Conscientiousness	Individuals high on this trait are responsible, organized, thoughtful, competent, orderly, and planful. Their sense of duty is high; they are motivated to be successful, demonstrate a high degree of self-discipline, and do not act impulsively.
Extraversion	Individuals high on this trait enjoy being around others; they are friendly, outgoing, assertive, gregarious, and gravitate toward excitement and high activity levels.
Agreeableness	Individuals high on this trait are generally cooperative and easy to get along with, trustworthy and straightforward; they connect with others and understand their feelings easily.
Neuroticism	Individuals high on this trait are anxious, high-strung, and can be prone to irritability, hostility, and depression. They are impulsive and self-conscious, and tend to worry and feel vulnerable.

Resource: The International Personality Item Pool.

The International Personality Item Pool (IPIP) website is designed to allow researchers easy access to measures of individual differences as outlined by the Big Five framework. The actual items (questionnaires) are available along with instructions for administering and scoring the tests, and other general personality-relevant information. No special permissions are needed to use these measurement tools; they are in the public domain. The website address is: http://ipip.ori.org/

What does it mean to say that personality is created as a result of interactions between temperament and environment? Let's take, as an example, an infant who is biologically (temperamentally) predisposed to be especially sensitive to the environment, perhaps startling easily and crying heartily. If this infant is raised in a volatile environment where sleeping schedules are unpredictable and parents are inconsistent or unavailable, these biological tendencies may develop into the personality characteristic of neuroticism. An individual high on the dimension of neuroticism tends to worry a lot and feel anxious, emotional, and high-strung. If that same temperamentally volatile infant is raised in a stable, predictable environment, they may develop into someone who is lower on neuroticism. They may still be emotionally sensitive and attuned to environmental cues, but not overly anxious or moody.

Personality predisposes individuals to interpret the world in particular ways and makes certain emotional reactions and behavioral responses likely. Therefore, it is not surprising that while personality traits do not *determine* health behaviors, they are stable over time and can be important predictors of behavior.

One personality characteristic in particular is strongly related to adherence and health behavior change. *Conscientiousness* (the tendency to be responsible, organized, and planful, with good impulse control) is associated with certain better health behaviors including limiting alcohol consumption, refraining from smoking, practicing safer sex, eating healthfully, exercising, and adhering to prescribed medications.[18-20] Someone who is high in conscientiousness will likely be organized enough to make good use of a daily diary or a chart of the foods eaten or steps walked. A person who is low on conscientiousness might view the regimentation and organization required for daily charting or meal planning as tiresome, and practice it sporadically or resist it altogether. For them, a different behavioral strategy might be a better choice.

Those high on the trait of agreeableness tend to be more adherent to medical recommendations and treatment plans.[21,22] They tend to be particularly influenced by the preferences of their healthcare professionals and are more willing to do what their providers ask them to do. They also tend to respond more favorably to suggestions that their health behaviors are important to those close to them, such as their family members.

In our example of personality development above, we looked at neuroticism—a trait that is also consequential to health behaviors. Those high on neuroticism are more anxious and tend to notice symptoms of ill health and worry about them.[23,24] These tendencies can be channeled to foster better health outcomes. As we saw in Chapter 5, health messages that invoke fear can, under some circumstances, be quite persuasive. A person who is high on neuroticism may already be somewhat afraid and worried, so convincing them of the importance of health behavior change might be relatively easy. Keep in mind, however, that *overwhelming* fear can be incapacitating; a practitioner may need to work with a very anxious patient to actually *diminish* their perceptions of threat. And for anxiety to be a good motivator, the individual must know how to minimize the likelihood of the feared outcome.

Personality is not the sole determinant of behavior, of course. In Chapter 4, we discussed ways in which messages might be tailored so that patients pay attention to them, understand them, and remember them. We noted the particular importance of customizing health messages with regard to health literacy and sociodemographic characteristics.[25] Knowing about personality and an individual's associated strengths and weaknesses can make it easier to tailor behavior-change strategies so that they complement the individual's natural tendencies. Many questionnaires are available for assessing personality dimensions, although some are lengthy and/or costly. In Table 6.1 we provide a link for accessing free assessment tools—for clinicians and those wishing to better understand personality.

Choosing the right environments

By the time they reach later adolescence, most people have a good deal of control over where and how they spend their time; a powerful strategy for successful change involves choosing the physical and social environments that support healthy behaviors. Research shows that when significant others (especially family members and close friends) are supportive of good health behaviors, individuals are better able to achieve them.[26,27] Bringing these individuals into the behavior change plan can enhance the effectiveness of any behavior change strategy. When friends, coworkers, and family members are supportive of one's efforts, the environments in which one functions in work, play, and family life can foster and promote health behavior. It is helpful for an individual to seek out environments where others are engaging in the targeted health behavior, thus creating a sort of "buddy system."[28] On the other hand, time spent among those engaging in behaviors one seeks to avoid (e.g., smoking, drinking alcohol, lounging on the couch for hours) can diminish the chances of achieving health goals.

The physical environment itself can also play an important role in health behavior change. When people have access to exercise equipment or pleasant areas in which to walk safely, for example, they are more likely to exercise;[26,29] supervised exercise classes can be more successful than "going it alone."[30] The triggers available in certain environments can "nudge" the individual's behavior in the right direction. The most recent edition of the book *Nudge*[31] outlines the theory and research underlying the concept of nudging behaviors in the right direction rather than using more heavy-handed approaches and directives. Rooted in behavioral economics, including the work of Amos Tversky, Robert Cialdini, and Nobel Laureate Daniel Kahneman, this approach advocates designing environments to encourage people to gently "slide into" desired behaviors. One classic example is the functional keyboard installed on a set of subway steps in Sweden.[32] People found it was fun to make music as they stepped, and 66% more people opted for the stairs instead of the escalator. Multiple studies have now shown that nudges can be effective; one meta-analysis found that nudges increased healthy nutritional choices by 15% on average.[33] Across domains, nudges shift behavior in meaningful ways, with effect sizes typically small to moderate.[34]

This does not mean that, for example, one must relocate or completely redesign one's environment in order to experience nudges to exercise. The whole point of the nudge approach is that *small changes* can facilitate good choices and may be all that is needed to foster better habits. To find a supportive environment for exercise, one might seek out nearby parks, low-traffic walking areas, or a gym in which one feels comfortable. Or, one might look into purchasing some inexpensive exercise equipment to use near the television when watching a favorite show. Keeping a pair of comfortable shoes in one's car or work locker might make it easy to take a brief walk during a lunch break. Nudges serve as reminders (much like traditional informational prompts and directives); they make it easy and appealing to choose healthy behaviors and create supportive environments for carrying them out. Structuring frequent nudges and prompts into one's environment can encourage the use of available opportunities for health behavior.[35-37] Table 6.2 provides some sample prompts and nudges, which can help remind individuals about the goals they have set and encourage them to continue pursuing them.

Prompts can be essential to beginning any health behavior; starting is often the most difficult step. Intentions to exercise, for example, can often be derailed by concerns about discomfort, disappointment, or embarrassment; these concerns can be avoided or managed well if the individual proceeds slowly and carefully, warming up and "taking it easy" at first. Reminders can help initiate the desired behavior, after which many contextual factors can help to motivate and support it. Healthcare providers may wish to focus some attention and rewards specifically on their patients' first steps and understand that getting started represents a significant move toward achieving the larger health-related goal.

Table 6.2 Sample Nudges, Prompts, and Associated Health Behaviors

Nudge/Prompt	Behavior
Setting dental floss on counter in the bathroom	Flossing
Reminder postcard from dentist's office	Dental cleaning
Shower card with pictures and descriptions	Breast self-exam
Mass media campaign	Seatbelt use
Keeping running shoes by the back door	Jogging
Public service announcement	Smoking cessation
Taping pictures of delicious-looking prepared vegetables on the refrigerator	Healthy whole food choices
Putting medication vial next to coffee maker	Taking pills each morning
Drug advertisements	Asking doctor about drugs
Keeping water flask nearby	Increase water intake

Balancing habits with mindfulness

When we confront novel situations and consider what actions we need to take toward our goals, we engage in decision-making. In Chapter 2, we briefly reviewed theoretical models of behavior change and noted that the process of decision-making relies on attitudes and beliefs, prevailing social norms, and expectations of a likely outcome. As Daniel considers whether to try meditation to lower his stress, he remembers reading a news report about research supporting meditation as an effective approach to hypertension. Daniel is willing to try scientifically tested remedies for stress management, and he would like to avoid antihypertensive medication if at all possible. In his circle of friends, meditating is *not* the norm, and it is sometimes ridiculed. He recognizes that he also holds some stereotypes about meditators, and does not think he fits the pattern. Finally, he considers his own likelihood of success, and anticipates that he will have difficulty meditating "correctly." Daniel decides that if he does give it a try, he will need some help—perhaps a guided meditation app, or maybe a podcast that can support him in his efforts.

Daniel's decision-making process illustrates how difficult it can be to start a new behavior. Many of our everyday actions occur in familiar situations and tend to be repetitive and characterized by predictability rather than constant decision-making.[38,39] We tend to eat, sleep, work, and play in basically the same patterns, whether they are good or bad. We tend to buy mostly the same grocery products, drive the same streets, engage in the same hobbies, hang out with the same people, and brush our teeth in the same pattern, day after day. Our habitual behaviors are usually efficient and take little thought; they are automatic and allow us to focus on other things while we are doing them. The advantage *and* the disadvantage are that they often are "mindless," meaning that they are conducted without a great deal of thought regarding whether or how to do them.[40]

Habits, mindlessly carried out, are desirable when they exemplify good health behaviors. Enacted with little effort, they leave the mind free to engage in other tasks. Some automatic behaviors, however, are not at all good for health; it is best, instead, to pursue those with mind*ful*ness. Consider Alexis. Her job as an administrator requires managing many tasks; she saves time in her day by eating lunch at her desk. She has found, however, that when she is "desktop dining" she eats more than she intended, and although her hunger is sated, she doesn't feel satisfied. She hardly even remembers what she ate, and when she gets home later in the evening, she mindlessly eats snack foods even though she's not really hungry.

The practice of mindfulness might help Alexis gain control of her eating habits. This would involve slowing down and engaging in the *experience*—paying attention to the texture and taste of her food, taking the time to savor it, and focusing on eating as a single event rather than combining it with some other activity or chore. Studies have shown that mindful eating does tend to decrease the number of calories consumed and fosters a greater sense of control in eating.[41] Of course, the effort necessary to create a positive habit (or to extinguish an undesirable one) will vary according to the complexity of the behavior itself, the characteristics of the person trying to make the change, and the distractions and barriers that occur while the change is being implemented.

Managing barriers to behavior change

In Chapter 5, we outlined several strategies for motivating behavioral changes; in this chapter we have focused on implementing and solidifying those changes. Thus far, we have emphasized techniques for initiating and maintaining good habits, here we further examine the potential *barriers* to change and consider some ways to forestall and mitigate their impact.

Two critical components of change are: *(1)* a person must *believe* in the importance of making the change, and *(2)* they must *feel competent* to do it (also known as self-efficacy). Self-efficacy takes time to develop, and is built on success at reaching smaller, more manageable goals that are components of larger, more complex ones. The person, ideally, feels: "Success is possible—I'm achieving it!"

Even when these two essential ingredients are in place, additional factors like an unsupportive social network can sabotage the individual's progress. Family members might continue to buy and consume junk food while one member tries to make healthy food choices; friends at work might smoke during breaks (and freely share their cigarettes). These present real obstacles for the person trying to maintain good health habits. The monetary costs of change might also be challenging. Buying workout clothes, organic produce, and prescribed medications might be difficult on a tight budget. One study found, for example, that while taste was the most important factor in food choices, cost was second in importance; after that, nutritional content and convenience were of concern.[42] Not surprisingly, cost was the greatest barrier to low-income groups and to younger people.

In the realm of exercise, barriers often include soreness and discomfort, particularly in the early stages of an exercise endeavor. Managing expectations is important, so that muscle soreness will not be surprising or discouraging. Encouraging patients to monitor and adjust their exercise to minimize discomfort, and to recognize its reduction as they become stronger, can be valuable.

Limited accessibility is another frequently encountered barrier, whether one is trying to gain access to healthcare, to a walking trail, or to accurate information about treatment options. Imagine a woman with low income, working long hours at a desk job, commuting on the bus and subway, and rarely getting home before dark. She cannot afford to join a gym, and feels unsafe walking in her neighborhood after work. Incorporating physical activity into daily routines will be a significant challenge. Creative solutions, such as taking a walk at lunchtime with coworkers, may be essential.

Each of these potential barriers represents a challenge; being aware and monitoring success in overcoming them are crucial to the process of change.

Self-monitoring and regulating

Learning skills to anticipate problems, cope with setbacks, and keep track of successes and failures can help achieve health goals. Using methods of reinforcement described in this chapter, an individual can take responsibility for, and internalize, good health behaviors and make them habitual. Over a long period of time, maintaining a system of rewards can be challenging; accurate record-keeping and self-monitoring, along with examination and modification of the plan, are essential. (See Chapter 8 for discussion of technologies that help to make this possible.) Research shows that paying attention to what has been successful in the past and using these same strategies when implementing new behavior changes, can do a great deal to promote success.[28] Without such self-monitoring and strategic adjustments, the road to behavior change will be difficult at best, and perhaps even impossible.

Earlier we met Daniel, who wanted to use meditation to help reduce stress. In Case Study 6.5 we explore his experience in more detail, as he worked to make meditation a part of his life.

Case Study 6.5 Daniel's Adoption of Meditation for Stress Reduction

Daniel was on his way to meet with his health behavior coach, Kairi. At their first meeting, nearly two months before, they had agreed that he was simply not dealing well with the stresses in his life—his job, problems with his stepdaughter, and the strain of his wife's chronic illness. Together, they decided that meditation might be helpful, and even enjoyable, to manage his stress and help control his high blood pressure. Daniel did not see himself as a "meditator," but he felt he would try it, before starting anti-hypertension medication.

At that first meeting, Kairi provided him with materials explaining various meditation techniques and a list of apps and resources to try out. Their time was limited, but Daniel was glad to have a plan of action. At their next meeting, they talked about Daniel's difficulties with meditation and devised a behavioral plan to help him overcome them. Daniel told Kairi that he really enjoyed the soothing music on the app he had chosen, and that the instructions were very easy and required little for him to do. Therein lay one of its problems, however! Daniel was a "doer" who was constantly thinking, problem-solving, and acting. He had trouble clearing his mind, and "letting thoughts flow like running water." Instead, he was distracted by thoughts of work and by his wife's and stepdaughter's conversations. Daniel had "stuck with the plan" to meditate daily for most of the first week, but then his frequency tapered off and he became considerably less optimistic that he could meditate.

Kairi's first suggestion was to find a more peaceful place to meditate. Daniel had been following the guided meditations in his study, but even with the door closed, his family members' conversations distracted him. He needed quiet in order to focus on his own thoughts, and decided to try wearing noise-canceling headphones and sit in a comfortable chair out in the backyard.

Daniel also needed to change the time frame for his meditation. He had been diligently trying to adhere to 30-minute meditation sessions, but they felt too long, so Kairi suggested trying just five minutes twice per day. This would enable him to become familiar with the process and maintain focus without becoming overwhelmed or frustrated. With Kairi's help, Daniel worked out a month-long schedule, gradually increasing the amount of time he spent in meditation; by the end of the month, he would be doing full 30-minute sessions. They also worked out a simple system of rewards that Daniel could use to reinforce his progress as he practiced meditation skills. These rewards would help him early on, before he was able to notice the reinforcing effects of stress reduction.

As he walked toward his third appointment, Daniel felt in control and optimistic about learning to meditate. He realized that it would be a long process, but he could already sense some changes in his reactions to stressful events in his life. He could now meditate for 30 minutes at a stretch; when intrusions interrupted his concentration, he could quickly reorient himself. He had been keeping track of what worked for him, and was able to taper off his rewards because he was starting to feel the direct benefits of relaxation and meditation. Daniel's case is a good example of how selecting appropriate environments, taking small steps toward a goal, rewarding those steps, and carefully self-monitoring and then adjusting strategies can lead to success in behavior change.

The Health Behavior Internalization Model

The Health Behavior Internalization Model is a theoretical framework that argues for the importance of both personal needs (such as for self-determination and security) and behavior-related needs (like competence and context) when trying to incorporate new health behaviors into a person's sense of self.[43] The process of internalization (or incorporation) of new behaviors can itself be motivating, and it can also serve as a mechanism for self-monitoring and maintenance of those behaviors. It is important to note that internalization will happen only when all internal and external factors are taken into account. Thus, religious beliefs, cultural food preferences, family support systems, peer networks, personality characteristics, and job-related stresses among others must all be integrated into any "plan" for adopting a new health behavior.

Bringing together many aspects of an individual's life to support behavior change helps to increase the chances for success. In Chapter 7, we will discuss how social support, social norms, and social pressures might motivate a person to take on the challenge of behavior change. We note here, briefly, that a health goal (e.g., increased cardiac fitness) can be motivated by family connections (e.g., wanting to be able to run and play with grandkids) or the desire to spare loved ones any worry about one's health. These are powerful external (social) factors. These same elements can also help one maintain health behaviors.

Even pets can help us maintain good habits. Elizabeth, whose dog Hemi is a four-time national agility finalist, was profiled in *Shape* magazine (December 2008). When she first started agility training with Hemi, she could tell that he had "the speed of a champion" but he wasn't winning because *she* wasn't quick enough. Her desire not to hold her dog back from *his* potential motivated fitness goals that she hadn't consistently pursued for herself. Many people find that they are motivated to take their dogs for walks or runs even if they aren't motivated to do it for themselves. These folks might stay in front of their computers or television sets if not for their canine companions who nag them for exercise and the chance to explore the neighborhood.

Successfully monitoring and directing our own health behaviors often require tracking our own progress. Self-monitoring can be more or less structured depending upon factors such as one's conscientiousness and the degree of chaos in one's schedule. Progress can be monitored if one has time and is inclined to make note of successes and challenges each day. Seeing behavioral patterns can be instructive,[28] and viewing personal progress can be quite motivating. Some find the activity tedious, however; for them, detailed self-assessment is unlikely to be helpful. In this case, fun technologies (see Chapter 8) might be useful, or perhaps just a few moments of reflection before sleep, quickly jotting down a + (successful/easy day), 0 (neutral) or − (unsuccessful/challenging day) on a bedside notepad might help monitor progress. It is important to remember that when it comes to behavior change, everyone has successes and failures; self-monitoring records make longer-term trajectories easy to see.

Managing ups and downs

Is there a trick to maintaining positive momentum through the occasional low points one encounters while building health habits? Fortunately, yes. A momentary "lapse" back into problematic behavior may, or may not, become a more serious "relapse" depending upon how one thinks about it. Berating and blaming oneself about a slip-up tends to be associated with a further slide into relapse.[44]

Imagine that one is trying to limit dietary sugar while attending a party. Several strategies might be helpful, such as eating a protein bar beforehand, using a small plate and choosing whole foods to eat, and engaging in conversation far away from the dessert table. Unfortunately, however, the party host has made the most wonderful apple pie and chocolate cake, and there are delicious chocolate truffles all around; one taste leads to many more.

Acknowledging utter failure at limiting sugar is one option, but catastrophic thinking can lead to some bad choices (like stopping for donuts on the way home and deciding that self-control for the entire weekend is a lost cause). Keeping the larger picture in mind, and thinking about the lapse as a learning experience, can help to re-initiate the target behaviors. It might be helpful to focus on the previous week's accomplishments—exercise done, sweets foregone—and accept that a lapse can be overcome. Reflecting on how one might have made better choices at the party and planning to do so in the future can support overall positive trends. Some examples of useful versus harmful responses to behavioral lapses can be found in Table 6.3.

Recognizing when one is likely to be most vulnerable and taking extra precautions during those times and in those situations is also a good strategy to avoid health behavior lapses. *Proactive coping* involves actively anticipating potential barriers or problems, garnering resources to help deal with these, and maintaining vigilance so that the situations can be dealt with quickly.[45] These prepared resources can be personal, or social, or external/concrete in nature, and they must fit the specific challenge. For example, knowing

Table 6.3 Lapses and Reactions

Behavioral Lapse	Harmful Reaction	Useful Reaction
Eating a large piece of pie at a party	"I've blown it now. Might as well pig out tonight and start over tomorrow."	"I wish I hadn't eaten quite such a big piece, but at least I didn't lose control entirely. I'm going to walk an extra mile tomorrow and that will help me get back on track."
Losing track of time while having coffee with friends, and missing kickboxing class	"Good grief, I guess this is a couch potato day. Since I'm obviously not exercising today anyway, I wonder if I can make it home in time to see the season opener of that new TV series."	"Too bad I missed class. I think I'll head over to the gym and see if there is another class I can take. If not, I can always do my own workout!"
Last-minute requests from the boss lead to missing yoga class	"Yoga helps me de-stress so it's too bad I missed it. Maybe I should just keep working at this pile of work on my desk. Getting things done might de-stress me. I don't care if I'm here until midnight!"	"I could have really used yoga after the stress of this afternoon! I'm going to go home and do an online yoga class; that's a pretty good substitute. Then maybe I'll have a nice cup of tea."
Forgetting to brush teeth before bed (recognizing that it's happened several times already this month)	"I'm already in bed and I'm so tired. It doesn't seem to matter anyway; I've forgotten to brush a bunch of times lately and I don't feel any cavities."	"Oh, glad I remembered! I'm lucky that my teeth are strong enough to withstand the bad care I've been giving them lately. I'm going to be extra diligent to make up for it."
Smoking a cigarette after a period of being smoke-free	"Once a smoker, always a smoker. I knew this whole stopping-smoking thing wasn't very realistic for me."	"One cigarette compared to what I used to smoke is nothing. I'm still making good progress. Let me think about how I was feeling before I decided to have that smoke. What was different from all the times I've resisted the urge?"
Drinking too much alcohol	"Well, I'm already pretty wasted and I'm not going to be driving home. Since that's the case, I might as well go all-out!"	"I'm feeling tipsy; if I want to wake up tomorrow without a raging headache, I'd better have some water and no more alcohol. Oh, and a multivitamin when I get home, too."

that a party atmosphere will be challenging, one might recruit a friend who will also be at the party to encourage healthy food choices and discourage overeating sugared treats. A social resource such as this may be more powerful in the party context than a more private monitoring method, such as self-administering "points" for good food choices. In the party environment, it might be easy to stop caring about the points and give in to temptation; a social monitor is more difficult to ignore. Depending on how well a particular strategy works, modifications can be made to future plans (such as scheduling extra workouts) as part of the proactive coping method.

Cognitive Behavioral Therapy and a habit of moving

Few people make it through life without ever having back pain; it is one of the most frequent reasons for medical visits, and among the most common patient complaints presented to primary care physicians. Back pain, primarily low back pain, affects 60–80% of adults in the United States at some time in their lives.[46] Healthcare costs (e.g., increased use of health services) and indirect costs (e.g., missed work and disability payments) due to back pain are estimated to be over $12 billion per year.[47] For most back pain sufferers, a flare-up is episodic and resolves in several weeks. But for about 8%, back pain becomes chronic—limiting activities, threatening work and family obligations, and increasing the likelihood of psychological distress.[48-50]

Many treatment options are available to back pain sufferers, but only a few have been shown in research to be effective. Bedrest is generally unhelpful;[51] surgery often has negligible success;[52] and medications have their own set of problems, including addiction.[53] Exercise, on the other hand, *does* work. There is a great deal of evidence that movement, careful exercise, and the psychological technique of Cognitive Behavioral Therapy (CBT) together work wonders in helping people manage back pain over the long term. Although moving can be difficult for those in pain, CBT can help them initiate and maintain habits of movement as well as patterns of thinking that can help them deal with their pain.

Cognitive Behavioral Therapy (CBT) is a psychological approach to behavior change. With CBT, the individual learns to self-reinforce specific thoughts and behavior patterns that are targeted to managing (in this case pain-related) problems. For example, CBT can be helpful to develop the habit of paying attention to one's energy level and appropriately pacing activity and resting to better manage pain. It can also help the individual control their thoughts to avoid catastrophic thinking (e.g., "If it hurts this much today, imagine how bad it will be tomorrow!"). Anxiety about worsening pain can cause an individual to opt out of valued activities and instead remain sedentary, which then increases pain and can lead to depression. CBT helps people maintain self-efficacy and believe in their ability to accomplish their goals (e.g., "I've solved a similar problem before, I can do it again"). Reducing anxiety and depression associated with pain and physical limitations can help those with back pain remain positive and solution-focused.

Exercising and keeping a positive attitude supported by CBT sound cliché, but they work well to manage chronic pain. Both depend upon basic principles of habit formation and maintenance and together they surpass many medical and surgical interventions in their efficacy and safety in back pain treatment.[54]

Summary

In this chapter, we examine the ways in which health behavior change and treatment adherence are shaped by an individual's habits. Sustained, incremental actions, while less dramatic than any promise of miracle cures, are essential for achieving and maintaining behavioral goals. A habit is "an acquired mode of behavior that has become nearly or completely involuntary"; there are implications of this involuntary unawareness for management and change. For good or ill, small daily habits, strung together, can become larger, more complex patterns of behavior; these might be desirable habits such as taking essential medications and developing a physically active lifestyle, or addictive or problematic behaviors such as smoking, drinking too much alcohol, or avoiding treatment. Nowhere is this more important than in the management of chronic disease, which accounts for most of the medical care delivered in the United States today.

In this chapter, we review a number of new developments in the "science of habit formation and maintenance" as well as the basic principles of classical and operant conditioning which form the basis of the decades-old field of behavioral psychology. We examine rewards for the maintenance of habits, as well as reinforcement schedules, behavioral contracts, contingency plans, and intrinsic versus extrinsic motivation. We consider common barriers encountered by those attempting to change their habits, as well as ways to overcome these barriers. We describe how the new habit science makes the "old habit science" more accessible and emphasizes agency, self-efficacy, daily actions, tiny habits, and nudges. In this chapter, we examine "demotivation" and the elimination of problematic behaviors, as well as the role of familiarity, environmental cues, and triggers. We also describe the power of self-monitoring, behavioral lapses and relapses, and the success of Cognitive Behavioral Therapy (CBT) and exercise in managing chronic back pain.

Tools for instruction and self-study

Learning objectives

By the end of this chapter, readers should be able to

1. Define a habit.
2. Evaluate the relative costs and benefits associated with different schedules of reinforcement.
3. Describe how intrinsic motivation can be influenced by extrinsic rewards.
4. Outline the elements of a behavioral contract, and describe why these contracts can be effective.
5. Compare and contrast nudges and tiny habits, including how they relate to one another and to more traditional approaches to shifting health behaviors.
6. Explain approaches to "demotivating" and eliminating bad habits.
7. Describe why cultural competency is important for clinicians who aim to help their patients change behaviors.

Review questions

1. How is a habit different from a behavior?
2. Give one example of how a habit could be created using classical conditioning principles.
3. Give one example of how a habit could be created using operant conditioning principles.

4. Name and describe the five types of reinforcement schedules. Which is most effective for encouraging an initial behavior? Which is most resistant to extinction? Why?
5. What is the difference between intrinsic and extrinsic motivation? What is the danger in relying too heavily on external rewards?
6. What is a "nudge" and what do data suggest regarding the effectiveness of nudges?
7. Describe how personality can be leveraged to create better habits. Provide one example.
8. Why is it that unlearning poor health habits is often extremely difficult? What is one strategy for demotivating and unlearning a bad habit?
9. What is cognitive-behavioral therapy (CBT), and how can it be used to promote the development of positive health behaviors?

Prompts for discussion and further study

1. Environments, including the reinforcements and punishments they contain, can be powerful influences on behavior and the development of habits. Are there environmental elements that go "too far" and would be considered unethical? Are there some behaviors/habits that are so important that any type of environmental constraint can be considered appropriate?
2. To what extent should public health policy involve nudges? Are there some behaviors that should be left up to the individual with no attempts at influence from public health officials? Which behaviors do you think are so relevant to the public good as to warrant policy change rather than more subtle nudges?
3. What are the ramifications of financial rewards for creating and maintaining good health habits? How would successful creation/maintenance be assessed?

Suggested reading

1. Duhigg C. *The Power of Habit: Why We Do What We Do in Life and Business*. Random House; 2012.

2. Fogg BJ. *Tiny Habits: The Small Changes That Change Everything.* Harvest-Harper Collins; 2020.
3. Clear J. *Atomic Habits: An Easy & Proven Way to Build Good Habits & Break Bad Ones.* Avery-Penguin; 2018.
4. Thaler RH, Sunstein CR. *Nudge: The Final Edition.* Yale University Press; 2021.
5. Pryor K. *Don't Shoot the Dog.* Simon and Schuster; 2019.
6. DiClemente CC. *Addiction and Change: How Addictions Develop and Addicted People Recover.* Guilford Publications; 2018.
7. Heyman GM. *Addiction: A Disorder of Choice.* Harvard University Press; 2009.
8. Miller WR, Forcehimes AA, Zweben A. *Treating Addiction: A Guide for Professionals.* Guilford Publications; 2019.

References

1. Weinstock RS, Trief PM, Burke BK, et al. Antihypertensive and lipid-lowering medication adherence in young adults with youth-onset type 2 diabetes. *JAMA Netw Open.* 2023; Oct 2; 6(10): e2336964. doi: 10.1001/jamanetworkopen.2023.36964.
2. Habit. *The American Heritage Dictionary of the English Language,* 5th edition. November 13, 2023. https://www.ahdictionary.com/word/search.html?q=habit
3. Habit. *Merriam-Webster.com Dictionary.* November 13, 2023. https://www.merriam-webster.com/dictionary/habit
4. Wood W, Neal DT. A new look at habits and the habit-goal interface. *Psychol Rev.* 2007; 114(4): pp. 843–863.
5. Skinner BF. *About Behaviorism.* New York, NY: Knopf; 1947.
6. Dapcich-Miura E, Hovell MF. Contingency management of adherence to a complex medical regimen in an elderly heart patient. *Beh Ther.* 1979; 10: pp. 193–201.
7. Haynes RB, Sackett DL, Gibson ES, et al. Improvement of medication compliance in uncontrolled hypertension. *Lancet.* 1976; 1(7972): pp. 1265–1268.
8. Myers MG, Cowley MA, Munzberg H. Mechanisms of leptin action and leptin resistance. *Annu Rev Physiol.* 2008; 70: pp. 537–556.
9. Nevin JA. Behavioral momentum and the partial reinforcement effect. *Psychol Bull.* 1988; 103(1): pp. 445–456.
10. Solanto MV, Jacobson MS, Heller L, Golden NH, Hertz S. Rate of weight gain of inpatients with anorexia nervosa under two behavioral contracts. *Pediatrics.* 1994; 93(6 Pt 1): pp. 989–991.
11. Ureda JR. The effect of contract witnessing on motivation and weight loss in a weight control program. *Health Educ Q.* 1980; 7(3): pp. 163–185.
12. Higgins ST, Budney AJ, Bickel WK. Applying behavioral concepts and principles to the treatment of cocaine dependence. *Drug Alcohol Depend.* 1994; 34(2): pp. 87–97.
13. Petry NM. A comprehensive guide to the application of contingency management procedures in clinical settings. *Drug Alcohol Depend.* 2000; 58(1–2): pp. 9–25.

14. Cupples SA, Steslow B. Use of behavioral contingency contracting with heart transplant candidates. *Prog Transplant.* 2001; 11(2): pp. 137–144.
15. Cullen KW, Baranowski T, Smith SP. Using goal setting as a strategy for dietary behavior change. *J Am Diet Assoc.* 2001; 101(5): pp. 562–566.
16. Rawsthorne LJ, Elliot AJ. Achievement goals and intrinsic motivation: a meta-analytic review. *Pers Soc Psychol Rev.* 1999; 3(4): pp. 326–344.
17. Cerasoli CP, Nicklin JM, Ford MT. Intrinsic motivation and extrinsic incentives jointly predict performance: a 40-year meta-analysis. *Psychol Bull.* 2014; 140(4): pp. 980–1008. doi: 10.1037/a0035661
18. Bogg T, Roberts BW. Conscientiousness and health-related behaviors: a meta-analysis of the leading behavioral contributors to mortality. *Psychol Bull.* 2004; 130(6): pp. 887–919.
19. Courneya KS, Hellsten LM. Personality correlates of exercise behavior, motives, barriers and preferences: an application of the five-factor model. *Pers Indiv Diff.* 1998; 24(5): pp. 625–633.
20. Molloy GJ, O'Carroll RE, Ferguson E. Conscientiousness and medication adherence: a meta-analysis. *Ann Behav Med.* 2014; 47(1): pp. 92–101. doi: 10.1007/s12160-013-9524-4
21. Vollrath ME, Landolt MA, Gnehm HE, Laimbacher J, Sennhauser FH. Child and parental personality are associated with glycaemic control in Type 1 diabetes. *Diabet Med.* 2007; 24(9): pp. 1028–1033.
22. Ediger JP, Walker JR, Graff L et al. Predictors of medication adherence in inflammatory bowel disease. *Am J Gastroenterol.* 2007; 102(7): pp. 1417–1426.
23. Kolk AM, Hanewald GJ, Schagen S, Gijsbers van Wijk CM. A symptom perception approach to common physical symptoms. *Soc Sci Med.* 2003; 57(12): pp. 2343–2354.
24. Williams PG, Wiebe DJ. Individual differences in self-assessed health: gender, neuroticism and physical symptom reports. *Pers Indiv Diff.* 2000; 28(5): pp. 823–835.
25. Rimer BK, Conaway M, Lyna P, et al. The impact of tailored interventions on a community health center population. *Patient Educ Couns.* 1999; 37(2): pp. 125–140. doi: 10.1016/s0738-3991(98)00122-0
26. Trost SG, Owen N, Bauman AE, Sallis JF, Brown W. Correlates of adults' participation in physical activity: review and update. *Med Sci Sports Exerc.* 2002; 34(12): pp. 1996–2001.
27. Zimmerman RS, Connor C. Health promotion in context: the effects of significant others on health behavior change. *Health Educ Behav.* 1989; 16(1): pp. 57–75.
28. Elder JP, Ayala GX, Harris S. Theories and intervention approaches to health-behavior change in primary care. *Am J Prev Med.* 1999; 17(4): pp. 275–284.
29. Humpel N, Owen N, Leslie E. Environmental factors associated with adults' participation in physical activity: a review. *Am J Prev Med.* 2002; 22(3): pp. 188–199.
30. Ainsworth BE, Youmans CP. Tools for physical activity counseling in medical practice. *Obes Res.* 2002; 10 Suppl 1: pp. 69S–75S.
31. Thaler RH, Sunstein CR. *Nudge: The Final Edition.* Yale University Press; 2021.
32. Bates C. Scaling new heights: piano stairway encourages commuters to ditch the escalators. The Daily Mail.com. October 11, 2009. https://www.dailymail.co.uk/sciencetech/article-1218944/Scaling-new-heights-Piano-stairway-encourages-commuters-ditch-escalators.html
33. Arno A, Thomas S. The efficacy of nudge theory strategies in influencing adult dietary behaviour: a systematic review and meta-analysis. *BMC Public Health.* 2016; 16: p. 676. doi: 10.1186/s12889-016-3272-x

34. Mertens S, Herberz M, Hahnel UJJ, Brosch T. The effectiveness of nudging: a meta-analysis of choice architecture interventions across behavioral domains. *Proc Natl Acad Sci U S A.* 2022; 119(1): e2107346118. doi: 10.1073/pnas.2107346118
35. Dolan MS, Weiss LA, Lewis RA, Pietrobelli A, Heo M, Faith MS. "Take the stairs instead of the escalator": effect of environmental prompts on community stair use and implications for a national "Small Steps" campaign. *Obes Rev.* 2006; 7(1): pp. 25–32.
36. French SA, Story M, Jeffery RW. Environmental influences on eating and physical activity. *Annu Rev Public Health.* 2001; 22: pp. 309–335.
37. Lombard DN, Lombard TN, Winett RA. Walking to meet health guidelines: the effect of prompting frequency and prompt structure. *Health Psychol.* 1995; 14(2): pp. 164–170.
38. Ouellette JA, Wood W. Habit and intention in everyday life: the multiple processes by which past behavior predicts future behavior. *Psychol Bull.* 1998; 124(1): pp. 54–74.
39. Townsend DJ, Bever TG. *Sentence Comprehension: The Integration of Habits and Rules.* Cambridge, MA: MIT Press; 2001.
40. Aarts H, Verplanken B, van Knippenberg A. Predicting behavior from actions in the past: repeated decision making or a matter of habit? *J Appl Soc Psychol.* 1998; 28(15): pp. 1355–1374.
41. Baer RA, Fischer S, Huss DB. Mindfulness-based cognitive therapy applied to binge eating: a case study. *Cognitive and Behavioral Practice.* 2005; 12: pp. 351–358.
42. Glanz K, Basil M, Maibach E, Goldberg J, Snyder D. Why Americans eat what they do: taste, nutrition, cost, convenience, and weight control concerns as influences on food consumption. *J Am Diet Assoc.* 1998; 98(10): pp. 1118–1126.
43. Bellg AJ. Maintenance of health behavior change in preventive cardiology: internalization and self-regulation of new behaviors. *Behav Modif.* 2003; 27(1): pp. 103–131.
44. Brownell KD, Marlatt GA, Lichtenstein E, Wilson GT. Understanding and preventing relapse. *Am Psychol.* 1986; 41(7): pp. 765–782.
45. Aspinwall LG, Taylor SE. A stitch in time: self-regulation and proactive coping. *Psychol Bull.* 1997; 121(3): pp. 417–436.
46. Deyo RA, *Watch Your Back.* Ithaca, NY: ILR Press, Cornell University; 2014.
47. Chronic back pain statistics in the US (2023). CFAH.org. November 17, 2023. https://cfah.org/back-pain-statistics/
48. Parthan A, Evans CJ, Le K. Chronic low back pain: epidemiology, economic burden and patient-reported outcomes in the USA. *Expert Rev Pharmacoecon Outcomes Res.* 2006; 6(3): pp. 359–369. doi: 10.1586/14737167.6.3.359
49. Shirey L, Rogers S. Chronic back pain. Georgetown University Health Policy Institute. December 8, 2023. https://hpi.georgetown.edu/backpain/#
50. Baumeister H, Knecht A, Hutter N. Direct and indirect costs in persons with chronic back pain and comorbid mental disorders—a systematic review. *Journal of Psychosomatic Research.* 2012; 73(2): pp. 79–85.
51. Waddell G, Feder G, Lewis M. Systematic reviews of bed rest and advice to stay active for acute low back pain. *Br J Gen Pract.* 1997; 47(423): pp. 647–652.
52. Deyo R, Chou R. Back pain. The evidence for nonsurgical management. *Surgical Management of Pain.* New York, NY: Thieme; 2014.

53. Martell BA, O'Connor PG, Kerns RD, et al. Systematic review: opioid treatment for chronic back pain: prevalence, efficacy, and association with addiction. *Ann Intern Med.* 2007; 146(2): pp. 116–127. doi: 10.7326/0003-4819-146-2-200701160-00006
54. Zofness R. *The Pain Management Workbook: Powerful CBT and Mindfulness Skills to Take Control of Pain and Reclaim Your Life.* Oakland, CA: New Harbinger; 2020.

Chapter 7
Health Behavior and Adherence in a Sociocultural Context

Health behaviors—indeed most behaviors—result from myriad influences. Personal beliefs, cognitive processes, and habits are vitally important, but equally so are the interpersonal, sociocultural, and socioeconomic contexts in which people live and function. Humans are social creatures whose actions affect, and are affected by, others to whom they look for information, acknowledgment, reinforcement, correction, and connection. Many elements of their complex social and economic environments affect risks to their health and quality of life. These elements are called the "social determinants of health," and we examine them in this and the remaining chapters of this book.

The importance of social context in human behavior is well recognized and is reflected in many theories of health behavior change. Let's review how social context contributes to theoretical models, particularly those labeled "social cognitive," and then examine more closely what these factors look like in action—from the personal (micro) level to the sociocultural (macro) level.

Social cognitive models

As we saw in Chapter 2, researchers and clinicians in a variety of health fields have developed theoretical models to explain people's beliefs about health and their motivations and strategies for addressing it. There, we discussed several prominent models including the Health Belief Model, the Theory of Planned Behavior (which, notably, includes subjective norms), the Transtheoretical Model of Change, the Precaution Adoption Process Model, and the Information-Motivation-Strategy Model. We also briefly examined social cognitive models, noting that we would return to them in this chapter.

As a group, social cognitive models propose that behavior is determined by both personal factors (such as expectations) and environmental elements. Both classical[1] and operant[2] conditioning processes can operate through environmental influences on behavior. Adults are usually more likely to modify their behavior in response to the judgment of other people (a secondary punishment) than in response to simply having a treat withheld from them (a primary punishment). Social cognitive models expand on the original "subjective expected utility theory"[3] by recognizing that we are all subject to social influence[4] and we usually do not base our health-related decisions[5] simply on rational cost-benefit analyses.

How does this social influence occur? In part, it happens through *social expectations*—what we think other people expect or want us to do. Some individuals are meaningfully influenced by their perceptions of the desires of other people in their lives; the beliefs and expectations of others are salient in determining their own health behaviors.[6] Invoking the beliefs or needs of others (e.g., "Your children would want you to take care of yourself" or "You need to stay healthy in order to protect those around you") can prompt efforts toward health-related goals. Even the simple mention of the name of someone who has an interest in a particular goal can influence a person's commitment to it.[7] This effect is most powerful when the relationship is close (although the effect can be diluted if too many goals are associated with one person).

In this chapter, we examine in more detail the various aspects of social cognitive models, including cultural elements that comprise the individual's social milieu and contribute to their cognitive processing. We'll begin with the earliest source of social influence—the family.

Family

Family members are the first educators of children, who are taught, explicitly or otherwise, how to interact with others and care for themselves. Many studies show that the family plays a primary role in developing health behaviors,[8] through explicit directives and through modeling.[9,10] These learned behaviors, such as dietary habits,[11,12] can continue into adulthood.

As such, it is important to provide support to families—both educational and resource-based. For example, California's "First 5"[13] program supports parents during the first five years of children's lives with many services including parenting classes, play groups, developmental screenings, crisis management, and support. Families can also benefit from nutritional programs (e.g., the USDA's Healthy Meals Incentives for schools and its Fresh Fruit and Vegetable Program).[14] Clinicians can and should link families with federal-, state-, or community-based resources whenever possible.

The family can also play an active role in individual health by supporting (or, conversely, by sabotaging) the individual's efforts to be healthy. Family members might bring home healthy whole foods or, on the other hand, continue to buy and consume "junk food" when one member is trying to make healthy eating choices. An individual might face either supportive encouragement or snide remarks when endeavoring to exercise regularly. Families also establish norms. An individual might feel more comfortable using herbal remedies than pharmaceuticals because their family members do so, or might walk regularly and encourage others in the family to join them. Social modeling affects the ease associated with making good (or bad) choices.

In the context of this often-pervasive influence of family, what can a clinician do? Studies find that the most common and effective ways to leverage family influences in favor of health are with supervision, modeling, and support.[15] Supervision (e.g., engaging a family member to remind a person about medications or to exercise) tends to work best with children and sometimes older adults who are more reliant on care. Modeling and support can be used broadly, and specific techniques may be idiosyncratic. Some examples can be found in Table 7.1, and clinicians can help individuals to think creatively about how they might encourage their family members or obtain assistance from them.

Social support

Encouragement and support can be garnered from a broad array of individuals. Those close to us (family or friends) might provide "social support," which health psychologists further define into three distinct types—concrete, informational, and emotional. Concrete (or instrumental) social support involves tangible or physical assistance, such as rides to medical

Table 7.1 Examples of Family Influences on Health Behavior

Mode of Influence	Example
Support	Fill weekly pill sorting box for family member with cognitive decline
	Create a dedicated space for exercise equipment
	Purchase healthful food options
	Attend sports competition of family member
	Empathize with health behavior challenges, praise successes
Supervision	Remind family member to brush and floss teeth before bed
	Remind that bedtime is approaching, encourage wind-down
	Limit video gaming time
Modeling	Cook and eat nutritious meals with family members
	Make a habit of an evening walk with children or other family members
	Turn off all screens and devices one hour before bedtime
	Join a gym together as a family

appointments or guest passes to the gym. Informational social support is that which offers the individual evidence, ideas, facts, and information that is needed for a health action, such as the name and contact details for a good optometrist or a web link for yoga sessions that can be done virtually. Emotional social support involves the offering of empathy and human connection, such as when a friend listens and makes supportive statements that remind the person that they are not alone in facing their chronic illness. Depending on the nature of an individual's challenges, various combinations of these forms of social support may be needed.

Social support is a demonstrably powerful aid to changing behavior and adhering to change over time. Important individuals in a person's life can influence them through expectations and (dis)approval, and can be helpful for monitoring behavior and supervising rewards. This social support is also valuable in other ways. Researchers have studied many health behaviors, including smoking cessation, diet and weight loss, medication adherence, and oral health, and have consistently identified social support[16-19] as important to an individual's perceived *sense of behavioral control*. People with stronger networks of social support feel more empowered to make behavioral changes; their sense of empowerment increases their intentions to change, leading to greater success at achieving their target behaviors.[20]

For example, among older individuals, interpersonal support (including peer sharing and learning) was found to have a significant effect on exercise adoption and maintenance.[21] It makes good sense for a clinician to assess the level of social support available to a patient because of the impact that such support (or its absence) can have on adherence. Meta-analytic research shows that the odds of nonadherence are significantly higher among patients who do not receive emotional support; the odds of adhering to treatment are three times higher for patients who have close, cohesive families.[22]

Social contexts can meaningfully support the development of intrinsic motivation by fostering individuals' sense of autonomy and competence. Social contexts can also hinder intrinsic motivation by exerting control and inhibiting internalization and behavioral integration.[23] Simply dictating to people what they should or should not do is not helpful. Rather, those in the social context can help by motivating the individual's commitment and supporting their sustained efforts, as well as by providing environments in which they can actively practice their behavioral skills.

Social support can sometimes be a two-edged sword. One meta-analysis of smoking cessation and partner support found that when partners provided "reminders" in the form of nagging and criticism, smokers were *more* likely to relapse and begin smoking again.[24] Family conflict has been found to be very problematic; the odds of nonadherence were twice as high among patients in high-conflict families than among those in families with low levels of conflict.[22] Family discord clearly threatens patient adherence, and caution should be used when involving others in any behavior change plan. Considerable thought should be given to the best method of utilizing social support while avoiding potentially destructive aspects of familial involvement.

Several clear recommendations for clinicians can be drawn from this vast literature. First, patients should be asked about the effect of their chronic diseases on their families and social networks, as well as any constraints with which they may be dealing. Second, patients should be asked about the role(s) of their family, if any, in treatment management. Third, clinicians should consider referrals to family counseling if necessary, and be ready with contact information. Of course, having mental health professionals available in the same practice would be ideal and is something we consider in more detail in Chapter 8. Finally, clinicians should help their patients make contact with community resources whenever possible—especially if patients appear not to have supportive family or friends or if they seem lonely. Case Study 7.1 offers two examples of how family and sociocultural context can influence patient adherence.

Case Study 7.1 Frank and Mrs. Tomasetti

Frank: "My girlfriend is against it."

Frank is 61 years old and has been driving for a car service for close to two decades. He likes his job because of all the interesting people he meets. But he knows it's not great to sit for such long periods of time and, as he's gotten older, he finds that his joints are incredibly stiff at the end of a shift. Frank is also overweight and was diagnosed with hypertension two years ago. At that time, he was given a prescription for medication—which he *still* has not filled!

Frank deftly maneuvers to the curb at the busy airport and hoists himself out of the car so that he can open the door for his passenger and stow her small suitcase in the vehicle. Deepa, a physician on her way to give a lecture at a medical conference, leans back against the seat and prepares for what might turn out to be a long ride, given the traffic.

"Oh, you're a doctor," Frank says, hoping for a backseat consultation. "Yeah… I was diagnosed with super high blood pressure about two years ago."

"And how's it been going, managing that?" Deepa asks, tired from her flight but trying to convey empathy and support.

"Great!" Frank responds, "I'm thinking about starting the medicine they gave me, but I want to do a little more research first. My girlfriend said those medicines can hurt you if you're not careful. She's pretty smart, so I usually listen to her. But I'm not so sure anymore; we might break up."

Deepa sighs. She has encountered many patients like Frank.

Analysis

Frank provides us with a good example of the power of social cognitive processing. He is clearly persuaded by important people in his life, although his girlfriend's influence appears to be waning as their relationship weakens. Her hesitancy about the medication did make him wary and he wants to do more research and make a good decision. Many people, including Frank, tend to be hesitant to do things that go against an individual or group with whom they are motivated to comply.

Mrs. Tomasetti: Cultural Factors and Nonadherence

Mrs. Tomasetti is famous—not on the internet or in the music business, but rather from the early days of the field of medical sociology; she was a woman whose noncompliance to behavioral management was enmeshed with her culture.[25] At age 55, Mrs. Tomasetti was overweight and had type 2 diabetes. She faithfully followed her complex regimen of glucose testing and medication, but her diet posed a significant danger to her health. She couldn't (or wouldn't) follow a low-carbohydrate, low-fat diet and her physicians were frustrated with her. A medical student assigned to her care spent some time talking with Mrs. Tomasetti and figured out that her ethnic background (Southern Italian) was of great significance; she valued food highly and believed that being overweight was a sign of health. She and her family enjoyed traditional pasta-based meals; cooking and eating with her family played a central role in her life. Mrs. Tomasetti was a good cook and spent much of her day preparing food for her children and grandchildren; family and friends loved to visit in her kitchen. For her, a restricted diet threatened full and spontaneous involvement in her social network.

Analysis

Eventually, Mrs. Tomasetti's adult children worked with her and her doctors to modify her recipes, reducing their fat content and adding more vegetables and lean meats. They also helped manage her tendency to snack between meals while cooking and visiting. Although her dietary nonadherence was heavily influenced by her cultural background and her strong need for social connection, her behavior was by no means immutable.

As we see in Case Study 7.1, health behavior is unlikely to change if it conflicts with a person's social context. If prescribed dietary recommendations are dramatically different from an individual's cultural norms and family preferences, they are likely to be resisted. This is especially true if important social interactions center around certain foods. Relatedly, in some families there are strong pressures to use natural, herbal remedies that have been relied upon for generations; family members may reject medications prescribed by a doctor. An individual's culture and family history can influence attention to and acceptance of health information, as well as efforts to follow preventive and treatment recommendations.

Culture: a deeper dive

As we saw in Chapter 4, effective communication demands an understanding of culture. Culturally informed healthcare, as detailed below, requires recognizing how culture shapes norms and shared values, and affects health literacy, provider-patient power dynamics, and access to and acceptance of medical treatment. There is a critical need for culturally informed treatment in ethnically diverse and low-income populations, where issues of diversity, equity, and inclusion (DEI) are of particular concern.

In this section, we first examine what we mean by *culture*, a term that refers to a variety of concepts. In the history of medical sociology, "culture" has been understood to consist of a group's adaptations to the social and physical environments that characterize their lives. Culture refers to shared behavioral patterns within groups including, but not limited to, gender, age cohort, ethnicity, religion, or social class. This concept allows us to see differences in behavioral trends between groups, and to see that cultural ideas and activities tend to be communicated from one generation to the next. Individuals are socialized to adhere to cultural norms and shared values, and a practitioner's awareness of the patient's culture can be critical to understanding their response to health and medical advice.[26] Culture offers us a way to view a person's social world and to understand their health and illness behavior. Culture affects basic health-related elements of life such as food preferences and preparation, patterns of eating, and traditional remedies for healing. As we saw in Case Study 7.1 with Mrs. Tomasetti, food restrictions can significantly disrupt cultural group associations.[27]

Nearly 50 years ago, medical sociologists proposed that medicine is a *clinical social science*, and they argued for the relevance of culture to medical treatment.[28] They described the case of a 26-year-old Guatemalan woman who had lived in the United States for ten years but whose cultural beliefs strongly influenced her perceptions of clinical reality, making her behavior confusing and distressing to her physicians and nurses. She was hospitalized and being nourished and hydrated intravenously because severe enteritis prevented her from eating or drinking anything for a time. During her hospital stay, she became emotionally withdrawn, angry, and uncooperative, believing that her medical problem was caused by the witchcraft of her fiancé's sister. She reasoned that by not giving her any food, her physicians had "written her off" as unlikely to live. Further, she believed that she was being prevented from regulating her hot/cold balance of nutrients, which was essential according to her traditional health beliefs and practices. This patient initially told no one about these beliefs because she feared ridicule. When finally encouraged to talk about her conception of her illness, however, she found that her ideas were treated with respect, even though her doctors did not share those beliefs and did not change her treatment. Her hostile attitude and withdrawn, uncooperative behavior ceased when she was reassured that the doctors had not given up on her.

Medical sociologists have also focused attention on socioeconomic status[29] as a cultural factor that can challenge understanding between providers and patients. Differences in their expectations for disease prevention activities may be based upon some very real barriers. Patients of lower socioeconomic class rarely have a private physician of their own as a source of medical care and preventive health education. When they do receive care, they are often considerably sicker than those who have enjoyed regular medical attention. As a result, practitioners might view patients in poverty as unlikely to make health-related behavioral changes or as having delayed care because they are not concerned enough about their health.

Decisions about the use of heroic measures, the institution of long-term treatments, and cost-benefit considerations in the allocation of medical resources tend to be affected by culture and social class,[30] as well. The more similar the patient's social class, cultural values, and interests are to those of the practitioner, the more positive the outcome of care is likely to be.[31] More physically attractive patients are believed to be better patients as well, and providers tend to be more dissatisfied with, and rejecting of, patients who are difficult to manage, assertive, uncooperative, or rebellious. Even in psychotherapy, a patient's perceived similarity to, and liking by, their therapist can be important in preventing drop-out from treatment.[32] Practitioners' decisions regarding psychiatric diagnoses can be influenced by the patient's culture and social class such that lower-class patients are more likely to be judged aberrant in their behaviors.[33] Health professionals' preferences for and expectations about patients can have a profound effect on patients' achievement of healthful outcomes.[33]

Social norms and comparisons

Somewhere between the personal (micro) level and the sociocultural (macro) level, the individual interfaces with groups that are personal, but with somewhat more distant connections. These groups can sometimes be surprisingly influential. Consider the following: "Nobody was wearing masks in the airport so I figured I didn't need to," said 65-year-old Emma. "I didn't want to look like a germaphobe." Several days later Emma tested positive for COVID-19 and, although she had a relatively mild case, she was still miserable for several days and missed an event she'd been looking forward to for weeks.

Health behaviors are often driven by social norms and the desire to "fit in" with how people around us are behaving. Emma didn't want to appear odd or to be the only one wearing a mask. She also figured that if it was important, others would be wearing masks. Unfortunately, other people may not be the best sources of information, and they might also be looking to others, including us, for clues about how to behave.

The field of social psychology offers us a rich body of research on the phenomenon of *conformity*, which occurs when individuals align their behaviors or attitudes with those of the people around them, or with society more generally. Conformity is likely when people aren't sure of the appropriate behavior or attitude to adopt, and they look for guidance and validation, comparing themselves to others and hoping to fit in. Conformity is different from obedience, which involves aligning behaviors or attitudes in response to a directive. Both conformity and obedience characterize some environments, however, and can have a meaningful influence on health behaviors. For example, school programs that are multifaceted (i.e., involve school policy as well as parent and community engagement) can effectively promote a wide range of health-relevant outcomes including better nutrition, physical activity, and sexual health.[34-36] Similarly, church communities not only provide peer groups with shared worldviews to offer social support, they also often prescribe and proscribe health behaviors. For instance, members of both the Church of Jesus Christ of Latter-day Saints and the Seventh-day Adventist Church are directed to avoid alcohol, smoking, and tobacco and are encouraged to eat vegetables, fruits, nuts, and grains. These dietary recommendations, and the socially supported adherence to them, are at least partly responsible for Loma Linda, California's designation as a "Blue

Zone," which is one of the regions of the world where people tend to live significantly longer than average.[37] More than one third of Loma Linda's population is Adventist.

Social comparison processes

Since psychologist Leon Festinger[38] first described his theory of social comparison processes, researchers have been interested in how people's emotions and behaviors are influenced by others. Particular attention has been paid to how different aspects of emotion, goal-setting, and motivation are associated with "upward" and "downward" comparisons. Upward comparisons are those in which a person compares themselves with someone else (either real or hypothetical) who is "above them," or "ahead of them," on a particular dimension. For example, one might compare oneself with someone who is more accomplished at a particular sport, more physically fit, or more successful at sticking to a healthy eating plan. Alternatively, downward comparisons are those in which the person looks to a reference group or person who falls "below" or "behind" them. One might, for example, compare oneself to those who never exercise or are more severely ill with the same disease. Downward comparisons are often linked to more positive emotional states than upward comparisons[39,40] because they tend to make us feel better about ourselves. Our own difficulties can be put into perspective and the things we are thankful for can be highlighted. But downward comparisons tend not to serve as potent motivators because they focus attention on obstacles that have already been surmounted or goals that have already been achieved.[41,42] Downward comparisons can cause us to become complacent about our health behaviors. We might be doing better than other people, even if we are still not doing very well. Upward comparisons can, instead, energize a person to action[41,42] by providing a picture of what "could be." Of course, if there is a wide gap between an individual's current state and the upward comparison point, the person might feel discouraged, especially if they see their own progress falling short of what others seem to have achieved.[43,44]

We cannot really know, of course, how any one individual will react to upward and downward comparisons to their own health behaviors. Various factors, such as the individual's self-esteem and perceived control over situations, can further complicate their emotional responses to any comparison[39] with others. Most studies, though, do find that downward comparisons help to ameliorate negative moods for those with low self-esteem,[45] and that people tend to select upward comparisons, even when these might challenge their self-esteem.[46]

Let's consider an example. Katia is feeling overwhelmed by all the changes she needs to make to get her blood sugar under control. She knows she must change her diet and start exercising, but her knees hurt when she tries to "power-walk," and she easily gets a side-ache and becomes short of breath. Katia has low self-esteem; she feels hopeless to overcome these obstacles to exercise, and she feels bad about herself because of it. At her first meeting of an exercise support group for those with diabetes, Katia met several people who are in worse shape than she is. During the group session, she listened to them talk about their own difficulties with exercise, and she began to feel that there might be some hope for her; she felt that her situation was not as bad as theirs. Her downward comparison improved her mood and allowed her to feel that exercise was something she could indeed do—if she persisted and took it a day at a time.

The role of upward and downward comparisons can be even further complicated by an individual's perceived control. Research shows that positive mood states are less likely to follow comparisons when individuals believe they have little control over their outcomes no matter what they do. If, during her group meeting, Katia had felt she couldn't exert any control over her exercise regimen and was firmly on track toward diabetes complications, she would have been much less likely to experience improved mood. Seeing her situation as less dire than others might have simply been discouraging, with the others representing her own future. Another member of Katia's group, Luis, is similar to Katia health-wise, but he makes an upward comparison. He focuses on a group member who exercises regularly and has achieved a hemoglobin A1c score in the normal range after only a year in the program. Luis feels that he has control over his outcomes, and he is motivated to similarly improve his own blood test results; he finds upward comparison to be invigorating and motivating. If Luis had low perceived control over his own diabetes-related outcomes, however, upward comparison would likely be disheartening rather than inspiring.

Research on social comparison underscores the importance of understanding a person's characteristics before encouraging specific types of comparisons in the adoption of health-related goals. Does the person currently have high self-esteem? Do they believe they have control over their behaviors and their outcomes? Are they optimistic? Easily discouraged? Intrinsically motivated? The answers to these questions are essential if healthcare professionals are to target the social comparisons that will be most effective. Social comparisons do not operate in a vacuum; they function against the backdrop of an individual's already-present tendencies, strengths, and weaknesses within the context of their life.

Social comparisons are also not "snapshots." People usually receive feedback over time about their capabilities relative to others as they strive to achieve their goals. An individual might consistently perform better than, worse than, or the same as their peers. They might then progressively decline in performance or, instead, grow in mastery relative to peers. Feedback about one's performance compared with others is important and can contribute to subsequent goal-setting and self-efficacy. For example, a patient might be told that they are quite physically fit for their age, or conversely that most people their age get more exercise than they do. Not surprisingly, feedback that one is doing well has an empowering effect and tends to be associated with greater self-efficacy, clearer thinking, and setting higher subsequent goals. On the other hand, feedback that suggests one is losing ground or not meeting expectations can accelerate a downward spiral; it can lower the individual's sense of self-efficacy and lead to deteriorating performance.[47]

Katia and Luis enjoy hanging out with another member of their group, Amir; the three of them often compare the number of daily steps they walk. Over time, Katia's trend has been toward poorer management. Even though she is still walking and recording her progress, she is not doing as well as Luis and Amir, and she is becoming less enthusiastic about recording and analyzing her steps. Luis's experience is the opposite. He demonstrates a consistent pattern of improvement that fosters his sense of self-efficacy, encourages him to set higher goals in the future, and increases his chances of future success. Amir's case is perhaps the most illustrative. His step count started quite a bit below the group average, yet his performance pattern demonstrates regular progress at each meeting. Although he may never catch up to Luis, his exercise success also increases his self-efficacy and his future goal-setting and performance.

So, what can be done to help Katia? Does her downward performance pattern doom her to ultimate failure? Not necessarily. An astute group leader might take a little extra time with Katia to offer feedback and help redirect her comparisons. Instead of pointing out how Katia is doing relative to her group's average, she might instead compare her performance to that of another comparison group, such as those in the general population (who, as we saw in Chapter 1, typically don't move very much). Or the group leader might point out that step-count fluctuations are common, and the overall trajectory is most important. This strategy may help increase Katia's self-efficacy and put her back on a more successful path.

Social media

The "lay referral network" is alive and well. It's no longer the lady down the street who works at a hospital laboratory—now it's the "hive mind of the internet," and it's everywhere. Sociologist Talcott Parsons once argued that the need for a lay referral network derived partly from lack of access to medical experts and partly from a lack of trust in them;[48] indeed, people sometimes place greater trust in their communities than in their health professionals. The modern lay referral network has expanded to include websites, blogs, podcasts, and various apps and forums that fall under the umbrella of "social media." This network has influence, for better or worse, on many health and medical choices. People tend to feel empowered by this new and unprecedented access to health information; sometimes, though, they feel overwhelmed. Many cannot distinguish between accurate and untrustworthy sources of health information and may treat misinformation as fact. Personal anecdotes, which many can relate to, often feel more believable (and more accessible) than scientific data and conclusions from empirical studies. Humans are social beings and stories of the experiences of other humans are compelling. But anecdotes are, by definition, idiosyncratic; when compared with aggregate data, they are less likely to represent general truths.

During the COVID-19 pandemic, confusing descriptions of viral transmission, the limited availability of proper masks, changes in leadership, and disorganized and conflicting recommendations for how to remain safe led to a lack of confidence in medical and public health systems (see Case Study 7.2 for an example). Layered on top of this was genuine fear as death tolls rose, hospitals became overwhelmed, and supermarket shelves emptied. Political and public health agendas became intertwined, and polarization was seen across much of the country and the globe. It was against this backdrop that social media gained ascendence; at times there were few consistent messages from trusted sources, and social media filled in the gaps.

Case Study 7.2 Travius

Travius is 22 and works for a pool cleaning and maintenance company. Back in 2021, when the new COVID-19 vaccine was first available, he was asked if he planned to get it. "I'll do my own research first," he said. Like many people, his research consisted of scrolling through social media, clicking on links that were recommended, and reading what his friends sent him. They had a lot to say, including: "Let the government test it on themselves"; "I'm not some kind of guinea pig"; and "They say it's a vaccine, but anyone who's informed knows it's about implanting a tracking device." The response that affected Travius the most was this: "This virus was created, and now they're selling the cure. It's all about money." Travius certainly knew that he should not believe everything he read or heard, so he tried to be sure that the websites he visited were trustworthy, or at least that he personally trusted them. He was *not* sure that the government recommendations were reliable; his trust in them was shaken when different government officials contradicted each other. Even doctors didn't seem to agree, and he did not know which ones to trust.

The more Travius tried to learn, the more confused he became. Finally, he did find someone who spoke in a way that made sense to him. This individual, who claimed to have a healthcare background, explained things in ways that were clear and engaging. He followed this individual's YouTube channel and after a while felt that he had a pretty good handle on what was going on with COVID-19. Unfortunately, he also decided that he didn't need a vaccine and would be putting himself at substantial risk if he got one. Health recommendations from the experts did not seem credible to him, and they went against what most of his friends were saying. As Dr. Peter Hotez explains in his book *The Deadly Rise of Anti-Science*, public health recommendations are likely to fail if they conflict with the person's social context.[49] They clearly failed with Travius.

The case study (7.2) of Travius reminds us that at every level, health information needs to be transmitted in ways that people can understand and remember. This information should not be conflicting or confusing for them. Information may tend to be rejected if it is *dictated* by authorities, but accepted if it is "networked by peers" in family and cultural systems and in social media.[50] Medical decision-making is a complicated process which requires, at its foundation, an acceptance of scientific evidence that might not be easy to understand. As we discussed in Chapter 4, effect sizes, risks, and probabilities would ideally be understood and effectively communicated in order for individuals to comprehend risk. But these concepts tend to be much more complex and nuanced than what is often communicated to the public about medical decisions. In the absence of technical understanding, a trusting relationship with someone who *does* understand these things is key. Medical professionals are such people. In surveys, patients list their physicians as their most highly trusted information source; nearly half say they would prefer to first go to their physician for specific health information.

What people say they want to do, however, tends not to be what they actually do. For a variety of reasons, nearly half go online first, instead of to their physician; only about 10% actually go to their physician first.[51] In fact, the internet is the most common source of initial health information.[52] Most people believe what they read on the internet, and those with worse health are more likely than healthier people to seek health information there.[53] Internet information also tends to prompt patients to argue with their physicians and insist on treatments that may not be indicated; some even embark on internet-guided treatments themselves. Fortunately, sicker patients are more likely to talk with their doctors about what they find online, and many use online searches to supplement their knowledge and help them to develop a list of questions for discussion in their medical visits.

On the internet, individuals can access a wide range of informational sources, all differing in quality and reliability.[54] People tend to display aversion to ambiguity;[55,56] put simply, they do not like uncertainty. When presented with conflicting informational sources, people tend to lose trust in the information altogether and place greater weight on their own prior subjective beliefs.[57] The larger the disparity across sources, the less they trust external information and the more they rely on their own personal evaluation of the situation.

This happened during the COVID-19 pandemic, where ambiguity and contradictory information drove people to rely more heavily on their own beliefs and those of people they trusted (many of whom were not experts). Generally, informational campaigns—such as those created by governments and by nonprofit and professional organizations—attempt to build on verifiable information in order to highlight potential health risks and reshape individuals' health beliefs. Informational ambiguity has the opposite effect, however; it reinforces the individual's prior beliefs and reduces trust and attentiveness to the available information. This would not be problematic if people tended to have accurate prior beliefs about health risks. Research consistently shows, however, that most individuals underestimate risks to their health. This phenomenon is termed "optimistic bias."[58,59]

While there are many positive aspects of social media, such as opportunities for connection to family members, friends, and communities, there are problematic aspects as well. In addition to the potential for health misinformation, social media use is associated with greater anxiety, depression, and emotional distress;[60,61] and cutting back on social media leads to better self-esteem in young people.[62,63]

As we have noted (especially in Chapter 3), perhaps the single best thing that clinicians can do to help their patients protect their health is to develop strong relationships with them. In the context of trusting partnerships, many aspects of health behavior change and treatment adherence can become easier. When patients need to make medical decisions, their clinicians can work through a structured decision-making process with them at the office (or provide assistance so that they can work on it on their own). Healthcare providers can offer guidance to patients as they navigate the process of "doing their own research" on the internet. If patients can be guided to sources that contain accurate information, their research will be much more useful to them. Patients should also be encouraged to share their findings and related questions with their doctors, nurses, PAs, pharmacists, and other health professionals so that clarity is ensured, and any misinformation can be identified and corrected. Finally, the risks associated with spending too much time on social media should be frankly discussed. Health professionals can do much to ensure that their patients navigate the internet and engage with social media in ways that are productive and safe.

In the next section of this chapter, we examine how health professionals also have perspectives, beliefs, and even hesitations that can play out in the medical encounter. Let us take the example of vaccinations—a topic about which there is a great deal of data and opinion.

Health professionals and vaccination-related decisions

Immunization is one of the most effective methods for dealing with many infectious diseases, although vaccine uptake is variable across vaccine types. In the United States, most children receive recommended vaccinations.[64,65]

However, many adults—including healthcare workers—opt out of seasonal influenza shots. Substantial numbers of individuals, especially adults under 30, are uncertain about the effectiveness[66] of vaccines, and vaccination rates are on the decline in some parts of the world.[67,68] This vaccine hesitancy is partly due to beliefs that vaccines are ineffective or unnecessary.[69,70] These views are not uncommon; for example, one study found that less than 58% of sampled adults recognized the importance of vaccinations.[71] But even when their protective benefit *is* recognized, concerns over risks often remain.[66,70,72] Interventions aimed at increasing vaccine uptake usually focus on enhancing knowledge about them, but are often ineffective and occasionally counterproductive.[73,74] While people's objective knowledge often improves as a result of these interventions (e.g., they might concede that vaccines do not cause autism), their attitudes and intentions often remain unchanged. We also know that social processes (e.g., social norms) can meaningfully influence the behavior of individuals; it is less clear, however, that interventions in the form of normative messages can actually improve vaccine acceptance.

Individuals' acceptance of vaccinations depends partly on their health professionals and the provider-patient relationship. Poor medical communication, for example, has been linked to decreased vaccination uptake.[75] The strength of the provider's recommendations, and the knowledge base and attitudes of healthcare professionals, have been found to play key roles in vaccine acceptance and hesitancy.[76,77] Although health professionals hold demonstrably more positive attitudes toward vaccines than does the general public, not all members of the healthcare team may be uniformly positive about vaccinations.[78–81] Because personal knowledge, attitudes, and beliefs can influence medical communications, these differences may affect the degree to which a cohesive message is conveyed to patients.[77,82] Although messages from their healthcare providers are likely to be meaningful to patients, achieving a shared perspective with their healthcare professional may be particularly important when more vaccinations are required (e.g., for elderly patients).

Messaging regarding vaccinations may vary across vaccine type and patient type. For example, parents of young children may be consistently informed of the importance of the Measles-Mumps-Rubella (MMR) vaccine. Discussions about Human Papillomavirus (HPV) immunization, however, may be less frequently initiated with parents of older children, perhaps because HPV is transmitted through sexual contact, and clinicians anticipate more "pushback" related to morality norms and expectations for teenagers. The provider's role may affect the frequency and nature of vaccine-related discussions. While physicians are typically seen as the primary medical authority, they may not have time to undertake detailed discussions about vaccine importance and vaccine safety. Other members of the healthcare team (e.g., nurses, nurse practitioners, physicians' assistants) often have more patient contact time and may be viewed as more approachable,[83] thus making them particularly vital to the building of vaccine confidence. Each member of the team, of course, brings to the medical encounter a set of personal beliefs, experiences, and behaviors that may influence the way they discuss and encourage patient immunization.

Not all vaccines are deemed equally valuable by providers. Research shows that when thinking of a hypothetical 67-year-old patient, 89% of physicians rated the influenza vaccine as "very important" and 80% rated the pneumococcal pneumonia vaccine as "very important" but only 63% gave that same rating to the Tetanus-Diphtheria-Pertussis (Tdap) vaccine.[78] This same study revealed that 29% of physicians found the vaccination schedule from the Advisory Committee on Immunization Practices confusing. Another study[84] found that primary care physicians sometimes did not understand the guidelines for administering certain vaccines and were more likely to administer the HPV vaccine if they had a good understanding of the guidelines. It was more difficult for them to make recommendations if their own knowledge was lacking. This study highlights that failures of communication can occur for providers not only with their own patients, but also with vaccine experts they depend upon to inform and guide their clinical practice.

A clinician's understanding of guidelines and vaccine schedules is not the only factor influencing their vaccination approach with patients. Physicians in one study were less likely to recommend the pneumococcal conjugate vaccine (PCV7) against pneumonia if they believed the patient could not afford it; they varied their recommendations based on state funding levels for the vaccine and the insurance status of the patient.[85] Physicians are also influenced by patient preferences. In one study, 80% of surveyed physicians believed patients would leave their practice if they pushed for vaccinations the patient did not want; 87% believed, however, that failing to administer vaccines would place families at risk.[86] Many physicians are in a difficult position, trying to maintain a trusting relationship with their patients while doing what is best for them.

Physicians are not the only influential members of the patient's social context in medical settings. Nurses directly administer vaccinations and can have a significant influence on patients' vaccination decisions.[87] Research shows that nurses' own vaccination records and perspectives on vaccines play an important role in their ability to effectively advocate for vaccinations. Indeed, not all nurses are positive about vaccinations;[88,89] their primary reasons for refusal involve concern about possible vaccine-associated side effects.[90-92] The more nurses know about vaccines, however, the more they accept vaccines themselves and present them positively to patients. Pharmacists can also play a key role in improving vaccine uptake. Whether they are acting as immunizers, advocates, or both, pharmacists' involvement is associated with better immunization rates.[93] These examples illustrate the importance of each member of the healthcare team, and of having team members deliver consistent messages to patients.

Although we have been focusing here on what happens in medical encounters (which might be viewed as a micro- or meso-level issue), these encounters are embedded in a larger sociocultural structure that includes a good deal of history and culture. Let us turn our attention to some of these overarching issues now.

Disparities and the death gap

Between 1997 and 2014 in the United States, there was a significant socioeconomic status gradient in life expectancy; regardless of sex and race/ethnicity, those who were poor and less educated lived substantially shorter lives.[94] This trend has continued and even accelerated in the years since then.[95]

It is not surprising that economic inequities translate into health disparities. Even with health insurance, many low-income workers delay medical care or avoid purchasing prescription medications because the copayments and deductibles remain financially prohibitive. Getting the car repaired so that one can get to work and earn an essential paycheck may take precedence when money is tight. Socioeconomic status impacts health behavior, healthcare, and environmental exposure, and the stress associated with inadequate resources can affect bodily systems (e.g., cardiovascular, immunologic) and cognitive processing.[96,97]

This gap is not just socioeconomic, it is also racial. These factors certainly overlap, but when socioeconomic variables are statistically controlled,

20–30% of the Black-White difference in life expectancy remains.[98] This may be partly explained by the "cardiovascular conundrum" described by Julian Thayer and colleagues. African Americans have greater heart rate variability and greater total peripheral blood vessel resistance, conditions that are linked to anger inhibition and emotion dampening in response to repeated instances of unfair treatment. Resultant higher rates of hypertension and cardiovascular disease are logical precursors to this life expectancy difference.[99] These researchers note that the same psychophysiological pathways may also be relevant to other groups who receive unfair treatment.

Research on issues of DEI show us that even medical encounters are not free from systematic biases and disparities; these macro-level elements are insidiously integrated into attitudes and beliefs, and regularly filter into dyadic interactions as can be seen in Case Study 7.3.

Case Study 7.3 Racial Bias and Pain Communication

Sapphire is 28 years old, and African American; she works as a certified nursing assistant in an assisted living facility. Sapphire loves her job, and she loves helping her patients. Unfortunately, she recently hurt her back trying to support an older patient with dementia who became dizzy and almost fell while getting out of bed.

Sapphire's access to medical care has been sporadic. She has insurance right now, although the co-payments are prohibitive; because of this, she tried for some time to get along without a medical visit for her back pain. But, after several months, she was still in too much pain to enjoy spending time with her family and friends. She could not exercise at all and had given up singing in her church choir and volunteering at the food bank.

So, Sapphire finally made an appointment with a primary care physician in her insurance panel. Dr. Sapolsky, an older gentleman, quizzed Sapphire about her health habits. She reported that she had no other health problems; she had never smoked, never drank alcohol, used no drugs, and tried to eat at least five servings of fruits and vegetables each day. Sapphire was of normal weight, and when her back didn't hurt she got plenty of exercise walking and hiking (and helping to move patients!).

> Dr. Sapolsky ordered an x-ray of her back, and had Sapphire go to the lab for some blood tests and a urinalysis. She returned the next day for the results and was disappointed by Dr. Sapolsky's response to her. He told her that the tests were all normal, and that the pain would likely go away soon. He seemed uninterested in her experience of pain, and when Sapphire told him that over-the-counter pain relievers were not helping with the pain, Dr. Sapolsky became defensive. He immediately told her that he would not prescribe anything stronger because of the potential for addiction; Sapphire felt like he was implying that she might abuse the medication. Although pain is the most common symptom presented to primary care physicians, Dr. Sapolsky appeared to know very little about pain management and had nothing to offer her. Worse, he doubted her experience of the pain, and offered no support or empathy in caring for her.

Racism, discrimination, and disparities in medical care

Medicine is not well-equipped to deal with pain that lasts. The pain of surgery or medical procedures can be banished with anesthesia and pain-killing drugs but when pain becomes entrenched, such as chronic low back pain following an injury, many physicians have no good answers; studies have identified multiple knowledge and practice gaps.[100-102] Inadequate management of pain is difficult for patients and doctors, who often have very limited time together. Miscommunications are common around the issue of pain, and are made worse by expectations and false beliefs about biological differences between racial and ethnic groups. The work of Hoffman and colleagues in 2016[103] provides a particularly good example. In this study, approximately half of White medical students and residents endorsed inaccurate "facts" about biological differences between Black and White people (e.g., that Black people have less sensitive nerve endings, that their blood coagulates more quickly, that they have thicker skin). Furthermore, those who held these beliefs rated Black patients' pain as less severe than that of White patients and made less accurate recommendations for the treatment of their pain. These findings help to explain the well-documented reality[104] of racial bias in pain assessment and treatment. Similar, inaccurate beliefs may contribute to other pain-assessment and treatment disparities—in particular, for women[105] and older people.[106]

Seeming insensitivity to patients' pain may have many sources, not the least of which might be lack of empathy. Some physicians simply cannot understand their patients' nonverbal cues of distress, and some have difficulty understanding the meaning behind patients' descriptions of their experience. Patients are likely to appear distressed, anxious, frustrated, and even somewhat angry both at being in pain and at their physician's dismissal of their concerns. In response, physicians might become defensive because they feel their patients want something from them, such as medications that the opioid crisis taught us can be dangerous, and which can be quite limited in their ability to effectively treat chronic pain.[107,108]

Consider for a moment that patients in pain might want something more than a prescription from their medical providers. Pain relief is greatly desired, of course, but patients are very likely also to benefit from simply being heard, understood, supported, and helped to problem-solve their pain challenges. The failure to offer empathy and understanding to patients is a truly tragic element of chronic pain management. The opioid crisis, where so many patients were given addictive drugs that did not effectively treat their chronic pain, was as much a failure of empathy and physician training as anything else. Many physicians did not have the tools, the knowledge, or the time to help their patients with chronic pain.[109]

Although we have focused our analysis on the assessment and management of pain, there exist many areas of healthcare in which racial and ethnic disparities can be found. Machine learning analyses of electronic health records (EHRs) showed that the EHRs of Black patients had 2.5 times the odds of containing at least one negative descriptor.[110] The authors of this study cautioned that such negative descriptors can perpetuate racial disparities in healthcare. Another especially profound area of difference between Blacks and Whites is that of maternal mortality rates, which are two to three times higher for Black mothers than for non-Hispanic White mothers.[111,112] In 2020, there were 19.1 deaths per 100,000 live births in non-Hispanic White women, contrasted with 55.3 for non-Hispanic Black women.[113] Some of this difference is due to preexisting morbidities, but another element involves implicit racial bias on the part of providers.[114] Patients' perceptions of discrimination[112] can compromise the provider-patient relationship and place the patient at risk in everything that occurs within the context of that relationship.

How can we reduce the implicit biases that are revealed in EHRs? How can we shift the narrative of discrimination against pregnant women of color to one of engagement and trust? Dr. Arghavan Salles and colleagues urge non-Black healthcare providers to take direct action including reviewing and revising existing institutional policies, advocating for transparency and professional development, and committing to recognizing race as a social construct.[115] When interacting with patients, there needs to be an emphasis on communication that embodies respect and compassion. Effective patient-provider communication has been shown to have a positive effect on pregnant African Americans' satisfaction with prenatal care and trust in their provider[116] and it should be the foundation of each medical interaction. Over time, these human connections may help to mend the fractures in medical trust.

A cultural distrust of medicine

The medical establishment has not always treated African Americans ethically. One of the most blatant examples of mistreatment is the U.S. Public Health Service's study of the natural history of syphilis at the Tuskegee Institute. It ran for four decades, ostensibly treating nearly 400 African American men who had syphilis but, in reality, merely tracking the progression of their disease.[117] These men did not consent to this "treatment"—they were lied to and used by the medical establishment and the U.S. government. Is it any wonder that many in the African American community are still wary of what they are told by medical professionals? Confidence has been eroded; and educational programs and health interventions targeting African Americans still suffer from this loss of trust.[118]

Trust is relevant at many levels, from the relationship between the patient and health professional to the broader system including the medical profession, public health, and even science itself. Distrust at any of these levels can foster intentional nonadherence. Even when there has been no overtly unethical action (such as communities of color have experienced), some patients might feel that healthcare providers do too many procedures and prescribe too many drugs. Research does confirm that some medical interventions have questionable utility and limited benefit, as well as being costly.[119-121] This may be particularly true in some geographic areas and for certain treatments.[122,123] This well-known problem is one of several possible drivers of patients' resistance to medical recommendations. Because they do not have the expertise to determine which treatments might be beneficial and which might be unnecessary or harmful, however, patients and those who socially influence them may overgeneralize and reject medical recommendations that would have been both safe and effective.

Relatedly, some accepted medical truths have been reversed (e.g., public health directives during the COVID-19 pandemic, and recent research showing that opioid medications do little to relieve chronic back pain). Awareness of such changes can leave some patients feeling skeptical of all medical advances and medical advice.[122] Their confidence in the validity of medical recommendations is challenged.

All these instances demonstrate just how fragile trust can be, and how easily a culture of distrust can develop. We are regularly inundated with information—scientific, conspiracy-oriented, politically slanted, anecdotal, and economically driven. It can be hard to sort it all out.

Unquestioning confidence in modern medicine is obviously unwarranted; adverse effects of medical treatment (AEMTs) do occur, including nosocomial infections, allergic reactions to and serious side effects of drugs, and mistakes such as incorrect medication dosing. Tragically, AEMTs account for as many as 5,200 deaths each year. While this number is less than that offered in the press (which often reports, incorrectly, that medical mistakes are the third leading cause of death in the United States), it is clear that ideally *none* of these events and errors would occur. Patients should be able to count on their medical care delivery being safe, and AEMTs can erode trust and undermine patients' acceptance of medical recommendations and their commitment to adhere to them. Several lines of evidence suggest that AEMTs have recently been decreasing modestly, and that many health systems are making concerted efforts to reduce these as much as possible and gain patients' trust in their healthcare.[124]

Trauma, stress, and health vulnerabilities

As we have seen so far in this chapter, the sociocultural context of an individual's life—their family, friends, social support networks, and cultural norms—can help to promote and maintain their efforts to achieve health. Of course, this context can also hinder their health behavior change and treatment adherence. Social media friends might argue against vaccinations;

cultural practices might directly conflict with prescribed treatments. As we saw earlier, the awareness and management of sociocultural factors by astute and sensitive health professionals can facilitate the positive use of this context and can mitigate its negative effects.

Racial, ethnic, and socioeconomic disparities are major determinants of health and health behavior, and are influenced by disadvantaged environments and the differential effects of exposure to environmental health risk. The increasingly recognized vulnerabilities of chronic stress, mental health challenges, and trauma are drivers of health through behavior change and treatment adherence. Many traumatic events and experiences can have long term effects on health, preventive health behaviors, and acceptance of medical treatment.[125] These include a broad array of elements such as childhood trauma and neglect, domestic and neighborhood violence, immigration-related trauma, dislocation, poverty, food insecurity, and intergenerational trauma.[126,127]

Chronic environmental stresses such as unsafe neighborhoods, as well as natural and weather-related disasters, can increase displacement and isolation and affect mental health. Climate change affects health directly (e.g., air pollution, water contaminations, and food availability), and causes disruptions and dislocations (individual and community) due to extreme weather events, fires, and floods. These can interfere with personal health management and treatment adherence; significant disparities exist in these effects as well. Record breaking hot and cold temperatures are not experienced in the same way by everyone, even those living and working in the same small geographic area. Heat deaths due to climate change, for example, are more numerous in communities of color and for those in poverty. Individuals who cannot stay indoors with heat or air conditioning, or whose jobs require heavy labor outdoors, are most affected. There are significant income disparities in the health effects of climate change. "When people die of heat, they are actually dying of poverty."[128]

Stress and traumatic experience can affect health and health behavior in several ways, most obviously *directly*. Traumatic experiences can cause stress-related diseases such as cardiovascular disease and diabetes, via well-understood physiological pathways.[129] Furthermore, stressful and traumatic events are more numerous and problematic for vulnerable individuals, causing persistent damage manifesting in chronic illness and faster aging. In these populations, the opportunities for mitigating unremitting stresses are considerably fewer, as individuals contend with stressful environments.[129]

Struggling against inequality, especially in the context of past and ongoing traumatic events, wears down bodily systems. Just coping requires exceptional effort. In her model of "weathering" (as in weathering a storm), University of Michigan professor of public health Arline Geronimus studied not only individuals of color and the urban poor, but also other marginalized communities including immigrants, LGBTQIA individuals, and those living in rural poverty, such as in Appalachia.[130] She found that "weathering" can be an almost constant task in marginalized groups, and the body is affected through cortisol and glucose metabolism, leading to obesity, cardiovascular disease, high levels of inflammation, preterm births, poorer immune functioning, and higher rates of death from cancer. Dysregulated cortisol is also tied to depression, anxiety, poor sleep, premature aging, and early death.[130] These ideas are consistent with the health effects associated with the "cardiovascular conundrum" described earlier in this chapter.

Misguided attempts to cope with trauma and stress can promote the adoption of health risk behaviors. Lifelong unhealthy behavior patterns and habits (e.g., overeating, smoking, alcohol use) might understandably be used to mitigate and manage negative emotions in the face of stress and trauma. Individuals with a history of childhood sexual abuse, for example, are at an increased risk for a range of adverse outcomes, including greater engagement in risky behaviors.[131-133] Looking at the big picture, of course, we have seen that in vulnerable communities, health risks are made considerably worse by the easy availability of tobacco, alcohol, and junk foods, and the challenges in accessing environments that support health. Walking, to be healthier or to cope better with stress, requires a safe and navigable neighborhood; steaming vegetables for dinner requires that one can purchase the vegetables, and have the time and opportunity to steam them. For many people, those very basic requirements are not met.

Stress and traumatic experiences can also affect health behavior change and treatment adherence by limiting information processing and interfering with the attention, focus, and recall necessary to motivate and support the planning and execution of behavior change. Long-term stress can make the habits of self-management and maintenance much more difficult. Past trauma or severe stress can also affect treatment adherence in other ways. Fear of needles, embarrassment with physical examinations, and claustrophobia in scanning machines, for example, can drive resistance to screening and diagnostic tests. Recollections of traumatic medical experiences from childhood can later influence adult tolerance of treatments that are uncomfortable.

Stress and trauma can also affect health behavior and adherence by increasing an individual's vulnerability to depression with its attendant passivity, disengagement, hopelessness, loss of personal agency, and diminished investment in the future. Meta-analytic research shows that adherence is diminished by as much as 27% when medical patients have untreated depression.[134,135] Up to 40% of chronically ill medical patients are depressed, and individuals of color and those in poverty are at greatest risk. Chronic illness and depression can trigger social isolation and derail the social support needed for following treatment regimens, jeopardizing health outcomes and threatening quality of life.[136-138] Case Study 7.4 illustrates some of these issues with a patient who rejects potentially valuable treatment.

Case Study 7.4 Cassandra

Cassandra is 52 years old and has suffered from Crohn's disease for nearly a decade. Although her immune system is attacking her healthy tissues, she has conscientiously managed a variety of oral medications that have been helpful. These include immunosuppressant and anti-inflammatory drugs, antibiotics, steroids, and, when needed, painkillers. She has also followed a restricted diet, eliminating dairy, gluten, and sugar. Now, however, all these approaches have become less effective. She needs something more.

Cassandra's doctor is excited to offer her a new option for treatment with a "biologic" medication. Administration of the treatment requires Cassandra to either go to the hospital infusion center to receive an intravenous infusion or take under-the-skin injections at home. Right away, Cassandra realizes that this will be very hard for her. She hates needles, and the idea of being connected to an IV bag with a needle in her arm, or injecting liquid into the fat on her abdomen or her hip, is almost too much to imagine.

During the medical visit, Cassandra remains poised and expresses gratitude to her doctor for finding another treatment option; she says that she will follow up on the prescription. But weeks go by, and Cassandra keeps erasing the emails and texts asking her to set up an appointment for treatment. She pretty much knows that she will never be able to take the regular injections, or even make it past the front door of the infusion center without having a panic attack. Unfortunately, she does not tell her doctor about her difficulties with needles. There are acceptable alternatives for administration such as special injection cartridges, but she never brings up the need for such accommodation, and her Crohn's disease continues to get worse, increasingly interfering with her life.

Cassandra grew up in poverty. Like many in her neighborhood, she and her family did not have access to good healthcare, and when she had streptococcus throat infections as a young child, she rarely got proper antibiotic treatment. Consequently, she developed rheumatic fever and was hospitalized at age 7. These days, children are usually cared for in children's hospitals or in special pediatric care units that try to reduce the stress of hospitalization. Care is taken to help children deal with their fears, and the environment is made as stress-free as possible. Cassandra was sent to the general hospital, however, and it was very scary. She was administered injections without adequate preparation, and her usual caregivers, primarily her mother and grandmother, were working and caring for her siblings; they could not stay at the hospital to comfort her. In the context of the many challenges of poverty and the disruptions of being ill, Cassandra became fearful of hospitals and indeed all medical delivery settings.

As an adult, she is particularly fearful of needles. Some years, she avoids getting the flu shot, and when she must have a blood test, she loses sleep the night before her appointment at the lab. Feeling scared and helpless, she often postpones the test; sometimes she arrives only to leave again before her turn is called. Cassandra's fear of needles, *trypanophobia*, is not uncommon. It can result from stressful or traumatic childhood experiences with needles and involves intense anxiety at the sight or thought of a medical procedure involving a needle.[139,140] Like many, Cassandra's reaction to the thought of going for an intravenous infusion, where she will be awake and aware of everything including the needle going into her arm, is so severe it leads her to a panic attack. Cassandra already knows she will experience dizziness and a racing heartbeat, and she might faint.

Chronic psychological stress, such as that in Cassandra's life, is also a culprit in the development and exacerbation of Crohn's and other forms of inflammatory bowel disease. Psychosocial stress models, animal analog studies, and longitudinal research all suggest that a vicious cycle can develop, where stress itself makes Crohn's disease worse, and the stress of treatment leads to its avoidance and the eventual exacerbation of the condition. Patients with Crohn's and related inflammatory bowel conditions also have a higher risk of developing symptoms of anxiety and depression compared with healthy individuals.[125] Although the precise mechanisms remain unclear, stress, anxiety, and depression are both causes and consequences of Crohn's disease progression and relapse.[125]

What health professionals can do

Health professionals can provide better care when they understand their patients' sociocultural context. This includes exploring the unique vulnerabilities that patients might face individually and in their social and cultural groups. Health professionals' awareness of stress, trauma, and mental health vulnerabilities such as anxiety and depression can be essential to the management of health behavior change and treatment adherence. Studies show, however, that few physicians take the time to ask. In one study, only 6% of a group of medical patients who (as assessed by pre-visit questionnaires) *actually were depressed* were asked anything about their emotional experience by their doctors.[141] This study analyzed audio-tape recordings of hundreds of primary care medical visits. By coding who said what to whom, this research found surprising evidence that primary care doctors avoided discussing emotional health with their patients, despite its importance for medical treatment outcomes.

One simple approach for a clinician to address the role of emotional challenges is to include in their conversation with their patient a two-item adult depression screening "questionnaire" (the Patient Health Questionnaire; PHQ-2).[142] These are the questions: "Over the past two weeks, have you felt down, depressed, or hopeless?" and "Over the past two weeks, have you felt little interest or pleasure in doing things?" These questions can open the conversation and establish a path for treatment and referral.

Providers, practicing in an already strained healthcare system, wonder what they can do with the limited time they have with their patients. Paying attention and talking with the patient may be the most important actions the provider can take. A chronic disease diagnosis can bring a sense of loss and grieving; the patient should not have to bear that alone. Attention, empathy, and encouragement of social support networks can help the patient toward acceptance and effective chronic disease management.

The centrality of mental healthcare is described in more detail in Chapter 8, where we consider models for integrating this important aspect into primary care medicine. Facilitating mental health referrals to effective treatments for stress and trauma are critical to care; these include Cognitive Behavior Therapy (CBT),[143] Acceptance and Commitment Therapy (ACT),[144] Eye Movement Desensitization and Reprocessing (EMDR) Therapy,[145] and clinical hypnosis.[139] These treatment modalities can be very valuable in mitigating the effects of stress and trauma on medical outcomes.

Culturally informed medical care and communication

As we saw earlier in this chapter, culture is multifaceted, including values, norms, beliefs, habits, history, and behaviors passed from generation to generation. Culture is linked to social structures such as religious groups, to racial/ethnic identity, and to geographic origins. Culture can often be identified through foods, language, and music, although it is much more than just these outward manifestations. Finally, culture is dynamic, with some aspects changing over time and others maintained and transmitted. As such, each individual's culture influences them, and combines with their personal experiences in unique ways.[146]

Culturally informed medical care acknowledges that cultural factors influence the delivery of healthcare. Addressing cultural factors helps to minimize discrimination and disparities in care. Training in this area aims for "cultural competency" and typically includes strategies for treating patients from various cultural backgrounds. In some cases, clinicians are encouraged to closely examine and reflect on the ways that their own cultural backgrounds affect their interactions with patients. This training has been shown to increase awareness of personal blind spots[147] and recognition that reducing bias is a lifelong task. Such blind spots and biases can be rooted in the healthcare provider's own cultural experience, including in the culture of medicine itself, where some views can be so firmly entrenched that group members no longer notice them.[148]

Culturally informed medical care is an important part of patient-centered care models, which are examined in detail in Chapter 8. These models describe team-based care that is compassionate and well-coordinated, and engages patients[149] while emphasizing health professional-patient relationships that are critical to the cultivation of trust in medical recommendations. These healthcare models offer much of what we have been describing in this chapter, and indeed throughout this book. A large body of research supports patient-centered care and contributes to trust and to better patient outcomes.[150-152]

Culturally informed care can also guide medical communication more broadly. Individuals' health-related choices are sometimes partly due to their misunderstanding of guidelines that would support their health outcomes. Scientific communications may be unintentionally vague and confusing, particularly within the sociocultural context of the individuals that these communications hope to reach. The National Academy of Sciences, in 2017, critiqued this "deficit model" of scientific communication, advocating for the central role of the first element of the information-motivation-strategy model—effective communication and understanding.[153] As we have seen throughout this book, of course, people sometimes do understand but fail to agree with, or be motivated to act upon, scientific findings. There is a clear need to incorporate what we know about culture, health literacy, psychology, and history into the communication of scientific findings[154] because information is filtered through sociocultural experience, and it is understood and acted upon in a sociocultural context.

Summary

In Chapter 7, we consider the many aspects of an individual's social-ecological context that can drive health behavior and treatment adherence. This context includes their social network expectations, friendship and family norms and supports, and cultural habits; it can significantly influence their commitment to health promotion and disease prevention activities. In this chapter, we examine how family and friends can support the long-term maintenance and management of chronic disease treatments, and consider ways in which a social network can support rejection of a treatment strategy or interfere with it by placing barriers in the patient's path. We examine how online access can open up a world of medical knowledge to patients or can unduly influence them with misinformation. In this chapter, we also address the social determinants of wellness, and the interpersonal and intrapersonal factors affecting adherence and health behavior change. We focus significant attention on the role of social media, which can be a driver of health decisions, for good or bad, and serve as a source of resistance to care and even a potential threat to mental health. We examine social, racial, ethnic, and economic inequalities/disparities in health, healthcare, health threats, and environmental risk in vulnerable populations. We consider the value of culturally informed medical care and the increasing recognition of vulnerabilities including mental health challenges and trauma as drivers of health and health behaviors.

Tools for instruction and self-study

Learning objectives

By the end of this chapter, readers should be able to

1. Explain the concept of social determinants of health.
2. Summarize how family and culture influence health behavior and adherence.
3. Demonstrate how social comparison and social norms influence health behavior.
4. Discuss how social media and the internet can affect people's access to health information and choices.
5. Explain how vaccination decisions are related to social factors, including physician-patient communication.
6. Discuss the mechanisms by which stress and trauma affect health behavior change and adherence.
7. Discuss disparities in health and healthcare, and how health professionals can address these through communication in the care setting.

Review questions

1. What is likely the earliest contributor to, and shaper of, health behaviors?
2. What are the three ways that family influence can be leveraged to improve health? Provide one example of each.
3. What are the three categories (forms) of social support? Provide a brief description and example of each.

4. Compare and contrast upward and downward comparisons. For what is each best suited, in a health context?
5. What is meant by the term "socioeconomic status gradient" or "SES gradient"?
6. What is a "lay referral network"? How is today's lay referral network different from that of 50 years ago?
7. What does Geronimus mean by the term "weathering"?
8. What does Thayer mean by the term "cardiovascular conundrum"?
9. How can stress and trauma, broadly defined, affect health behavior change and treatment adherence?

Prompts for discussion and further study

1. Can implicit biases be unlearned? If not, why not? If so, what might be the best approach(es) for doing this?
2. Have you ever been in less-than-complete agreement with a healthcare provider? If so, what did you do? Why did you react in this way? What do you believe were the consequences of your response?
3. As a health professional, how would you approach conversations with your patients about issues of stress, trauma, and mental health?

Suggested reading

1. Perry BD, Winfrey O. *What Happened to You? Conversations on Trauma, Resilience, and Healing.* Macmillan; 2021.
2. Villarosa L. *Under the Skin: The Hidden Toll of Racism on American Lives* (Pulitzer Prize Finalist). Anchor; 2022.
3. Mullan J. *Decolonizing Therapy: Oppression, Historical Trauma, and Politicizing your Practice.* Norton; 2023.
4. Trzeciak S, Mazzarelli A, Booker C. *Compassionomics: The Revolutionary Scientific Evidence that Caring Makes a Difference.* Studer Group, 2019.
5. Fadiman, A. *The Spirit Catches You and You Fall Down: A Hmong Child, Her American Doctors, and the Collision of Two Cultures.* Farrar, Straus, & Giroux; 2012.

References

1. Pavlov I. *Conditioned Reflexes: An Investigation of the Physiological Activity of the Cerebral Cortex*. London: Oxford University Press; 1927.
2. Bandura A. *Principles of Behavior Modification*. New York: Holt, Rinehart, & Winston; 1969.
3. Edwards N. The theory of decision making. *Psychol Bull*. 1954; 51: pp. 380–417.
4. Mittelmark MB. The psychology of social influence and healthy public policy. *Prev Med*. 1999; 29(6 Pt 2): pp. S24–S29. doi: 10.1006/pmed.1998.0468
5. Whitehead D. A social cognitive model for health education/health promotion practice. *J Adv Nurs*. 2001; 36(3): pp. 417–425. doi: 10.1046/j.1365-2648.2001.01973.x
6. Wallston KA, Strudler Wallston B, DeVellis R. Development of the Multidimensional Health Locus of Control (MHLC) Scales. *Health Educ Monogr*. 1978; 6(1): pp. 160–170. doi: 10.1177/109019817800600107
7. Shah J. Automatic for the people: how representations of significant others implicitly affect goal pursuit. *J Pers Soc Psychol*. 2003; 84(4): pp. 661–681. doi: 10.1037/0022-3514.84.4.661
8. Spear HJ, Kulbok PA. Adolescent health behaviors and related factors: a review. *Public Health Nurs*. 2001; 18(2): pp. 82–93. doi: 10.1046/j.1525-1446.2001.00082.x
9. Stewart M, Brown JB, Donner A, et al. The impact of patient-centered care on outcomes. *J Fam Pract*. 2000; 49(9): pp. 796–804.
10. Michaelson V, Pilato KA, Davison CM. Family as a health promotion setting: a scoping review of conceptual models of the health-promoting family. *PLoS One*. 2021; 16(4): e0249707. doi: 10.1371/journal.pone.0249707
11. Lien N, Lytle LA, Klepp K. Stability in consumption of fruit, vegetables, and sugary foods in a cohort from age 14 to age 21. *Prev Med*. 2001; 33: pp. 217–226.
12. Mikkilä V, Räsänen L, Raitakari OT, Pietinen P, Viikari J. Consistent dietary patterns identified from childhood to adulthood: the cardiovascular risk in young Finns study. *Br J Nutr*. 2005; 93: pp. 923–931.
13. First 5 California website. Retrieved May 6, 2024. https://www.first5california.com/en-us/
14. Meals for schools and childcare. USDA Food and Nutrition Services website. Retrieved May 6, 2024. https://www.fns.usda.gov/school-meals
15. Ho YL, Mahirah D, Ho CZ, Thumboo J. The role of the family in health promotion: a scoping review of models and mechanisms. *Health Promot Int*. 2022; 37(6): daac119. doi: 10.1093/heapro/daac119
16. DiMatteo MR. Variations in patients' adherence to medical recommendations: a quantitative review of 50 years of research. *Med Care*. 2004; 42(3): pp. 200–209.
17. Fiore MC. US public health service clinical practice guideline: treating tobacco use and dependence. *Respir Care*. 2000; 45(10): pp. 1200–1262.
18. Williams GC, McGregor HA, Zeldman A, Freedman ZR, Deci EL. Testing a self-determination theory process model for promoting glycemic control through diabetes self-management. *Health Psychol*. 2004; 23(1): pp. 58–66.
19. Lemstra M, Nwankwo C, Bird Y, Moraros J. Primary nonadherence to chronic disease medications: a meta-analysis. *Patient Prefer Adherence*. 2018; 12: pp. 721–731.

20. Courneya KS, McAuley E. Cognitive mediators of the social influence-exercise adherence relationship: a test of the theory of planned behavior. *J Behav Med.* 1995; 18(5): pp. 499–515.
21. McMahon SK, Lewis BA, Guan W, et al. Effect of intrapersonal and interpersonal behavior change strategies on physical activity among older adults: a randomized clinical trial. *JAMA Netw Open.* 2024; 7(2): e240298 doi: 10.1001/jamanetworkopen.2024.0298
22. DiMatteo MR. Social support and patient adherence to medical treatment: a meta-analysis. *Health Psychol.* 2004; 23(2): pp. 207–218. doi: 10.1037/0278-6133.23.2.207
23. Ryan RM, Deci EL. Self-determination theory and the facilitation of intrinsic motivation, social development, and well-being. *Am Psychol.* 2000; 55(1): pp. 68–78.
24. Faseru B, Richter KP, Scheuermann TS, Park EW. Enhancing partner support to improve smoking cessation. *Cochrane Database Syst Rev.* 2018; 8(8): CD002928. doi: 10.1002/14651858.CD002928.pub4
25. DiMatteo MR, DiNicola DD. *Achieving Patient Compliance.* New York: Pergamon Press; 1982.
26. Becker MH, Maiman LA. Strategies for enhancing patient compliance. *J Community Health.* 1980; 6(2): pp. 113–135. doi: 10.1007/BF01318980
27. Mechanic D. *Medical Sociology*, 2nd ed. New York: Free Press; 1978.
28. Kleinman A, Eisenberg L, Good B. Culture, illness, and care: clinical lessons from anthropologic and cross-cultural research. *Ann Intern Med.* 1978; 88(2): pp. 251–258. doi: 10.7326/0003-4819-88-2-251
29. Young JT. Illness behaviour: a selective review and synthesis. *Sociol Health Illn.* 2004; 26(1): pp. 1–31. doi: 10.1111/j.1467-9566.2004.00376.x
30. Miller WD, Peek ME, Parker WF. Scarce resource allocation scores threaten to exacerbate racial disparities in health care. *Chest.* 2020; 158(4): pp. 1332–1334. doi: 10.1016/j.chest.2020.05.526
31. Gehrman E. Shared identity and the doctor-patient relationship. *Harvard Medicine Magazine.* February 2024.
32. Herman SM. The relationship between therapist-client modality similarity and psychotherapy outcome. *J Psychother Pract Res.* 1997; 7(1): pp. 56–64.
33. Dougall I, Vasiljevic M, Wright JD, Weick M. How, when, and why is social class linked to mental health and wellbeing? A systematic meta-review. *Soc Sci Med.* 2024; 343: p. 116542.
34. Shackleton N, Jamal F, Viner RM, Dickson K, Patton G, Bonell C. School-based interventions going beyond health education to promote adolescent health: systematic review of reviews. *J Adolesc Health.* 2016; 58(4): pp. 382–396.
35. Lima-Serrano M, Lima-Rodríguez JS. Impact of school-based health promotion interventions aimed at different behavioral domains: a systematic review. *Gac Sanit.* 2014; 28(5): pp. 411–417.
36. Busch V, de Leeuw JR, de Harder A, Schrijvers AJ. Changing multiple adolescent health behaviors through school-based interventions: a review of the literature. *J Sch Health.* 2013; 83(7): pp. 514–523. doi: 10.1111/josh.12060
37. Loma Linda, California: a group of Americans living 10 years longer. Blue Zones website. Retrieved May 6, 2024. https://www.bluezones.com/explorations/loma-linda-california/#

38. Festinger L. A theory of social comparison processes. *Hum Relat.* 1954; 7(2): pp. 117–140.
39. Buunk BP, Collins RL, Taylor SE, VanYperen NW, Dakof GA. The affective consequences of social comparison: either direction has its ups and downs. *J Pers Soc Psychol.* 1990; 59(6): pp. 1238–1249. doi: 10.1037//0022-3514.59.6.1238
40. Park SY, Baek YM. Two faces of social comparison on Facebook: the interplay between social comparison orientation, emotions, and psychological well-being. *Comp Hum Behav.* 2018; 79: pp. 83–93.
41. Gibbons FX. Social comparison as a mediator of response shift. *Soc Sci Med.* 1999; 48(11): pp. 1517–1530. doi: 10.1016/s0277-9536(99)00046-5
42. Croyle RT. Appraisal of health threats: cognition, motivation, and social comparison. *Cog Ther Res.* 1992; 16(2): pp. 165–182.
43. Buunk BP, Ybema JF. Social comparisons and occupational stress: the identification-contrast model. In: Buunk BP, Gibbons FX, Buunk A, eds. *Health, Coping, and Well-Being*. New York: Psychology Press; 1997; pp. 359–388.
44. Van der Zee K, Buunk B, Sanderman R, Botke G, Van den Bergh F. Social comparison and coping with cancer treatment. *Pers Indiv Diff.* 2000; 28(1): pp. 17–34.
45. Aspinwall LG, Taylor SE. Effects of social comparison direction, threat, and self-esteem on affect, self-evaluation, and expected success. *J Pers Soc Psychol.* 1993; 64(5): pp. 708–722. doi: 10.1037//0022-3514.64.5.708
46. Gerber JP, Wheeler L, Suls J. A social comparison theory meta-analysis 60+ years on. *Psychol Bull.* 2018; 144(2): pp. 177–197. doi: 10.1037/bul0000127
47. Bandura A, Jourden FJ. Self-regulatory mechanisms governing the impact of social comparison on complex decision making. *J Pers Soc Psychol.* 1991; 60(6): p. 941.
48. Parsons T. *Talcott Parsons on Institutions and Social Evolution: Selected Writings*. University of Chicago Press; 1985.
49. Hotez PJ. *The Deadly Rise of Anti-Science: A Scientist's Warning*. Johns Hopkins University Press; 2023.
50. Wallace-Wells D. It's time to talk about pandemic revisionism, David Wallace-Wells interviews Katelyn Jetelina [internet podcast]. The Ezra Klein Show. *New York Times.* August 29, 2023. https://www.nytimes.com/2023/08/29/podcasts/transcript-david-wallace-wells-interviews-katelyn-jetelina.html
51. Hesse BW, Nelson DE, Kreps GL, et al. Trust and sources of health information: the impact of the Internet and its implications for health care providers: findings from the first Health Information National Trends Survey. *Arch Intern Med.* 2005; 165(22): pp. 2618–2624. doi: 10.1001/archinte.165.22.2618
52. Swoboda CM, Van Hulle JM, McAlearney AS, Huerta TR. Odds of talking to healthcare providers as the initial source of healthcare information: updated cross-sectional results from the Health Information National Trends Survey (HINTS). *BMC Fam Pract.* 2018; 19(1): p. 146. doi: 10.1186/s12875-018-0805-7
53. Rice RE. Influences, usage, and outcomes of Internet health information searching: multivariate results from the Pew surveys. *Int J Med Inform.* 2006; 75(1): pp. 8–28. doi: 10.1016/j.ijmedinf.2005.07.032
54. Benigeri M, Pluye P. Shortcomings of health information on the Internet. *Health Promot Int.* 2003; 18(4): pp. 381–386. doi: 10.1093/heapro/dag409

55. Ellsberg D. Risk, ambiguity, and the Savage axioms. *Quarterly Journal of Economics.* 1961; pp. 643–669.
56. Viscusi WK, Magat WA. Bayesian decisions with ambiguous belief aversion, *Journal of Risk and Uncertainty.* 1992; 5: pp. 371–387.
57. Cameron TA. Updating subjective risks in the presence of conflicting information: an application to climate change. *Journal of Risk and Uncertainty.* 2005; 30(1): pp. 63–97.
58. Kreuter MW, Strecher VJ. Changing inaccurate perceptions of health risk: results from a randomized trial. *Health Psychol.* 1995; 14(1): pp. 56–63. doi: 10.1037/0278-6133.14.1.56
59. Weinstein ND. Unrealistic optimism about future life events. *J Pers Soc Psychol.* 1980; 39: pp. 806–820.
60. Keles B, McCrae N, Grealish A. A systematic review: the influence of social media on depression, anxiety and psychological distress in adolescents. *International Journal of Adolescence and Youth.* 2020; 25(1): pp. 79–93.
61. Shensa A, Sidani JE, Dew MA, Escobar-Viera CG, Primack BA. Social media use and depression and anxiety symptoms: a cluster analysis. *Am J Health Behav.* 2018; 42(2): pp. 116–128. doi: 10.5993/AJHB.42.2.11
62. Thai H, Davis CG, Stewart N, Gunnell KE, Goldfield GS. The effects of reducing social media use on body esteem among transitional-aged youth. *J Soc Clin Psychol.* 2021; 40(6): pp. 481–507.
63. Thai H, Davis CG, Mahboob W, Perry S, Adams A, Goldfield GS. Reducing social media use improves appearance and weight esteem in youth with emotional distress. *Psychology of Popular Media.* 2023; 13(1): pp. 162–169.
64. Immunization coverage. World Health Organization website. July 18, 2023. https://www.who.int/news-room/fact-sheets/detail/immunization-coverage
65. Brewer NT. What works to increase vaccination uptake. *Acad Pediat.* 2021; 21(4): pp. S9–S16.
66. Funk C, Kennedy B, Hefferon M. Vast majority of Americans say benefits of childhood vaccines outweigh risks. Pew Research Center. February 2, 2017. http://www.pewresearch.org
67. Palache A, Oriol-Mathieu V, Abelin A, Music T; Influenza Vaccine Supply task force (IFPMA IVS). Seasonal influenza vaccine dose distribution in 157 countries (2004–2011). *Vaccine.* 2014; 32(48): pp. 6369–6376. doi: 10.1016/j.vaccine.2014.07.012
68. de Figueiredo A, Simas C, Karafillakis E, Paterson P, Larson HJ. Mapping global trends in vaccine confidence and investigating barriers to vaccine uptake: a large-scale retrospective temporal modelling study. *Lancet.* 2020; 396(10255): pp. 898–908. doi: 10.1016/S0140-6736(20)31558-0
69. Bish A, Yardley L, Nicoll A, Michie S. Factors associated with uptake of vaccination against pandemic influenza: A systematic review. *Vaccine.* 2011; 29: pp. 6472–6484. doi: 10.1016/j.vaccine.2011.06.107
70. Martin LR, Petrie KJ. Understanding the dimensions of anti-vaccination attitudes: the Vaccination Attitudes Examination (VAX) Scale. *Ann Behav Med.* 2017; 51(5): pp. 652–660. doi: 10.1007/s12160-017-9888-y

71. MacDougall DM, Halperin BA, MacKinnon-Cameron D, et al. The challenge of vaccinating adults: attitudes and beliefs of the Canadian public and healthcare providers. *BMJ Open*. 2015; 5(9): p. e009062. doi: 10.1136/bmjopen-2015-009062
72. Dubé E, Laberge C, Guay M, Bramadat P, Roy R, Bettinger J. Vaccine hesitancy: an overview. *Hum Vaccin Immunother*. 2013; 9(8): pp. 1763–1773. doi: 10.4161/hv.24657
73. Nyhan B, Reifler J. Does correcting myths about the flu vaccine work? An experimental evaluation of the effects of corrective information. *Vaccine*. 2015; 33(3): pp. 459–464.
74. Nyhan B, Reifler J, Richey S, Freed GL. Effective messages in vaccine promotion: a randomized trial. *Pediatrics*. 2014; 133(4): pp. e835–e842. doi: 10.1542/peds.2013-2365
75. Leask J, Kinnersley P, Jackson C, Cheater F, Bedford H, Rowles G. Communicating with parents about vaccination: a framework for health professionals. *BMC Pediatr*. 2012; 12: p. 154. doi: 10.1186/1471-2431-12-154
76. Gilkey MB, Calo WA, Moss JL, Shah PD, Marciniak MW, Brewer NT. Provider communication and HPV vaccination: The impact of recommendation quality. *Vaccine*. 2016; 34(9): pp. 1187–1192. doi: 10.1016/j.vaccine.2016.01.023
77. MacDonald NE, SAGE Working Group on Vaccine Hesitancy. Vaccine hesitancy: Definition, scope, and determinants. *Vaccine*. 2015; 33: pp. 4161–4164.
78. Hurley LP, Bridges CB, Harpaz R, et al. Physician attitudes toward adult vaccines and other preventive practices, United States, 2012. *Public Health Rep*. 2016; March; 131(2): pp. 320–330. doi: 10.1177/003335491613100216
79. Maridor M, Ruch S, Bangerter A, Emery V. Skepticism toward emerging infectious diseases and influenza vaccination intentions in nurses. *J Health Commun*. 2017;22(5): pp. 386–394. doi: 10.1080/10810730.2017.1296509
80. Schuler M, Schaedelin S, Aebi C, et al. Attitudes of Swiss health care providers toward childhood immunizations. *Pediatr Infect Dis J*. 2017; 36(6): pp. e167–e174. doi: 10.1097/INF.0000000000001522
81. Schrading WA, Trent SA, Paxton JH, et al; Project COVERED Emergency Department Network. Vaccination rates and acceptance of SARS-CoV-2 vaccination among U.S. emergency department health care personnel. *Acad Emerg Med*. 2021; 28(4): pp. 455–458. doi: 10.1111/acem.14236
82. Collange F, Verger P, Launay O, Pulcini C. Knowledge, attitudes, beliefs and behaviors of general practitioners/family physicians toward their own vaccination: A systematic review. *Hum Vaccin Immunother*. 2016; 12(5): pp. 1282–1292. doi: 10.1080/21645515.2015.1138024
83. Collins S. Explanations in consultations: the combined effectiveness of doctors' and nurses' communication with patients. *Med Educ*. 2005; 39(8): pp. 785–796.
84. Kulczycki A, Qu H, Shewchuk R. Primary care physicians' adherence to guidelines and their likelihood to prescribe the human papillomavirus vaccine for 11- and 12-year-old girls. *Women's Health Issues*. 2016; 26(1): pp. 34–39. doi: 10.1016/j.whi.2015.07.012
85. Davis MM, Ndiaye SM, Freed GL, Kim CS, Clark SJ. Influence of insurance status and vaccine cost on physicians' administration of pneumococcal conjugate vaccine. *Pediatrics*. 2003; 112(3 Pt 1): pp. 521–526. doi: 10.1542/peds.112.3.521

86. Kempe A, O'Leary ST, Kennedy A, et al. Physician response to parental requests to spread out the recommended vaccine schedule. *Pediatrics*. 2015; 135(4): pp. 666–677. doi: 10.1542/peds.2014-3474
87. Grandahl M, Larsson M, Tydén T, Stenhammar C. School nurses' attitudes towards and experiences of the Swedish school-based HPV vaccination programme—A repeated cross-sectional study. *PLoS One*. 2017; 12(4): e0175883. doi: 10.1371/journal.pone.0175883
88. Rhudy LM, Tucker SJ, Ofstead CL, Poland GA. Personal choice or evidence-based nursing intervention: nurses' decision-making about influenza vaccination. *Worldviews Evid Based Nurs*. 2010; 7(2): pp. 111–120. doi: 10.1111/j.1741-6787.2010.00190.x
89. Shahrabani S, Benzion U, Yom Din G. Factors affecting nurses' decision to get the flu vaccine. *Eur J Health Econ*. 2009; 10(2): pp. 227–231. doi: 10.1007/s10198-008-0124-3
90. Zhang J, While AE, Norman IJ. (2011). Nurses' knowledge and risk perception towards seasonal influenza and vaccination and their vaccination behaviours: A cross-sectional survey. *Int J Nurs Stud*. 2011; 48(10): pp. 1281–1289. doi: 10.1016/j.ijnurstu.2011.03.002
91. Paris C, Bénézit F, Geslin M, et al. COVID-19 vaccine hesitancy among healthcare workers. *Infect Dis Now*. 2021; 51(5): pp. 484–487. doi: 10.1016/j.idnow.2021.04.001
92. Huang D, Ganti L, Graham EW, et al. COVID-19 Vaccine Hesitancy Among Healthcare Providers. *Health Psychol Res*. 2022; 10(3): 34218. doi: 10.52965/001c.34218
93. Le LM, Veettil SK, Donaldson D, et al. The impact of pharmacist involvement on immunization uptake and other outcomes: An updated systematic review and meta-analysis. *J Am Pharm Assoc*. 2022; 62(5): pp. 1499–1513.e16. doi: 10.1016/j.japh.2022.06.008
94. Singh GK, Lee H. Marked disparities in life expectancy by education, poverty level, occupation, and housing tenure in the United States, 1997–2014. *Int J MCH AIDS*. 2021; 10(1): pp. 7–18. doi: 10.21106/ijma.402
95. Ghorayshi A. An unsettling drop in life expectancy for men. *New York Times*. November 13, 2023. https://www.nytimes.com/2023/11/13/health/men-life-expectancy-drops.html
96. Adler NE, Newman K. Socioeconomic disparities in health: pathways and policies. *Health Affairs*. 2002; 21(2): pp. 60–76.
97. Mullainathan S, Shafir E. *Scarcity: Why Having Too Little Means So Much*. Times Books; 2013.
98. Geruso M. Black-white disparities in life expectancy: how much can the standard SES variables explain? *Demography*. 2012; 49(2): pp. 553–574.
99. Thayer JF, Carnevali L, Sgiofo A, Williams DP. Angry in America: psychophysiological responses to unfair treatment. *Ann Behav Med*. 2020; 54(12): pp. 924–931. doi: 10.1093/abm/kaaa094
100. Pasricha T. Why doesn't my doctor believe I'm in pain? *The Washington Post*. September 25, 2023. https://www.washingtonpost.com/wellness/2023/09/25/chronic-pain-management-doctor/

101. Provenzano DA, Kamal KM, Giannetti V. Evaluation of primary care physician chronic pain management practice patterns. *Pain Physician*. 2018; 21(6): pp. E593–E602.
102. Phelan SM, van Ryn M, Wall M, Burgess D. Understanding primary care physicians' treatment of chronic low back pain: the role of physician and practice factors. *Pain Med*. 2009; 10(7): pp. 1270–1279. doi: 10.1111/j.1526-4637.2009.00717.x
103. Hoffman KM, Trawalter S, Axt JR, Oliver MN. Racial bias in pain assessment and treatment recommendations, and false beliefs about biological differences between blacks and whites. *Proc Natl Acad Sci USA*. 2016; 113(16): pp. 4296–4301. doi: 10.1073/pnas.1516047113
104. Shavers VL, Bakos A, Sheppard VB. Race, ethnicity, and pain among the U.S. adult population. *J Health Care Poor Underserved*. 2010; 21(1): pp. 177–220. doi: 10.1353/hpu.0.0255
105. Hoffmann DE, Tarzian AJ. The girl who cried pain: a bias against women in the treatment of pain. *J Law Med Ethics*. 2001; 29(1): pp. 13–27.
106. Kaye AD, Baluch A, Scott JT. Pain management in the elderly population: a review. *Ochsner J*. 2010; 10(3): pp. 179–187.
107. Stannard C. Where now for opioids in chronic pain? *Drug Ther Bull*. 2018; 56(10): pp. 118–122.
108. Volkow N, Benveniste H, McLellan AT. Use and misuse of opioids in chronic pain. *Annu Rev Med*. 2018; 69: pp. 451–465. doi: 10.1146/annurev-med-011817-044739
109. Warraich H. *The Song of Our Scars: The Untold Story of Pain*. New York: Basic Books; 2022.
110. Sun M, Oliwa T, Peek ME, Tung EL. Negative patient descriptors: documenting racial bias in the electronic health record. *Health Aff (Millwood)*. 2022; 41(2): pp. 203–211. doi: 10.1377/hlthaff.2021.01423
111. Singh GK. Trends and social inequalities in maternal mortality in the United States, 1969–2018. *Int J MCH AIDS*. 2021; 10(1): 29.
112. Lister RL, Drake W, Scott BH, Graves C. Black maternal mortality-the elephant in the room. *World J Gynecol Womens Health*. 2019; 3(1): doi: 10.33552/wjgwh.2019.03.000555
113. Maternal mortality rates in the United States, 2020. Centers for Disease Control and Prevention website. Retrieved February 10, 2024. https://www.cdc.gov/nchs/data/hestat/maternal-mortality/2020/maternal-mortality-rates-2020.htm
114. Hall WJ, Chapman MV, Lee KM, et al. Implicit racial/ethnic bias among health care professionals and its influence on health care outcomes: a systematic review. *Am J Public Health*. 2015; 105(12): pp. e60–e76.
115. Salles A, Arora VM, Mitchell KA. Everyone must address anti-black racism in health care: Steps for non-black health care professionals to take. *JAMA*. 2021; 326(7): pp. 601–602.
116. Dahlem CH, Villarruel AM, Ronis DL. African American women and prenatal care: perceptions of patient-provider interaction. *West J Nurs Res*. 2015; 37(2): pp. 217–235.
117. The U.S. Public Health Service Untreated Syphilis Study at Tuskegee. Centers for Disease Control and Prevention website. Retrieved May 6, 2024. https://www.cdc.gov/tuskegee/about.html

118. Thomas SB, Quinn SC. The Tuskegee Syphilis Study, 1932 to 1972: implications for HIV education and AIDS risk education programs in the black community. *Am J Public Health*. 1991; 81(11): pp. 1498–1505.
119. Gatchel RJ, Mayer TG, Chou R. What does/should the minimum clinically important difference measure?: A reconsideration of its clinical value in evaluating efficacy of lumbar fusion surgery. *Clin J Pain*. 2012; 28(5): pp. 387–397.
120. Chou R, Qaseem A, Owens DK, Shekelle P. Clinical Guidelines Committee of the American College of Physicians. Diagnostic imaging for low back pain: advice for high-value health care from the American College of Physicians. *Ann Intern Med*. 2011; 154: pp. 181–189.
121. Welch GH, Schwartz L, Woloshin S. *Over-diagnosed: Making People Sick in the Pursuit of Health*. Beacon Press; 2012.
122. Prasad VK, Cifu AS. *Ending Medical Reversal: Improving Outcomes, Saving Lives*. Johns Hopkins University Press; 2015.
123. Birkmeyer JD, Reames BN, McCulloch P, Carr AJ, Campbell WB, Wennberg JE. Understanding of regional variation in the use of surgery. *Lancet*. 2013; 382(9898): pp. 1121–1129. doi: 10.1016/s0140-6736(13)61215-5
124. Gorski D. Are medical errors really the third most common cause of death in the U.S.? (2019 edition). Science-Based Medicine website. February 4, 2019. https://sciencebasedmedicine.org/are-medical-errors-really-the-third-most-common-cause-of-death-in-the-u-s-2019-edition/
125. Ge L, Liu S, Li S, et al. Psychological stress in inflammatory bowel disease: Psychoneuroimmunological insights into bidirectional gut-brain communications. *Front Immunol*. 2022; 13: p. 1016578. doi: 10.3389/fimmu.2022.1016578
126. Hughes K, Bellis MA, Hardcastle KA, et al. The effect of multiple adverse childhood experiences on health: a systematic review and meta-analysis. *Lancet Public Health*. 2017; 2(8): pp. e356–e366. doi: 10.1016/S2468-2667(17)30118-4
127. Sowder KL, Knight LA, Fishalow J. Trauma exposure and health: A review of outcomes and pathways. *Journal of Aggression, Maltreatment & Trauma*. 2018; 27(10): pp. 1041–1059.
128. Warren TH. Rising heat deaths are not just about the temperature. *New York Times*. July 23, 2023.
129. Johnson A, Gomez C. Stress is weathering our bodies from the inside out. *Washington Post*. Oct 17, 2023.
130. Geronimus AT. *Weathering: The Extraordinary Stress of Ordinary Life in an Unjust Society*. Little, Brown Spark; 2023.
131. Samuels E, Khalife S, Alfonso CA, Alvarez R, Cohen MA. Early childhood trauma, posttraumatic stress disorder, and non-adherence in persons with AIDS: a psychodynamic perspective. *J Am Acad Psychoanal Dyn Psychiatry*. 2011; 39(4): pp. 633–650. doi: 10.1521/jaap.2011.39.4.633
132. Senn TE, Carey MP, Vanable PA. Childhood and adolescent sexual abuse and subsequent sexual risk behavior: Evidence from controlled studies, methodological critique, and suggestions for research. *Clin Psychol Rev*. 2008; 28: pp. 711–735.
133. Brown LK, Hadley W, Stewart A, et al. The Project Style Study Group. Psychiatric disorders and sexual risk among adolescents in mental health treatment. *J Consult Clin Psychol*. 2010; 78: pp. 590–597.

134. DiMatteo MR, Lepper HS, Croghan TW. Depression is a risk factor for noncompliance with medical treatment: meta-analysis of the effects of anxiety and depression on patient adherence. *Arch Intern Med.* 2000; 160(14): pp. 2101–2107. doi: 10.1001/archinte.160.14.2101.
135. Grenard JL, Munjas BA, Adams JL, et al. Depression and medication adherence in the treatment of chronic diseases in the United States: a meta-analysis. *J Gen Intern Med.* 2011; 26(10): pp. 1175–1182. doi: 10.1007/s11606-011-1704-y
136. DiMatteo MR, Haskard-Zolnierek KB. Impact of depression on treatment adherence and survival from cancer. In: Kissane D, Maj M, Sartorius N, eds. *Depression and Cancer.* World Psychiatric Association and Wiley/Blackwell; 2011; pp. 101–124.
137. DiMatteo MR, Haskard KB, Williams SL. Health beliefs, disease severity, and patient adherence: a meta-analysis. *Med Care.* 2007; 45(6): pp. 521–528. doi: 10.1097/MLR.0b013e318032937e
138. Carney RM, Freedland KE. Depression in patients with coronary heart disease. *Am J Med.* 2008; 121: pp. S20–27.
139. Anbar RD, Farnan R, Lancaster ME. Age regression in the treatment of needle phobia: a case report. *Am J Clin Hypn.* 2023; 11: pp. 1–6. doi: 10.1080/00029157.2023.2261517
140. Duncanson E, Le Leu RK, Shanahan L, et al. The prevalence and evidence-based management of needle fear in adults with chronic disease: A scoping review. *PLoS One.* 2021; 16(6): e0253048. doi: 10.1371/journal.pone.0253048
141. Williams SL. Emotional distress among patients in primary care: Analysis of physician-patient communication. University of California, Riverside, unpublished dissertation. 2008.
142. Kroenke K, Spitzer RL, Williams JB, Löwe B. The Patient Health Questionnaire Somatic, Anxiety, and Depressive Symptom Scales: a systematic review. *Gen Hosp Psychiatry.* 2010; 32(4): pp. 345–359.
143. Tompkins MA, Beck J (foreword). *The Cognitive Behavioral Therapy Workbook: Evidence-Based CBT Skills to Help You Manage Stress, Anxiety, Depression, and More.* New Harbinger Publications; Workbook edition; 2024.
144. Hayes SC, Smith S. *Get Out of Your Mind and into Your Life: The New Acceptance and Commitment Therapy.* 1st ed. New Harbinger Publications; 2005.
145. Shapiro F. *Eye Movement Desensitization and Reprocessing (EMDR) Therapy: Basic Principles, Protocols, and Procedures.* 3rd ed. Guilford Press; 2017.
146. Cultural respect. National Institutes of Health website. Retrieved May 6, 2024. https://www.nih.gov/institutes-nih/nih-office-director/office-communications-public-liaison/clear-communication/cultural-respect
147. White AA 3rd, Logghe HJ, Goodenough DA, et al. Self-awareness and cultural identity as an effort to reduce bias in medicine. *J Racial Ethn Health Disparities.* 2018; 5(1): pp. 34–49. doi: 10.1007/s40615-017-0340-6
148. Shanafelt TD, Schein E, Minor LB, Trockel M, Schein P, Kirch D. Healing the professional culture of medicine. *Mayo Clin Proc.* 2019; 94(8): pp. 1556–1566. doi: 10.1016/j.mayocp.2019.03.026
149. Institute of Medicine. *Crossing the Quality Chasm: A New Health System for the 21st Century.* Washington, DC: National Academies Press; 2001.
150. Mead N, Bower P. Patient-centredness: a conceptual framework and review of the empirical literature. *Soc Sci Med.* 2000; 51(7): pp. 1087–1110.

151. Rathert C, Wyrwich MD, Boren SA. Patient-centered care and outcomes: a systematic review of the literature. *Med Care Res Rev.* 2013; 70(4): pp. 351–379. doi: 10.1177/1077558712465774
152. Stewart M, Brown JB, Donner A, McWhinney IR, Oates J, Weston WW, Jordan J. The impact of patient-centered care on outcomes. *J Fam Pract.* 2000; 49(9): pp. 796–804.
153. National Academies of Sciences, Engineering, and Medicine. *Communicating Science Effectively: A Research Agenda.* Washington, DC: National Academies Press; 2017.
154. Scrimshaw SC. Science, health, and cultural literacy in a rapidly changing communication landscape. *PNAS.* 2019; 116(16): pp. 7650–7655.

Chapter 8
Using Teams and Technology to Deliver Better Care

Time is of the essence in medical care delivery; healthcare effectiveness and outcomes depend upon using time efficiently and successfully. In this chapter, we examine the expanding role of multidisciplinary healthcare teams in providing quality medical care within the constraints of time and resources, and the influence, value, and challenges of technologies that were only imagined just a few years ago but are commonplace today.

The past decade has seen an astonishing expansion in the role of technology in healthcare. Innovations are developing at a rapid pace and, because of the internet, more medical information than ever in history is available to patients. For better or worse, with the help of their social networks and artificial intelligence (AI)-based tools, patients can self-diagnose, self-treat, and learn (often through direct-to-patient advertising) about brand new pharmaceutical therapies, surgical interventions, and medical devices.

As we will see in this chapter, new mobile medical technologies are improving patients' access to and communication with health professionals. Patients can check in by email, text, and audio- or video-chat and even provide many digital metrics (e.g., heart rate, blood pressure, blood glucose, sleep quality) remotely. Patients and their doctors can consult with distant specialists about complex and difficult problems; the entire healthcare team can pool their expertise through emails and videoconferencing, keeping track of everything about the patient's case in an enhanced and searchable Electronic Medical Record (EMR). AI can help providers record and organize what occurs in the medical visit, make better diagnoses, and develop better communication skills and bedside manner. Personal digital tools can help patients plan and remember medication doses, develop and maintain activity schedules, and receive encouraging messages as they strive for health behavior change and treatment adherence.

Health Behavior Change and Treatment Adherence. Second Edition. M. Robin DiMatteo, Leslie R. Martin, and Kelly B. Haskard-Zolnierek, Oxford University Press. © Oxford University Press (2025).
DOI: 10.1093/oso/9780197778586.003.0008

Medical teams

Few patients receive as much time with their physicians as they would like; and many physicians share this concern. Despite having different amounts of time allocated for various types of visits, physicians across the U.S., the U.K., and Germany report feeling that they need more time[1] with their patients. While brief office visits do pose a challenge for effective healthcare delivery,[2] research is showing that a division of labor among the members of the healthcare team can help make the most of medical interactions.

Although much of the existing research on medical interactions has focused on physicians, medical care delivery involves multiple providers who spend considerable time in direct patient care; indeed, the complexity of today's medical care makes functioning without a team-oriented approach extremely difficult. Efforts to contain healthcare costs and maintain quality encourage many healthcare organizations to utilize a variety of clinical professionals to provide patient care under the physician's direction.[3-7]

A *healthcare team* generally consists of a diverse group of clinicians who together communicate about and participate in the management of a patient's care.[8] A patient with recently diagnosed but advanced diabetes might have a team consisting of a physician, a nurse practitioner, a nutritionist, a pharmacist, a medical educator, and a behavioral specialist. In the care of hypertension, the team might be smaller and include a primary care physician, a medical assistant, and perhaps a biofeedback specialist to help the patient manage stress.

Simply having the necessary group members in place, however, does not ensure that they will function as a cohesive team. An ideal healthcare team has: *(1)* clear and measurable team goals, *(2)* clearly defined systems for accomplishing those goals, *(3)* clear and precise division of tasks, *(4)* adequate training of all team members, and *(5)* effective communication amongst the team members. Many of the important communication principles from Chapter 3 also apply to interactions among healthcare team members.[5,7]

Research suggests that well-functioning healthcare teams foster greater satisfaction and better healthcare outcomes; shared responsibility among primary care physicians and other team members has been shown to be quite successful in chronic disease management.[7,9-11] Not surprisingly, miscommunication within healthcare teams can increase medical errors. Verbal instructions are particularly vulnerable to error and are more likely to be given in situations in which health professionals are distracted and hurried.[12] Written instructions are essential to patient safety; protocols that include responsibility for pursuing, receiving, and disseminating information using a common vocabulary can ensure precise and accurate communication. A full understanding of how people can optimally work together in groups can be essential to the success of healthcare teams. Research demonstrates, for example, that optimal team size tends to have an inverted U-shaped relationship with effectiveness; teams that are too small or too large may be disadvantaged.[13] The ideal size of a healthcare team depends upon the setting and circumstances, but research suggests that about six members may be ideal.[14] To maximize cost effectiveness, a team's tasks should be completed by those with the most basic level of training that would equip them for the task, freeing providers who have higher levels of expertise to focus on tasks for which they are specially trained.[3] There is good research evidence that nurse practitioners as members of the healthcare team generally deliver care that is equivalent to that delivered by primary care physicians.[15] Perhaps because of their training, nurse practitioners tend to excel at chronic disease management and behavioral counseling.[6,7] Successful implementation of a team approach can, of course, be challenged by personal conflicts and issues related to power-sharing.[16] Forming teams of health professionals who communicate and work well together is crucial.

Despite the challenges of implementing coordinated and efficient team-based care, there are many ways that members of the healthcare team can help patients with adherence and health behavior change. A trusted pharmacist, for example, can discuss medication details with a patient, and an experienced nurse can help overcome individual or system-related barriers to adherence. Let us examine some ways in which a team approach can make the most of limited time in the medical visit.

Planning and agenda-setting for the medical visit

When Tamara prepares for her annual exam with her primary care physician, she makes a list of her concerns. She has been experiencing low back pain and headaches. She worries that her blood pressure may be too high, and medication might be necessary, and she has been struggling with worsening anxiety. Like many patients, Tamara has multiple issues to address in a single appointment.

Patients and health professionals often have different, though unstated, agendas for their medical visits. Research shows that a brief training program, in which physicians were taught to elicit their patients' agendas and organize and negotiate priorities, significantly increased patients' satisfaction that their concerns had been addressed.[17] Regardless of the composition of the healthcare team, pre-visit counseling by a physician or other team member can help set the agenda for the visit, ensuring that the issues most important to health professional *and* patient are addressed.[18] Agenda-setting involves prioritizing issues to be discussed so that the most important items are covered during the visit; negotiation may be necessary in response to differing priorities of clinician and patient.[2] Agenda-setting is a critical, but often overlooked, component of efficient care delivery; training members of the healthcare team to do it well can improve the quality of communication in the medical visit.[19]

Consistent follow-up care can improve objective clinical outcomes and subjective experiences. Research shows that when compared with standard diabetes care, patients' blood glucose levels and self-reported health were better when a nurse case manager, a dietitian, and an exercise counselor followed up after their initial consultation.[4] Simple methods such as telephone post-visit follow-up and appointment reminders[20] can be effective in identifying problems early and demonstrating the healthcare team's commitment and concern for the patient.[21,22]

Models of care for the whole person

So much in healthcare is dependent upon psychological factors. Up to three quarters of primary care medical visits involve psychological or behavioral issues, including adherence and chronic disease management, mental health concerns such as anxiety and depression, and health behavior challenges like smoking cessation, stress management, physical activity, and dietary change. The biopsychosocial approach[23] is an essential model for primary care medicine, but its implementation requires a team and the incorporation of mental healthcare into medical practice. Because of time pressures and lack of personnel, however, the biopsychosocial model is often ignored in practice unless there are systems and frameworks to support it.

Several important team-based approaches have been developed and integrated into primary care medicine to provide these frameworks. These approaches are supported by the goals and provisions of the 2010 Affordable Care Act (also known, colloquially, as Obamacare). Here, we examine the basic elements of four models of primary care practice: the Chronic Care Model (CCM),[24] the Collaborative Care Model (CoCM),[25] the Primary Care Behavioral Health (PCBH) model, and the Patient-Centered Medical Home (PCMH) model, which is an overarching framework and represents an important development in primary care medicine. We also consider some of the research supporting their effectiveness in containing healthcare costs and improving access and healthcare outcomes. These models are dynamically integrated into ongoing medical practice; they offer solutions to the challenges of providing healthcare for the whole patient in their social context.

Let us start with the big picture and a foundational anecdote that highlights the central importance of care for the whole patient. Dr. Edward Wagner (developer of the Chronic Care Model, an organizing framework for improving chronic illness care) recounted an analogy to illustrate that in the management of chronic disease, a "patient as consumer" approach can have drawbacks. When a well-meaning health professional is simply "informative," managing a chronic disease becomes a bit like sending the patient off to fly a small airplane, mostly on their own. It is a bit like giving the person one flying lesson and telling them that once in a while the flight tower will ask for their location. It is like saying "Here's a manual on flying.... good luck!" Never an approach in aviation, this strategy is all too common in medicine where busy practitioners may support the concept of "patient involvement" but have little time to offer patients a structure in which to manage their own care.[24]

In the United States, most patients receive healthcare in medical practices that are outside of large integrated healthcare systems; they often face significant challenges in receiving the time, education, and follow-up required to manage their chronic illnesses effectively. Something as simple as reorganizing a daily medication schedule after a dosing change can sometimes require instruction and assistance, especially if multiple medications are involved.

The Chronic Care Model[24] involves both biological and behavioral management at the patient level (as well as at the system level, as described in Chapter 9). It requires healthcare team intervention and involves: *(1)* helping patients make decisions about their treatment in conjunction with their healthcare team; *(2)* helping patients self-manage their chronic conditions, including diet, exercise, and adherence to medications; and *(3)* connecting patients to community resources that can help provide both practical and emotional support. There exists strong evidence that this general model of chronic disease care works well; it keeps people out of the hospital and the emergency department by preventing medical crises and by intervening early, when problems are developing. As we have considered earlier in this book, many chronic diseases cause a loss of functioning, a change in capacity, and the need to alter future plans; many require regular medication and changes in daily habits. The Chronic Care Model, originally developed to help elder patients deal with depression, is focused on helping patients with all of these challenges, and it promotes care of the whole person including prevention and management of mental health concerns and improvement in their quality of life.

There are two "primary care integrated practice models" that support this approach to chronic illness management and are formally recognized by the U.S. Center for Medicare and Medicaid Services: the Collaborative Care Model (CoCM)[25] (which includes care management for patients with mental health conditions), and the Primary Care Behavioral Health (PCBH) model (which includes behavioral and mental health specialists on the primary medical care team).[26,27] Blending the two is currently the most widely implemented approach in integrated care.[28]

The Collaborative Care Model is an evidence-based approach to medical practice that strives to bring physical and mental healthcare together within the same primary care provider's office.[25] In one location, at their primary care medical practice, patients can receive mental health screening and collaborate with multiple providers in making care decisions. Referrals to psychiatric consultations and treatments are facilitated, and follow-up is provided for the duration of treatment. The CoCM is most effectively combined with the Primary Care Behavioral Health model. In the PCBH model, behavioral health is part and parcel of primary care; a clinical psychologist or other licensed mental health professional (e.g., clinical social worker; counseling psychologist) serves as a member of the primary healthcare team.[26,27] This behavioral health consultant educates patients, makes recommendations to the physician, provides support to the rest of the healthcare team, and normalizes psychological services for patients and team members. Patients are aware that the team members share a common medical record and meet regularly to take joint responsibility for integrated patient care.[28,29]

The Patient-Centered Medical Home is a model of primary care that was developed and supported as part of the Affordable Care Act; with certain provisions, a medical practice can be formally designated as a PCMH. Financial incentives are offered in the context of state Medicaid programs to improve primary care delivery and lower healthcare costs. PCMHs are based on a primary care delivery model with a personal physician, as well as enhanced access to care, a focus on the patient as a whole person in their social context, coordination of care, and an emphasis on quality and safety; payment mechanisms reward primary care practices that provide this patient-centered care.[30] The CoCM and PCMH models are often combined together to offer the biopsychosocial approach to patient care that the Patient Centered Medical Home requires. The patient as a whole person is cared for in these models, and mental health services and behavioral management are coordinated in an integrated manner within the practice.[31]

In order to be designated as a Patient-Centered Medical Home, a practice is required to assess *patient satisfaction* using appropriate assessment tools such as the Consumer Assessment of Healthcare Providers and Systems (CAHPS) provided by the U.S. Agency for Healthcare Research and Quality. These surveys ask patients to report on and evaluate their experiences with healthcare in the PCMH.[30,32] The requirements and guidelines for certification place significant emphasis on providing patients with education and counseling to help them develop and maintain self-management goals for adherence to treatment, adopt healthy lifestyles, and manage complex medication regimens, among other aspects of care.[33-35] There is an emphasis on facilitating patients' self-management, self-efficacy, and behavior change, and on training medical professionals in communication skills to help their patients with adherence and the achievement of treatment goals. This approach also works to identify depression, which (as we have seen earlier) can significantly interfere with patient adherence. Research shows that the quality of care achieved by these measures results in documented improvements in outcomes and healthcare cost savings.

The cost-effectiveness of including mental health professionals on healthcare teams is becoming more evident, and many teams benefit greatly.[36,37] In both adult practice and pediatrics,[38-40] this systemic approach successfully addresses primary prevention, disease management, pain and stress management, and screening for mental health challenges such as anxiety and depression. Consultations with psychologists and psychiatrists, for more intensive or specialized behavioral health services and substance use disorders care, are available and integrated into primary care practice.

These models of primary care practice, in whole or in part, are gradually becoming mainstream, supported by policy, public funding, education, private enterprise, and the growing awareness of the need to care for a patient as a whole person. Many resources and ideas for funding opportunities are available from the U.S. Department of Health and Human Services, the National Committee for Quality Assurance, the Commonwealth Fund, and various centers of integrative medicine that implement these models in clinical practice.

Group visits

One of the simplest ways that primary care providers can build new elements of psychosocial care into their practices is with supportive and educational group visits. When multiple patients with similar chronic diseases or other shared health concerns can meet together in a small group, several positive outcomes are likely to result. Because general information needs to be stated once rather than repeated for each patient, more time is available for discussing issues in depth and from a variety of perspectives. Members can bring multiple viewpoints and experiences to the group, allowing the emergence of creative ideas and strategies for solving and coping with health-related problems. The opportunity to interact with others who share similar struggles can contribute to effective coping by showing each participant that there are others "in the same boat" and helping to build their confidence through the processes of social comparison and vicarious experience.[41]

Group visits can be a component of practice in PCMH and other models of chronic care management. Patient groups may be led by a physician or by another member of the healthcare team such as a psychologist, or by both. In all cases, careful thought must be given to the form and function of the group. How many people will comprise the group? Will everyone have the same health issue, and will they be at about the same age and stage in the healthcare process? How will group members be recruited? Will the format be mostly informative, employing a lecture style, or will there be a guided "support-group" type discussion (or some combination of the two)? Will the same person lead the group at each meeting, or will different individuals take responsibility depending upon the topic?

Outcomes associated with such group visits are generally positive. Comprehensive reviews of the research consistently show that glycemic control and blood pressure improve with group visits, and these shared consultations are also associated with a better patient experience, greater self-efficacy, and higher satisfaction, especially among older patients.[42,43] Studies also demonstrate trends toward fewer hospital admissions and overall cost effectiveness associated with shared consultations.[44] Case Study 8.1 provides an example of a group visit in diabetes care.

Case Study 8.1 Group Health Education in Action

Dr. Bailey specializes in diabetes care. Today, she spends about 10 minutes with each of her patients, going over test results and discussing blood glucose management techniques. She must structure her time in each visit carefully so as not to be late for the next appointment. Feelings of guilt arise when one of her patients has questions that she can't take time to answer. Instead, she asks her patient to schedule another appointment to go over these remaining issues. Dr. Zimmer also provides diabetes care, and today he meets with five of his patients at the same time in a group meeting. These patients have all agreed to have others know they are working on management of their diabetes; they are aware that although they may choose to share their personal information in the group, Dr. Zimmer will not disclose anything about them to others. Before the group meeting, he has reviewed all their test results and is prepared to follow up with two of the patients after the meeting for brief one-on-one counseling. The group meeting lasts a bit over 30 minutes, and group members share tips and techniques for managing their blood sugar levels. They discuss the barriers they face in successfully managing their treatment regimens, and they provide support for one another. Dr. Zimmer guides the discussion, shares some advice, and provides encouragement. At the end of the session everyone feels that they have benefited from the meeting.

Technologies in health and healthcare

The proliferation of technologies in many fields over the past decade has been astounding. Automated safety features in newer cars remind us to stay in our lanes, wake us up if we start to doze, and apply the brakes if we fail to do so in time to avoid a crash. In some areas of the country, certain cars even have "driverless" features, allowing the operator to relax and let the vehicle take charge. Automated systems manage electrical grids and financial transactions; sophisticated technologies track goods, allowing them to be shipped in record time. And the significant expansion of technology in medicine, psychology, and behavior change via digital health offers more opportunity than ever for patients to be healthy. Technological developments increase the information available to patients and potentially reduce the costs of medical care. As we will see in this section, healthcare technologies, just like other automated systems, can offer advantages that were barely imagined a decade ago.

The use of technologies in medical care can, of course, have unintended negative consequences. For example, while technologies in health can increase the amount of information available to patients, many people do not know how to sort out the useful from the incorrect, and what to do with the sheer volume of facts. Technologies might also, in theory, lead to better healthcare access for the impoverished and those who live in rural communities. In practice, however, many people may be effectively cut out of the digital revolution in medicine because they have no access to, or cannot afford, high bandwidth internet. Technologies that help physicians improve their diagnoses might tempt some to cut corners in differential diagnosis or in provider-patient communication. Internet-based mental healthcare for complex problems like depression, addictions, and the management of distress in chronic illness might offer mobile support from a mental health professional, but reduce connections to in-person providers, family, and community support.

Definitions of key terms in the digital health sphere

Nearly 100 definitions of digital health have been proposed,[45] and often the terms "digital health," "mobile health (mHealth)," and "eHealth" are used interchangeably, leading to greater uncertainty about their meaning. Digital health involves "the convergence and utilization of digital sciences and technologies for healthcare improvement and the digital transformation of medicine (p. 10)."[46] Many other concepts and terms fall under the broad umbrella of "digital health," including eHealth, telehealth and telemedicine, and mHealth.[47] Here we consider each of these as distinct applications of digital health.

eHealth involves "the use of information and communication technologies for health."[48] The electronic health record was a pioneer in the eHealth realm.[49] However, other examples of eHealth include using the internet to find health information, electronic decision aids, virtual support groups, automated pharmacy systems, and medication packaging technology.

Telehealth is a facet of eHealth and is "the use of telecommunications technology in healthcare delivery, information, and education."[50] The term "telemedicine" is often used synonymously with telehealth[47] but specifically involves the use of technology (phone or video) to deliver medical care at a distance.[51]

mHealth involves use of mobile technologies such as smartphones, mobile applications (apps), and wearable devices to enhance healthcare delivery and improve health behavior change through enhanced connectivity.[46] Thus, in the realm of health behavior change and treatment adherence, mHealth includes smartphone apps to promote adherence using "push notifications" for reminders and logs of past medication taking, as well as many other features. Mobile apps for health behavior change can involve goal setting surrounding diet or exercise, monitoring of health behaviors, and social support by connecting with other app users.

In the following sections, we will separate the different components of digital health—eHealth, telehealth/telemedicine, AI technologies for medical communication, and mHealth—and discuss tools and approaches for behavior change and treatment adherence that are encompassed within each.

eHealth

Various components of eHealth are currently making significant contributions to health and healthcare by vastly increasing the availability of information, decision-making tools, automated systems, and opportunities for communication, problem-solving, and support. Let's examine them here.

Information-seeking and management using the internet and artificial intelligence

The internet can be a valuable source of timely medical information, potentially improving medical decision-making and reducing the isolation and stigma of illness as well as its costs. Additionally, online searching for health information can foster greater patient engagement in health maintenance and care and improve knowledge and decision-making.[52] In one study,[53] 68% of patients reported using online web-based applications after their medical visit to seek further information about their health beyond that given by their provider. These patients reported using the internet to self-diagnose or confirm the diagnosis, learn more about their condition, research various treatments beyond what they were offered, and find other people with similar experience. Sometimes they used it to find another doctor. In this study, looking for information online after the visit was associated with curiosity, worry, a lower level of trust, and greater disappointment in some aspects of their physicians' behavior. As we saw in Chapter 4, patients are often eager for health information, and if their providers do not offer enough to them, they are likely to seek that information themselves. Effective communication of information is essential for patients to understand the reasons for health directives; joint decision-making with their providers depends upon patients being informed.

Some patients search online as a substitute for seeking medical care because insurance premiums, co-payments, and/or deductibles might be unaffordable. Providers might be unavailable, or the desire, time, and opportunity to consult a professional are limited. Online searches and self-diagnoses might also allow an individual to find information to support and maintain their own explanatory model for illness and treatment. For example, a patient who believes that hypertension only occurs when they feel "hyper," tense, or pressured, might find evidence to support nonadherence to medication. Explanatory models affect beliefs about the severity of illness, the appropriateness of treatment, and the consequences of not adhering; some support for nearly every perspective can be found on the internet.[54,55] As we saw in Chapter 7, social influencers and misinformation on social media can affect patients' medical choices. Patients may do "their own research" and be motivated to comply with ideas that are posted by online "friends" instead of those offered by their providers.

Much online health information may be limited in its accuracy, and choosing reliable sources can be challenging. Many health and medical websites are unreliable when evaluated according to the clinical practice guidelines set out by the U.S. Public Health Service. In general, it may be most effective to consult reliable web sources such as university-based medical centers and foundations, as well as online sites such as offered by the National Institutes of Health, the Agency for Healthcare Research and Quality, and clearinghouses such as the American Heart Association.[56,57]

There exists so much online health information (both reliable and unreliable) that patients can be overwhelmed and misled. A patient can misunderstand a crucial point and be drawn to details and explanations that seem intuitively right but are incorrect. This misinformation can then make effective communication between the patient and their provider more difficult. Patients may also be affected by direct-to-patient advertising of pharmaceuticals and are more likely to ask their doctors specifically for medications they saw advertised. Studies suggest that the provider-patient relationship can sometimes become more difficult and tense because of this advertising,[58,59] although most providers report a neutral effect on the quality of their clinical interactions.

As we saw in Chapter 4, understanding health information, particularly about personal risks and medical choices, can be challenging. The internet offers a vast array of health perspectives; without guidance to comprehend, evaluate, manage, and apply them, many patients feel overwhelmed. Particularly in the face of uncertainty about troubling symptoms, some patients ask AI to sort out medical information and help them self-diagnose. They use AI-based tools like OpenAI's ChatGPT, Google Gemini, and Microsoft Bing for medical diagnoses and for help with making healthcare decisions. These tools in their basic forms are free (although there are premium paid versions). They can respond to a patient's questions, render a "diagnosis" in seconds, and offer clear and easy-to-understand explanations which seem, at least to a patient who has limited medical knowledge and experience, reasonable and accurate.

An AI tool might be quite helpful for learning about a specific condition, such as its causes, symptoms, likely prognosis, and usual treatments. An AI tool can provide information about a medication such as its uses and side effects. Ideally AI tools can be used to summarize information from reliable websites, and sources that involve published medical and scientific studies. Explanations can be made in nonmedical (layperson) terms, and patients can use AI tools to develop lists of questions to ask their providers.

For several reasons, however, people might do better *not* asking an AI tool for a diagnosis. First, in their present form, AIs synthesize web information that could be limited, skewed, incorrect, outdated, or even purposefully misinformative. Also, the weighting of information could be suboptimal, such that a cosmetics company influencer could be given the same weight in a medical decision as the National Academy of Medicine. Finally, AIs do not take into account the individuality of the patient, their medical and family history, lifestyle, risk factors, and so on, which would be necessary for generating accurate medical advice.

Automated healthcare systems and health information technology

Increasingly, people want (or even expect) the achievement of their healthcare needs to be convenient. Automated systems for making appointments and checking test results, along with downloadable forms that patients can access and complete prior to their appointments, increase efficiency and are generally well received by patients.[60,61] Automated and semi-automated systems also reduce errors, such as when online prescription systems decrease mistakes in dosage amounts or drug names.[62] These systems can make filling prescriptions more accurate and can make adherence easier for patients by providing them with information and offering electronic refill reminders.

Patients also tend to be more open to disclosing, and less influenced by social desirability pressures, when responding to a computerized assessment than when interacting in person or over the phone. This is particularly true if the shared information is embarrassing or portrays them in a poor light. A patient might feel uncomfortable describing sexual functioning or even food consumption to another person but may respond comfortably to a computerized assessment; decreased anxiety and embarrassment can produce more accurate recall and greater honesty in reporting.

Technology can also be used to help reconcile the patient's vocabulary with that of the practitioner, which can be quite different when the same medical issue is described.[63] One effort to create an open access consumer health vocabulary list is the Biomedical Informatics Center at George Washington University. Another resource for patients is https://medlineplus.gov/, provided by the National Library of Medicine. There has been considerable growth and change in eHealth technology systems for patient vocabulary; some of the more recent efforts involve natural language processing.[64]

Automated systems can change the interaction between patients and the healthcare team, but they do not reduce its importance. A patient who accesses laboratory results online will likely still need to discuss them with their clinician. Some patients may prefer not to access certain types of test results (e.g., regarding a serious illness or involving complicated data),[65] instead preferring to have their clinician deliver this information. Testing for HIV, for example, is often done using a rapid format so that patients can learn their results and be counseled about them during the same visit.[66]

Automated systems have some potential drawbacks as well. Patients might receive information that is not useful to them, become confused,[67] or even believe, erroneously, that information delivered electronically is always reliable and useful.[68] Thus, some guidance will likely be needed before most patients will be able to appropriately use automated systems.

Decision aids

In Chapter 4, we discussed decision-making aids that can help patients understand options, benefits, and risks related to their medical conditions and possible treatments. Some of these aids require simple materials (e.g., paper and pen, or a decision board); many others rely on more sophisticated technology to engage the patient.

Videos can provide patients with information and a variety of perspectives, particularly when time limitations in the medical encounter prohibit a thorough discussion.[69] For example, a brief (22-minute) video on prostate-specific antigen (PSA) screening provides balanced information on the test and discusses why one would or would not want to have it. The video includes a testimonial from a physician who regularly undergoes PSA screening and another from a physician who chooses not to do so.[70] Patients who viewed the video were better informed about PSA screening, more satisfied with the information they received, and more interested in collaborative decision-making than were those who did not see the video.[71] Interestingly, only 60% of patients who viewed the video chose screening, compared with 98% of those who did not view it.

Some internet-based decision aids are interactive, allowing patients to control the ordering of information they acquire and select additional information on particular subtopics. They can view educational videos, hear from people who face similar choices, and join support or discussion groups—options similar to those of in-person group visits.[72] For some medical choices, patients might also access information about the likelihood of various outcomes. Studies suggest that with these tools, patients become more actively involved in making medical decisions, feel less decisional conflict, and are more satisfied than when they simply consult with their physicians.[73,74] Internet-based consumer health-decision support tools tend to be even better than simple audiovisual presentations; their flexibility allows patients at varying levels of knowledge to access the type of information best for them.

Virtual support groups

Support groups and peer communities for people with shared health concerns are not new, although the "virtual" or "online" variety has more recently gained popularity. Systematic evaluation of these "online health communities" can be difficult because they are often embedded in more complex systems and have seldom been subjected to rigorous empirical study. Virtual support groups can take many forms: online discussion groups and chat rooms, newsgroups, email lists, and voice bulletin board systems. This variability and the continually developing technology make research in this area challenging. Individuals who have grown up with, or adapted well to, electronic communication tend to be most comfortable with online approaches; this suggests increasing popularity and usefulness of these methods in the healthcare context over time. One detailed analysis of computer-mediated support groups indicated a generally positive relationship between virtual social support and well-being.[75] However, there is less evidence of physical health improvements related to participation in online social support groups,[76] and patient preferences may drive individual participation in virtual support groups.[77] Particularly in situations where in-person interactions are not possible (e.g., during the COVID-19 pandemic), virtual interactions are crucial.[78] Ultimately, additional research attention needs to focus on evaluating online support groups in medical care; they are becoming ubiquitous, and a better understanding of them is essential.

Medication packaging technology

Some of the simplest technological interventions are aimed at improving patient adherence using innovations like a special device that records when a medication bottle is opened. This type of tracking system has been available for many years and has been shown to improve adherence rates somewhat, although not dramatically.[79] One study of patients with hypertension found that combining the use of these containers with home blood pressure testing devices and cards on which to record blood pressure resulted in nearly 100% adherence over 12 weeks.[80] This is particularly impressive because patients were unaware of the adherence monitoring, but believed they were simply evaluating new products for those with high blood pressure.

Technologies for medical communication and medical care

Not very long ago, patients had to get themselves to the doctor. Face-to-face conversations took place as physicians conducted physical exams and assessed the appearance of their patients in the context of various vital signs and important metrics such as temperature, heart rate, blood pressure, respiration rate, and oxygen saturation. If the patient complained of a skin rash, it needed to be examined in person. Emotional concerns, while possible to discuss over the phone, were often better dealt with in the context of a warm personal conversation. Of course, getting to the doctor could be inconvenient and, for some, it was quite difficult or even impossible.

So much has changed in the delivery of healthcare in the past decade. A patient can now step right outside their workplace for a few minutes and, using their smartphone, have a video visit with a provider. This provider might never have met and examined the patient in person, but nevertheless knows a great deal about them because their electronic medical record is populated with the results of blood tests and scans, previous medical visit notes, and specialty consultation reports. Photos, such as of the patient's skin rash, might be there too, uploaded by the patient for the provider to review. Some additional digital metrics (such as sleep and exercise parameters) might also be available from wearable medical devices. Despite even great physical distance between them, the patient and provider can have effective conversations with many symptoms reviewed and many questions asked and answered. These digital health elements offer the patient the best chance for comprehensive, cost-effective healthcare.

Telehealth and telemedicine

Telemedicine allows patients to receive medical care at their convenience through remote methods. Telemedicine allows healthcare to be accessible to more patients, while minimizing the transmission of infectious diseases.[81]

The use of telemedicine has increased rapidly in recent years, especially since the COVID-19 pandemic.[82] According to the CDC, in 2021, 37% of adults in the United States had used telemedicine in the past 12 months.[51]

Telemedicine and the provider-patient relationship, health behavior, and treatment adherence
Telemedicine and other technologies have great potential to improve the quality of communication and medical care outcomes, build trust in provider-patient relationships, help with decision-making, and foster health behavior change and treatment adherence.

Acceptance of virtual medical visits (also called e-visits, video visits, telehealth visits, and telemedicine visits) is growing significantly. In one study, 36% of patients said they prefer a virtual medical visit to an in-person visit.[83] Patients are quite satisfied with the quality of the care they receive from e-visits,[84] as well as with the ease, convenience, lack of travel required, low cost, and communication quality of telemedicine visits. As telemedicine usage increases, it is important that we determine whether and how provider-patient communication differs in telemedicine compared to in-person visits. One study compared oncology patients' telehealth and in-person visits during the COVID-19 pandemic; most patients found their providers communicated as well during telehealth as they did during in-person visits.[85] Factors affecting satisfaction with telemedicine include provider-patient communication,[86] rapport-building, information giving, and guidance.[87]

Virtual medical visits and mobile healthcare technologies can significantly improve healthcare access, especially for rural populations and those lacking transportation, as well as for busy people who cannot get to the clinic. Mobile education programs can build trust and improve physician-patient communication.[88] Telemedicine can be helpful for long-term care of chronic conditions; one review of 34 interventions showed significant improvements in chronic disease self-management and adherence.[89] When patients interact with their providers by emails and texts, and in virtual visits, they remain in their own environments; the sense of power conveyed by a provider in the clinic or hospital environment may be somewhat reduced, and a more equal and collaborative relationship fostered.

Limitations of telemedicine
In the context of electronic communication, some patients may feel less connected to their provider and more concerned about their providers'

attentiveness.[90] The opportunity for both parties to communicate information through nonverbal and vocal channels may be reduced by limited or poor internet connections and slower speeds. Virtual medical visits can also highlight disparities in care for some patients who may have limited access to broadband internet and/or few opportunities for privacy. Patients who have never used telemedicine or use the internet infrequently might be resistant to it.[91] Certain populations, such as older patients,[92] may be uncomfortable with telemedicine. Providers and their patients might diverge considerably in their comfort with technology, highlighting age, generational, and experiential differences between them. Demaryius and Dr. Hathaway demonstrate this challenge well in Case Study 8.2.

Case Study 8.2 A Different Type of Tech Issue

Dr. Fred Hathaway is just a few years short of retirement, but he still loves his job as a primary care doctor. He is, by all accounts, an excellent diagnostician with decades of experience in patient care. He keeps up with all the latest relevant research and puts considerable time and effort into giving his patients the best possible treatments. But when he must do remote visits, Dr. Hathaway cannot seem to work Zoom for anything!

Many of Dr. Hathaway's patients are older, and they like the electronic medical record even less than he does. Some are suspicious of the technology, so Dr. Hathaway always prints out instructions and tells them to call the office whenever they have questions.

Demaryius Jackson is in his early 20s and one of Dr. Hathaway's younger patients. He is surprised when Dr. Hathaway calls him on the telephone to discuss the questions he had sent in an email. Whenever a patient emails him, Dr. Hathaway makes it a point to personally call the patient back. He likes talking with patients, and he is a good communicator and teacher.

This approach seems antiquated to Demaryius, especially when Dr. Hathaway asks him to "grab a pencil and paper" to write something down. Like most young adults, Demaryius thrives on technology and uses it effectively to accomplish his professional and personal goals. He wishes he had a tech-savvy physician and thinks that despite Dr. Hathaway's exceptional medical skills and experience, he is "just a bit clueless."

Although innovative technology has great potential to improve communication and medical care outcomes, patients and physicians might differ from each other "culturally" in their embrace of and comfort with that technology and in their responses to the opportunities, advantages, and challenges of digital medicine. Digital platforms (such as for email exchanges, test results, and medical record entries) can facilitate provider-patient communication, but only to the extent that both parties are comfortable with these technologies and can learn to use them effectively. A match in perspectives and preferences might increase providers' and patients' comfort with each other and reduce the chances of misunderstanding. If such a match cannot be achieved, a discussion about it might still be useful. Some health systems might offer patients various choices, including telephone, video or in-person visits, and various options for communication.

Only a few years ago, the EMR was resisted by many physicians and patients, who disliked having a computer in the exam room. Many patients were distressed that their physician consulted a computer for information and entered data during the medical visit, devoting attention to a keyboard and screen instead of connecting interpersonally with them. With appropriate sight lines and face-to-face attention, acceptance has increased and the value of the EMR to safety and outcomes has been recognized.

Some of the most useful features of digital health communications involve their ability to change quickly, allowing them to offer individually tailored content that can be regularly updated.[93,94] Interactive media forms are powerful because of their flexibility, and some patients find the novelty of these media to be attractive and compelling.[95] Patients can seek out interactive technologies and use them entirely on their own, without their medical professionals. Noom is one currently popular example of a method for managing nutrition and healthy weight. Some technologies involve clinicians employed by the app, such as BetterHelp, which enables individuals to quickly connect with licensed therapists via video conferencing, phone calls, live chats, or text messaging. In both of these examples, technology enables people to surmount barriers to care and to more easily access the assistance they need.

Although constantly changing technology can be difficult for some who have limited experience, the capability to regularly update and individualize health related content is a major strength of eHealth communications.[96,97] Research suggests that this flexibility can positively influence a wide range of health-related outcomes.[98–100]

Artificial intelligence in patient care

In the new world of AI, which is changing almost daily as we write this, there might be an important role for Large Language Model (LLM) chatbots in helping physicians to better serve the needs of their patients. Here, we consider a few important and intriguing issues.

There is some evidence that AI chatbots can be helpful in giving patients medical advice. One cross-sectional study evaluated the quality of ophthalmology advice generated by a chatbot (ChatGPT) compared with advice written by an ophthalmologist.[101] In this study, ophthalmologists' responses to questions posted in an online medical forum were judged by eight board certified ophthalmologists who compared them with chatbot responses on several criteria: the presence of incorrect information, agreement with medically accepted answers, likelihood to cause harm, and the potential extent of any harm. Results showed that judges were correct in distinguishing AI responses from human ones 61.3% of the time. They judged the quality of the chatbot responses to be as good as the human answers: the likelihood of containing incorrect or inappropriate material was no different, and there was also no difference in the likelihood of harm from the replies offered. Thus, a chatbot appeared to respond as accurately as did ophthalmologists to questions about eye health. This study also found that evaluators preferred the chatbot responses to physicians' responses in 78.6% of the cases. In terms of empathy, 4.6% of physician replies were rated as empathic; 45.1% of the chatbot responses were rated as empathic.

AI can help to free up time for physicians in the medical visit, allowing them more opportunity to connect with their patients on an interpersonal level. Many physicians complain about the significant time and attention needed for paperwork, including entering data into patients' medical records and writing case notes. An AI digital scribe is fully automated,[102] and serves as a valuable assistant that can take over these tasks. It can record real time doctor-patient consultations, allow the physician to converse without note-taking, generate notes for treatment and billing, and incorporate new findings with the existing medical record. Research is supporting the accuracy and efficiency of AI scribes, as well as their value in improving doctor-patient relationships and physicians' quality of life.

In Chapter 3, we examined the central importance of bedside manner and empathy in caring for patients. In the stressful, fast-paced job of a physician, however, consistently offering empathic responses might be a tall order. Furthermore, doctors, like people in general, vary in their empathic abilities; some find it easier than others to choose just the right words to say.

Can a chatbot help improve a doctor's bedside manner, or augment the doctor's interpersonal care? *Should it* be allowed to do so? In considering these questions, let's first imagine that in our analysis we substitute different words for "chatbot": "nurse practitioner," "physician's assistant," or the "medical team therapist." The notion of a member of the medical team fulfilling an important interpersonal function in caring for patients seems perfectly acceptable, even desirable. In high-volume medical practices and health delivery systems, physician-extenders are quite common. They typically have more time to chat with the patient, get to know them better than the physician does, learn about their concerns, and even explore and troubleshoot their adherence challenges. The involvement of additional, caring (human) health professionals in medical care delivery probably seems like an encouraging step toward humanizing healthcare.

But what if the element that humanizes interactions is, in fact, not human? In one study, researchers selected 200 anonymous medical questions posted in 2022 to Reddit r/AskDocs that had been answered online by anonymous volunteer physicians with verified credentials.[103] The researchers then posed the same questions verbatim to ChatGPT. A team of physicians compared the responses (with the identity of the respondent, human doctor or chatbot, hidden). The results showed that (consistent with findings from the ophthalmology study described earlier) evaluators preferred the chatbot's responses to the real doctor's responses 80% of the time. The chatbot responses were longer than those of the real physician (averaging 180 versus 52 words) and were ranked higher in quality of information. The chatbot responses were also kinder; 45% were rated as empathic or very empathic, compared with only 5% of the physicians' responses.

Might chatbots be used by physicians to help them compose responses to their patients' emails? Or help physicians by generating some nice ideas of something to say to the patient when greeting them? Can an AI teach a physician to have better bedside manner by simply modeling things to say? (See Case Study 8.3 for an example.) Might physicians learn the language of empathy from an AI, just as one might learn a foreign language from an online language program? Should doctors use chatbots to improve their bedside manner? Soon, the answer to these questions will likely be "yes."

> **Case Study 8.3 Example of AI Compared to Human Physician Communication**
>
> Here we consider some interesting differences between what a busy, exhausted doctor might be inclined to say, and an abbreviated version of what we think an AI might suggest for a more sensitive, empathic, helpful response.
> *Scenario 1.* The patient says: "I am feeling better about my diagnosis. I have thought about it a lot and I am ready to start the next step in my treatment." Here are potential responses from the tired doctor and from the (not tired) AI.
> From the doctor: "Great. Go by the lab and get this bloodwork done, then take this medication as prescribed and I will see you in a month."
> From the AI: "I am heartened to learn that you are feeling better about your diagnosis; this is excellent news. So, our next steps are the following: some bloodwork at the lab which I have ordered for you, and some medication that you can pick up at the pharmacy. I would like you to start taking it as soon as possible. As always, please let me know if you have any questions, and I look forward to seeing you in one month."
> *Scenario 2.* The patient wants to investigate diet and holistic alternative medicine/herbal treatments for her high blood pressure. Here are potential responses from the doctor, who is frankly tired of hearing about herbal treatments, and the AI, which does not mind at all.
> From the doctor: "You have to take your treatments as prescribed; alternative medicine can be dangerous."
> From the AI: "I can see that you still have some questions or concerns about the medication we prescribed. I would like us to talk about the medicine and explore the choices you have available to you. Frankly, we

> need to make sure that your blood pressure is well controlled so that we can lower your risk of stroke; a stroke is a significant danger without medication."

Can AI help with medical diagnosis?

Often, when we think of AI, we imagine machines that can take in information, reason, and problem-solve like humans; as of this writing, this has not yet been achieved. Currently available is "general AI"—Large Language Models that involve artificial neural networks for general purpose language generation and processing. More specifically in medicine, what is most valuable and available now is "narrow AI," in which various AI technologies perform specific diagnostic tasks, particularly in specialties such as radiology, pathology, ophthalmology, and cardiology.[104] Narrow AI is also showing promise in emergency room diagnosis[105] and researchers expect that AI might soon contribute to some aspects of chronic disease management and clinical decision-making.[106]

The progress of AI in the diagnostic work typically done by primary care physicians has been considerably slower. ChatGPT does not deal well with the complexity of human factors associated with decision-making in primary care. In Fall 2023, ChatGPT failed to pass the UK's National Primary Care examinations (the test required to become a general practitioner), suggesting that AI cannot (yet) deal with diagnostic complexities as well as a human physician can.[107] Sometimes ChatGPT has been found to offer extended explanations stated in an authoritative way despite being inaccurate. This is a phenomenon known as "hallucination," and nonexperts often cannot identify the mistakes. (In the legal world, an attorney was found to have submitted an LLM-generated court brief citing a previous case that actually did not exist.)[108] An AI source trained on a general database, such as the entire World Wide Web, is much more likely to offer incorrect medical results compared with one trained on a medical research database such as the National Library of Medicine, which compiles all published medical research.

Physicians can, with care, effectively use LLM to provide clinical support, not just in diagnosis but in a broad range of ways.[109] AI is good at brainstorming, which could be invaluable when dealing with a puzzling diagnosis as an adjunct to the physician's own research, clinical reasoning, and input from colleagues. AI can help the physician consider conditions they might not have seen since medical school (or ever). Providers can cross-check scientific references to be sure they are real and remain aware that AI models have a bias to agree with everything they are told. Ideally, physicians can think of AI as another tool or member of the team (with flaws).

How do physicians and patients feel about AI?

Years ago, physicians in practice were resistant to the notion of physician extenders like physician assistants, and worried that patients would feel slighted, the extenders would give bad information to patients, and they might be worse (or better) than the physician at connecting with and educating patients. Patients' acceptance of physician extenders and the team approach is now generally quite high;[110-112] at the head of their teams, physicians still make the final decisions and control the content of care offered by extenders. In a similar way, at the present time some physicians might be open to a limited role of AI in their medical practice; many do remain skeptical, however.[113]

Despite generally positive attitudes toward AI in medicine, patients are *not* eager to replace their physicians with chatbots. In a 2019 study,[114] many patients were uncomfortable with the idea of care provided by an AI, even one that "out-performs human doctors" because they believe their medical needs are unique and cannot be adequately addressed by algorithms. When healthcare was described as provided by AI rather than by a human provider, patients were less likely to choose to utilize the service and wanted to pay less for it. They also preferred having a human provider perform the service even if that meant there would be a greater risk of an inaccurate diagnosis or a complication. A 2023 Pew Research Center survey found that 60% of patients felt uncomfortable with the idea of their medical provider using AI to assist in arriving at a diagnosis or recommend treatment. Patients expressed concern that LLM models can appear confident even when they are not accurate. Some people accepted AI involvement only if the physician remained in charge of the ultimate care decisions.[115] The recent appearance of AI on the landscape of medical training is also raising some important questions. Students are expected to experience a rapid increase in medical knowledge, which might double many times during their four years of medical school. Given this expectation, what might be the best role for AI during their residency training and in their future practices? How can they use AI to reduce errors, increase their productivity, replace repetitive tasks, and assist in workflow? How can they use it to make better diagnoses, choose better treatments, and communicate better with their patients? How is their medical education preparing them? These are important questions, and the research on them is presently sparse. One study reviewed 39 research articles to determine plans by medical schools for incorporating AI into the medical curriculum; most of the 39 articles stated the need for more research, but few offered any findings, plans, or solutions.[116]

Use with caution

AI has tremendous potential to change medical practice, improve communication and clinical decision-making, increase healthcare quality, and reduce costs. But there is a call to temper enthusiasm. Caution should be exercised in using AI, according to the 2023 guidelines of the World Health Organization, which recommended rigorous oversight to ensure that AI in healthcare is being used in safe, effective, and ethical ways.[117]

AI systems are still largely untested in healthcare, and these technologies might carry with them problems that have not yet been anticipated. Because there is currently little oversight for machine learning applications in medicine and few guidelines regarding standards of practice, legal liabilities may be significant. AI systems could generate and disseminate highly convincing health disinformation that is difficult for the public, and sometimes even professionals, to identify as inaccurate and misleading. There are concerns about privacy. LLMs are typically trained on data for which consent has not been given. AI tools use patients' personal data that might be quite sensitive and could be used to harm them; most LLM training does not comply with the Health Insurance Portability and Accountability Act (HIPAA). Google is pilot-testing an LLM called Med-PaLM 2, which is specifically developed for healthcare applications and has more safeguards in place.[118]

Mobile health (mHealth) technologies for healthcare and treatment adherence

The use of mHealth tools to promote health behavior and patient adherence is changing healthcare.[119] Mobile applications for managing disease and altering health habits are ubiquitous. Nearly 90% of U.S. mobile phone owners have a smartphone,[120] and more than 350,000 healthcare apps are available across the globe.[121]

It is important to consider psychological factors related to mHealth use and how they can improve adherence and health behavior change. Apps can encourage patients with chronic diseases to be actively involved in their care.[122] Some apps use rewards to encourage and motivate users[123] and thereby change health attitudes and behaviors. Others use encouraging motivational communication to improve chronic illness self-management.[124] One study followed hypertensive patients who used a wireless blood pressure self-monitoring mobile phone that incorporated reminders, an educational mobile app, and a web-based disease management program. Patients experiencing this intervention were more motivated to increase their health-related activation and achieved greater reductions in blood pressure and cigarette use than did those without the intervention.[125]

Mobile apps can also offer support networks and help with adherence and behavior change. For example, apps for physical activity often have a network of users comparing data (e.g., completion times, distances, and speeds for activities such as runs, walks, and cycling). Users can create customized training plans, earn points, and achieve recognition in the app for meeting various challenges. Other apps help users stick to eating and exercise plans by giving them an easy food diary to complete on the app and integrating wearable devices that track exercise; some apps encourage positive feedback from peers by posting users' progress to the app community. Apps designed to improve adherence may remind patients to take their medication and allow a preselected support group to access the patient's medication-taking history. Several studies have integrated individuals' social networks into mobile health apps. For example, researchers designed a mobile app for diabetes patients that incorporated peer support through a discussion forum.[126] Others developed an app involving networking with peers to promote physical activity in older cancer survivors.[127]

More mHealth options are becoming available all the time. One review identified over 150 medication adherence apps that medical providers can recommend to their patients.[128] These apps variously incorporate reminders, medication-taking history, information about the medication, and reminders about healthy lifestyle and medical appointments. A systematic review of 11 studies of mobile adherence apps showed that they increased adherence and had high user satisfaction.[129]

Bluetooth-connected smart pill bottles can also be activated with cell phone apps using sounds and lights to remind patients to take their medications. (These are more sophisticated than the simple pill bottle trackers described earlier.) These apps also track medication taken, and offer alarm notifications to medical providers, caregivers, or loved ones regarding missed doses.[130] "Digital pills" are even available to promote patient adherence through automatic collection of information about medication ingestion.[131,132] Ethical and privacy concerns are, of course, paramount in the use of these and other data collection approaches.

Studies of electronic reminder devices for medication show that they are modestly successful at improving adherence; there is limited evidence, however, that they improve clinical outcomes.[133] When adherence involves complex behaviors, such as multiple medications in antiretroviral therapy for HIV, results tend to be mixed. When the behavior required is less complicated (e.g., eye drops for glaucoma; daily asthma medications; oral contraceptives), electronic reminders tend to be more effective.[134-136]

Many websites can help patients with their healthcare regimens, although most focus on medication adherence. Some of these include the FDA's Safe Use Initiative, and the National Association of Community Health Centers' blood pressure monitoring guides. Many others are aimed at helping health professionals more effectively support their patients' adherence. The Agency for Healthcare Research and Quality has tools to assess health literacy and to help with medication therapy management; Million Hearts (as part of the Centers for Disease Control and Prevention) provides a list of tools for providers to support their patients' adherence. The United States Pharmacopeia has a library of 81 medicine descriptions, instructions, and warnings along with pictograms of each, which can be quite useful when working with patients who are low in health literacy or whose first language is not English. These resources can help patients and clinicians improve some of the skills that are so important to achieving medication adherence.

How mHealth tools support habits and behavior change

As we saw in Chapter 6, success at behavior change depends upon the development and maintenance of habits. How well an individual adheres to a medication schedule, for example, will depend upon principles such as associative learning (e.g., pairing a medication dose with a habitual behavior, such as teeth-brushing, to serve as a reminder). Operant reinforcement (whether from oneself, another person, or an app) further strengthens the habit. As we have seen earlier, in the behavioral management of one or more chronic medical conditions, scheduling of multiple medications can become challenging especially when doses and timing are adjusted; recent developments in technologies have made these tasks easier. Apps can not only organize and provide reminders for medications, but they can also order refills and schedule the delivery of prescriptions. Automated text messaging can provide helpful reminders in the care of a broad range of illnesses.[137] For those who are motivated and have decided to make certain behavioral changes, technologies can help with self-management. Some complex systems can even support cognitive behavior modification using self-monitoring, self-evaluation, and self-reinforcement for behavior change.[138,139]

It is important to keep in mind, however, that no matter how nimble and entertaining an app might be, the achievement of long-term change requires the individual to commit to goal-directed behavior.[140] A sedentary individual might choose to be helped by an app, or might decide to work with a trusted health professional or a supportive coach or friend—but they must *want* to change. Whatever choice is made, behavior change requires that the individual thinks ahead, has goals, and specifies the behaviors necessary to achieve those goals. They need to define endpoints and plan out contingencies, try to predict problems, use environmental behavioral cueing, and incorporate aids to memory and self-monitoring. For patients who can become comfortable with new technologies, like Jalisa in Case Study 8.4, apps can be very helpful with all these steps.

Case Study 8.4 Using a Digital App to Self-Monitor Eating Behavior and Exercise

Jalisa has always been quite skeptical of smartphone fitness apps and other digital tools for detailed self-monitoring. For years, she used her own homemade charts to keep track of her medication and physical therapy exercises; small check marks on a pad of paper were enough reward for her. The detail available with electronic methods seemed excessive, so when she did eventually try a digital app, she turned off all the many tracking and notification options available. She focused on the two health behaviors that seemed to have the greatest impact on her life and health: recording daily exercise and keeping track of her intake of junk food. Jalisa most wanted to stop her mindless snacking.

Monitoring our behavior can help to change it simply through the process of self-awareness; studies demonstrate that the form or level of detail of the self-monitoring is less important than consistent, daily recording. Jalisa used to think that compulsively documenting every morsel of food eaten and every physical activity was an unnecessary distraction in her life. Recently, though, she has come to see some value in keeping track of her two most problematic health behaviors—sitting too much and mindlessly consuming bags of corn chips.

The app that Jalisa chose is a simple one. When she wants to munch on crunchy corn chips, she counts out a serving for herself and records the number of chips and their total calories, so she can determine how much of her daily nutritional intake is going to junk food. Jalisa is proud of herself for taking control of her behavior.

The app has multiple components available that might help Jalisa with her motivation. She decided to allow the app to send her some notifications including reminders to take daily vitamins and to get up and move around each hour. The app offers her suggestions for a movement activity (such as links to an online yoga or dance class), as well as alternatives to snack food, such as a serving of nuts instead of chips. After a few weeks, Jalisa finds that being mindful and paying attention to what she is eating is becoming more of a habit. She also does some exercise every day, partly because she wants to record something in her app. She might not feel much like walking, but she experiences a sense of accomplishment seeing her time and exercise intensity tracked. Jalisa also connects to her close friends and family on the app; when she exercises, her chosen "circle" can post encouraging comments, and she can do the same for them. It helps Jalisa to know that her loved ones are virtually cheering her on as she makes exercise a daily habit.

Digital apps for behavior change do tend to be helpful. This is true partly because people who use them typically *want* to change; they have already solved one of the greatest challenges, motivation. There is no app that could get Jalisa going if she had zero motivation, but her app can

> help build on even a flicker of it. Her app can also help fine-tune her self-monitoring, remind her of the choices that she makes every day, reward her actions, and prompt mindfulness. Many apps can be entertaining, educational, and problem-solving; some offer explicit reinforcements for good choices (e.g., congratulations for choosing almonds for a snack or virtual celebrations for hitting a step or heart rate goal). Jalisa used to think that apps like this were unnecessary at best, and annoying at worst. But as better eating and exercise have become more of a challenge in her busy day, and the apps have gotten more personalized, Jalisa finds the technology is very useful to her.

Summary

In Chapter 8, we examine the importance of healthcare teams in providing direction and support for patients' health behavior change and treatment adherence. We examine models of integrated care for the patient as a whole person in the Patient-Centered Medical Home, the Chronic Care Model, the Collaborative Care Model, and the Primary Care Behavioral Health model. These integrated and blended approaches to primary care practice incorporate behavioral health and mental healthcare into primary care medicine; psychologists and other licensed mental health professionals serve as members of the primary healthcare team. In this chapter, we examine tools and options for practice, and see the many ways in which integrated care, with an emphasis on a team-based approach, is fast becoming a force in medicine. In Chapter 8, we offer a detailed analysis of the expanding role of and options for digital technologies in medicine, psychology, and behavior change. We examine the ubiquity of medical information available to patients through web searches, and patients' efforts to understand their medical conditions, interpret information offered to them, and even diagnose their own conditions by using AI-based tools. In this chapter we examine the role of mobile technologies that improve access to and communication with health professionals, as well as the benefits and challenges of virtual medical visits, telehealth, and other technologies in (and in support of) medical interactions. We consider the potential role of AI in patient care, particularly in helping providers improve their bedside manner and, sometimes, their diagnostic skills. We survey new technological aids to health behavior change and adherence, including apps for behavioral self-management.

Tools for instruction and self-study

Learning objectives

By the end of this chapter, readers should be able to

1. Explain the potential benefits a patient can incur from having a healthcare team.
2. Discuss the role of a psychologist on the healthcare team.
3. Identify the components of the Chronic Care Model, and describe various elements of integrated primary care practice.
4. Explain the challenges of seeking health information online.
5. Compare and contrast the concepts of eHealth, telehealth, and mHealth.
6. Explain how AI can play a role in doctor-patient communication.
7. Discuss examples of how mHealth tools can facilitate adherence and health behavior change.

Review questions

1. Briefly, define what is meant by "healthcare team." What are ideal characteristics for a team? What might be an ideal size and composition of the team?
2. What is the purpose of pre-visit counseling?
3. Describe the role of behavioral medicine and mental healthcare in the various models of primary care practice. What important patient care challenges are addressed?
4. What is a Patient-Centered Medical Home and what advantage might it provide in patient care?
5. What are two benefits of group medical education visits?
6. What are some advantages and disadvantages of direct-to-consumer advertising of pharmaceutical medications and medical devices and procedures?

7. In terms of empathic communication with patients, how do physicians and AI chatbots compare?

Prompts for discussion and further study

1. Can doctors be trained to communicate as well as a chatbot?
2. Should physicians rely on chatbots to educate their patients, or to empathize with and be kind to their patients?
3. What are some of the benefits of digital apps to help monitor health behaviors? What are some potential costs?

Suggested reading

1. Hunter CL, Goodie JL, Oordt MS, Dobmeyer AC. *Integrated Behavioral Health in Primary Care: Step-by-Step Guidance for Assessment and Intervention.* 3rd ed. American Psychological Association; 2024.
2. Dobmeyer AC. *Psychological Treatment of Medical Patients in Integrated Primary Care.* American Psychological Association; 2017.
3. Lee P, Goldberg C, Kohane I. *The AI Revolution in Medicine: GPT-4 and Beyond.* Pearson; 2023.
4. Topol E. *Deep Medicine: How Artificial Intelligence Can Make Healthcare Human Again.* Basic Books; 2019.
5. Topol E. *The Patient Will See You Now: The Future of Medicine Is in Your Hands.* Basic Books; 2015.

References

1. Konrad TR, Link CL, Shackelton RJ, et al. It's about time: physicians' perceptions of time constraints in primary care medical practice in three national healthcare systems. *Med Care.* 2010; 48(2): pp. 95–100. doi: 10.1097/MLR.0b013e3181c12e6a.
2. Bodenheimer T, Laing BY. The teamlet model of primary care. *Ann Fam Med.* 2007; 5(5): pp. 457–461.
3. Baldwin DC. *The role of interdisciplinary education and teamwork in primary care and health care reform.* Rockville, MD: Health Resources and Services Administration, Bureau of Health Professions; 1994.
4. Bogden PE, Abbott RD, Williamson P, Onopa JK, Koontz LM. Comparing standard care with a physician and pharmacist team approach for uncontrolled hypertension. *J Gen Intern Med.* 1998; 13(11): pp. 740–745.

5. Grumbach K, Bodenheimer T. Can health care teams improve primary care practice? *JAMA*. 2004; 291(10): pp. 1246–1251.
6. Kottke TE, Brekke ML, Solberg LI. Making "time" for preventive services. *Mayo Clin Proc*. 1993; 68(8): pp. 785–791.
7. Wagner EH. The role of patient care teams in chronic disease management. *BMJ*. 2000; 320(7234): pp. 569–572.
8. Starfield B. *Primary Care: Concept, Evaluation, and Policy*. New York: Oxford University Press; 1992.
9. Foy R, Hempel S, Rubenstein L, et al. Meta-analysis: effect of interactive communication between collaborating primary care physicians and specialists. *Ann Intern Med*. 2010; 152(4): pp. 247–58. doi: 10.7326/0003-4819-152-4-201002160-00010
10. Schmutz JB, Meier LL, Manser T. How effective is teamwork really? The relationship between teamwork and performance in healthcare teams: a systematic review and meta-analysis. *BMJ Open*. 2019; 9(9): e028280. doi: 10.1136/bmjopen-2018-028280
11. Hoff T, Prout K, Carabetta S. How teams impact patient satisfaction: a review of the empirical literature. *Health Care Manage Rev*. 2021; 46(1): pp. 75–85. doi: 10.1097/HMR.0000000000000234
12. Donchin Y, Gopher D, Olin M, et al. A look into the nature and causes of human errors in the intensive care unit. *Crit Care Med*. 1995; 23(2): pp. 294–300.
13. Cohen SG, Bailey DE. What makes teams work: group effectiveness research from the shop floor to the executive suite. *J Manag*. 1997; 23(3): pp. 239–290.
14. Starfield B. *Primary Care: Balancing Health Needs, Services, and Technology*. New York: Oxford University Press; 1998.
15. Horrocks S, Anderson E, Salisbury C. Systematic review of whether nurse practitioners working in primary care can provide equivalent care to doctors. *BMJ*. 2002; 324(7341): pp. 819–823.
16. Lencioni PM. Make your values mean something. *Harv Bus Rev*. 2002; 80(7): pp. 113–117, 126.
17. Haas LJ, Glazer K, Houchins J, Terry S. Improving the effectiveness of the medical visit: a brief visit-structuring workshop changes patients' perceptions of primary care visits. *Patient Educ Couns*. 2006; 62(3): pp. 374–378.
18. Baker LH, O'Connell D, Platt FW. "What else?" Setting the agenda for the clinical interview. *Ann Intern Med*. 2005; 143(10): pp. 766–770.
19. Rodriguez HP, Anastario MP, Frankel RM, et al. Can teaching agenda-setting skills to physicians improve clinical interaction quality? A controlled intervention. *BMC Medical Education*. 2008; 8: p. 3.
20. Macharia WM, Leon G, Rowe BH, Stephenson BJ, Haynes RB. An overview of interventions to improve compliance with appointment keeping for medical services. *JAMA*. 1992; 267(13): pp. 1813–1817.
21. Von Korff M, Gruman J, Schaefer J, Curry SJ, Wagner EH. Collaborative management of chronic illness. *Ann Intern Med*. 1997; 127(12): pp. 1097–1102.
22. Wasson J, Gaudette C, Whaley F, Sauvigne A, Baribeau P, Welch HG. Telephone care as a substitute for routine clinic follow-up. *JAMA*. 1992; 267(13): pp. 1788–1793.
23. Engel, G. The need for a new medical model: a challenge for biomedicine. *Science*. 1977; 196(4286): pp. 129–136.

24. Wagner EH, Austin BT, Davis C, Hindmarsh M, Schaefer J, Bonomi A. Improving chronic illness care: translating evidence into action. *Health Aff (Millwood)*. 2001; 20(6): pp. 64–78. doi: 10.1377/hlthaff.20.6.64
25. Eghaneyan BH, Sanchez K, Mitschke DB. Implementation of a collaborative care model for the treatment of depression and anxiety in a community health center: results from a qualitative case study. *J Multidiscip Healthc*. 2014; 7: pp. 503–513. doi: 10.2147/JMDH.S69821
26. McDaniel SH, deGruy FV 3rd. An introduction to primary care and psychology. *Am Psychol*. 2014; 69(4): pp. 325–331. doi: 10.1037/a0036222
27. Fiscella K, McDaniel SH. The complexity, diversity, and science of primary care teams. *Am Psychol*. 2018; 73(4): pp. 451–467. doi: 10.1037/amp0000244
28. Reiter JT, Dobmeyer AC, Hunter CL. The Primary Care Behavioral Health (PCBH) Model: an overview and operational definition. *J Clin Psychol Med Settings*. 2018; 25(2): pp. 109–126. doi: 10.1007/s10880-017-9531-x
29. Ratliff A, Unützer J, Katon W, Stephens KA. *Integrated Care: Creating Effective Mental and Primary Health Care Teams*. 1st ed. John Wiley & Sons; 2016.
30. What is integrated behavioral health care? Agency for Healthcare Research and Quality website. Retrieved April 24, 2024. https://integrationacademy.ahrq.gov/products/behavioral-health-measures-atlas/what-is-ibhc
31. Baird M, Blount A, Brungardt S, et al. The development of joint principles: integrating behavioral health care into the patient-centered medical home. *Ann Fam Med*. 2014; 12(2): 183. doi: 10.1370/afm.1634
32. CAHPS Patient Experience Surveys and Guidance. Agency for Healthcare Research and Quality website. Retrieved April 24, 2024. https://www.ahrq.gov/cahps/surveys-guidance/index.html
33. Hoff T, Weller W, DePuccio M. The patient-centered medical home: a review of recent research. *Med Care Res Rev*. 2012; 69(6): pp. 619–644. doi: 10.1177/1077558712447688
34. Schneider EC, Zaslavsky AM, Landon BE, Lied TR, Sheingold S, Cleary PD. National quality monitoring of Medicare health plans: the relationship between enrollees' reports and the quality of clinical care. *Med Care*. 2001; 39(12): pp. 1313–1325. doi: 10.1097/00005650-200112000-00007
35. Davies E, Shaller D, Edgman-Levitan S, et al. Evaluating the use of a modified CAHPS survey to support improvements in patient-centred care: lessons from a quality improvement collaborative. *Health Expect*. 2008; 11(2): pp. 160–176. doi: 10.1111/j.1369-7625.2007.00483.x
36. Ross KM, Klein B, Ferro K, McQueeney DA, Gernon R, Miller BF. The cost effectiveness of embedding a behavioral health clinician into an existing primary care practice to facilitate the integration of care: a prospective, case-control program evaluation. *J Clin Psychol Med Settings*. 2019; 26(1): pp. 59–67. doi: 10.1007/s10880-018-9564-9
37. Balasubramanian BA, Cohen DJ, Jetelina KK, et al. Outcomes of integrated behavioral health with primary care. *J Am Board Fam Med*. 2017; 30(2): pp. 130–139. doi: 10.3122/jabfm.2017.02.160234
38. deGruy FV, McDaniel SH. Proposed requirements for behavioral health in family medicine residencies. *Fam Med*. 2021; 53(7): pp. 516–520. doi: 10.22454/FamMed.2021.380617

39. Fisher L, Dickinson WP. Psychology and primary care: new collaborations for providing effective care for adults with chronic health conditions. *Am Psychol.* 2014; 69(4): pp. 355–363. doi: 10.1037/a0036101
40. Hoffses KW, Ramirez LY, Berdan L, et al. Topical review: building competency: professional skills for pediatric psychologists in integrated primary care settings. *J Pediatr Psychol.* 2016; 41(10): pp. 1144–1160. doi: 10.1093/jpepsy/jsw066
41. Noffsinger EB, Scott JC. Understanding today's group-visit models. *Permanente Journal.* 2000; 4(2): pp. 99–112.
42. Booth A, Cantrell A, Preston L, Chambers D, Goyder E. What is the evidence for the effectiveness, appropriateness, and feasibility of group clinics for patients with chronic conditions? A systematic review. *Health Services and Delivery Research.* 2015; 3: pp. 1–372.
43. Quiñones AR, Richardson J, Freeman M, et al. Educational group visits for the management of chronic health conditions: a systematic review. *Patient Educ Couns.* 2014; 95(1): pp. 3–29. doi: 10.1016/j.pec.2013.12.021
44. Edelman D, McDuffie JR, Oddone E, et al. *Shared Medical Appointments for Chronic Medical Conditions: A Systematic Review.* Washington: Department of Veterans Affairs (US), 2012. www.hsrd.research.va.gov/publications/esp/shared-med-appt.pdf
45. Fatehi F, Samadbeik M, Kazemi A. What is digital health? review of definitions. *Stud Health Technol Inform.* 2020; 275: pp. 67–71. doi: 10.3233/SHTI200696
46. Istepanian RSH. Mobile health (m-health) in retrospect: the known unknowns. *Int J Environ Res Public Health.* 2022; 19(7): 3747. doi: 10.3390/ijerph19073747
47. Sood S, Mbarika V, Jugoo S, et al. What is telemedicine? A collection of 104 peer-reviewed perspectives and theoretical underpinnings. *Telemed J E Health.* 2007; 13(5): pp. 573–90. doi: 10.1089/tmj.2006.0073
48. eHealth. World Health Organization website. Retrieved April 24, 2024. https://www.who.int/ehealth/en/
49. Chan J. Exploring digital health care: eHealth, mHealth, and librarian opportunities. *J Med Libr Assoc.* 2021; 109(3): pp. 376–381. doi: 10.5195/jmla.2021.1180
50. Gajarawala SN, Pelkowski JN. Telehealth benefits and barriers. *J Nurse Pract.* 2021; 17(2): pp. 218–221. doi: 10.1016/j.nurpra.2020.09.013
51. Lucas JW, Villarroel MA. Telemedicine use among adults: United States, 2021. NCHS Data Brief, no 445. Hyattsville, MD: National Center for Health Statistics. 2022. doi: 10.15620/cdc:121435
52. Tan SS, Goonawardene N. Internet health information seeking and the patient-physician relationship: a systematic review. *J Med Internet Res.* 2017; 19(1): e9. doi: 10.2196/jmir.572
53. Bell RA, Hu X, Orrange SE, Kravitz RL. Lingering questions and doubts: online information-seeking of support forum members following their medical visits. *Patient Educ Couns.* 2011; 85(3): pp. 525–528.
54. Haidet P, O'Malley KJ, Sharf BF, Gladney AP, Greisinger AJ, Street RL Jr. Characterizing explanatory models of illness in healthcare: development and validation of the CONNECT instrument. *Patient Educ Couns.* 2008; 73(2): pp. 232–239.
55. Helman CG. Communication in primary care: the role of patient and practitioner explanatory models. *Soc Sci Med.* 1985; 20(9): pp. 923–931.

56. Miller LM, Bell RA. Online health information seeking: the influence of age, information trustworthiness, and search challenges. *J Aging Health*. 2012; 24(3): pp. 525–541. doi: 10.1177/0898264311428167
57. Doupi P, van der Lei J. Rx medication information for the public and the WWW: quality issues. *Med Inform Internet Med*. 1999; 24(3): pp. 171–179. doi: 10.1080/146392399298375
58. Gilbody S, Wilson P, Watt I. Benefits and harms of direct-to-consumer advertising: a systematic review. *Qual Saf Health Care*. 2005; 14(4): pp. 246–250. doi: 10.1136/qshc.2004.012781
59. DeFrank JT, Berkman ND, Kahwati L, Cullen K, Aikin KJ, Sullivan HW. Direct-to-consumer advertising of prescription drugs and the patient-prescriber encounter: a systematic review. *Health Commun*. 2020; 35(6): pp. 739–746. doi: 10.1080/10410236.2019.1584781
60. Goldzweig CL, Orshansky G, Paige NM, et al. Electronic patient portals: evidence on health outcomes, satisfaction, efficiency, and attitudes: a systematic review. *Ann Intern Med*. 2013; 159(10): pp. 677–687. doi: 10.7326/0003-4819-159-10-201311190-00006
61. Versluis A, Schnoor K, Chavannes NH, Talboom-Kamp EP. Direct access for patients to diagnostic testing and results using ehealth: systematic review on ehealth and diagnostics. *J Med Internet Res*. 2022; 24(1): e29303. doi: 10.2196/29303
62. Roumeliotis N, Sniderman J, Adams-Webber T, et al. Effect of electronic prescribing strategies on medication error and harm in hospital: a systematic review and meta-analysis. *J Gen Intern Med*. 2019; 34(10): pp. 2210–2223.
63. Keselman A, Smith CA. A classification of errors in lay comprehension of medical documents. *J Biomed Inform*. 2012; 45(6): pp. 1151–1163. doi: 10.1016/j.jbi.2012.07.012
64. Gu G, Zhang X, Zhu X, et al. Development of a consumer health vocabulary by mining health forum texts based on word embedding: semiautomatic approach. *JMIR Med Inform*. 2019; 7(2): e12704. doi: 10.2196/12704
65. Baun C, Vogsen M, Nielsen MK, Høilund-Carlsen PF, Hildebrandt MG. Perspective of patients with metastatic breast cancer on electronic access to scan results: mixed-methods study. *J Med Internet Res*. 2020; 22(2): e15723. doi: 10.2196/15723
66. Centers for Disease Control and Prevention. Update: HIV counseling and testing using rapid tests—United States, 1995. *MMWR Morb Mortal Wkly Rep*. 1998; 47(11): pp. 211–215.
67. Turner A, Morris R, McDonagh L, et al. Unintended consequences of patient online access to health records: a qualitative study in UK primary care. *Br J Gen Pract*. 2022; 73(726): pp. e67–e74. doi: 10.3399/BJGP.2021.0720
68. Kunst H, Groot D, Latthe PM, Latthe M, Khan KS. Accuracy of information on apparently credible websites: survey of five common health topics. *BMJ*. 2002; 324(7337): pp. 581–582.
69. Butcher L. Shared decision-making aids improving, winning support among both patients & physicians for treatment choices. *Oncology Times*. 2008; 30(10): 23.
70. Barry MJ. Health decision aids to facilitate shared decision making in office practice. *Ann Intern Med*. 2002; 136(2): pp. 127–135.
71. Wilkins E, Lowery J, Hamill J. The impact of shared decision making in prostate specific antigen (PSA) screening. *Med Decision Making*. 1999; 19: p. 525.

72. Schwitzer G. A review of features in Internet consumer health decision-support tools. *J Med Internet Res.* 2002; 4(2): E11.
73. Morgan MW, Deber RB, Llewellyn-Thomas HA, et al. Randomized, controlled trial of an interactive videodisc decision aid for patients with ischemic heart disease. *J Gen Intern Med.* 2000; 15(10): pp. 685–693.
74. Murray E, Davis H, Tai SS, Coulter A, Gray A, Haines A. Randomised controlled trial of an interactive multimedia decision aid on hormone replacement therapy in primary care. *BMJ (Clinical Research Ed).* 2001; 323(7311): pp. 490–493.
75. Rains SA, Wright KB. Social support and computer-mediated communication: a state-of-the-art review and agenda for future research. *Ann Intl Comm Assoc.* 2016; 40(1), pp. 175–211. doi: 10.1080/23808985.2015.11735260
76. Wright KB. Communication in health-related online social support groups/communities: a review of research on predictors of participation, applications of social support theory, and health outcomes. *Rev Comm Research.* 2016; 4: pp. 65–87.
77. van Eenbergen MC, van de Poll-Franse LV, Heine P, Mols F. The impact of participation in online cancer communities on patient reported outcomes: systematic review. *JMIR Cancer.* 2017; 3(2): e15. doi: 10.2196/cancer.7312
78. Sanger S, Duffin S, Gough RE, Bath PA. Use of online health forums by people living with breast cancer during the COVID-19 pandemic: thematic analysis. *JMIR Cancer.* 2023; 9(1): e42783.
79. Checchi KD, Huybrechts KF, Avorn J, Kesselheim AS. Electronic medication packaging devices and medication adherence: a systematic review. *JAMA.* 2014; 312(12): pp. 1237–1247. doi: 10.1001/jama.2014.10059
80. McKenney JM, Munroe WP, Wright JT, Jr. Impact of an electronic medication compliance aid on long-term blood pressure control. *J Clin Pharmacol.* 1992; 32(3): pp. 277–283.
81. Haleem A, Javaid M, Singh RP, Suman R. Telemedicine for healthcare: capabilities, features, barriers, and applications. *Sens Int.* 2021; 2: p. 100117. doi: 10.1016/j.sintl.2021.100117
82. Shaver J. The state of telehealth before and after the COVID-19 pandemic. *Prim Care.* 2022; 49(4): pp. 517–530. doi: 10.1016/j.pop.2022.04.002
83. SteelFisher GK, McMurtry CL, Caporello H, et al. Video telemedicine experiences in COVID-19 were positive, but physicians and patients prefer in-person care for the future. *Health Aff (Millwood).* 2023; 42(4): pp. 575–584. doi: 10.1377/hlthaff.2022.01027
84. McGrail KM, Ahuja MA, Leaver CA. Virtual visits and patient-centered care: results of a patient survey and observational study. *J Med Internet Res.* 2017; 19(5): e177. doi: 10.2196/jmir.7374
85. Street RL Jr, Treiman K, Kranzler EC, et al. Oncology patients' communication experiences during COVID-19: comparing telehealth consultations to in-person visits. *Support Care Cancer.* 2022; 30(6): pp. 4769–4780. doi: 10.1007/s00520-022-06897-8
86. Kruse CS, Krowski N, Rodriguez B, Tran L, Vela J, Brooks M. Telehealth and patient satisfaction: a systematic review and narrative analysis. *BMJ Open.* 2017; 7(8): e016242. doi: 10.1136/bmjopen-2017-016242

87. Elliott T, Tong I, Sheridan A, Lown BA. Beyond convenience: patients' perceptions of physician interactional skills and compassion via telemedicine. *Mayo Clinic Proceedings: Innovations, Quality & Outcomes.* 2020; 4(3): pp. 305–314.
88. Wu D, Lowry PB, Zhang D, Tao Y. Patient trust in physicians matters—understanding the role of a mobile patient education system and patient-physician communication in improving patient adherence behavior: field study. *J Med Internet Res.* 2022; 24(12): e42941. doi: 10.2196/42941
89. Niznik JD, He H, Kane-Gill SL. Impact of clinical pharmacist services delivered via telemedicine in the outpatient or ambulatory care setting: a systematic review. *Res Social Adm Pharm.* 2018; 14(8): pp. 707–717. doi: 10.1016/j.sapharm.2017.10.011
90. Andreadis K, Muellers K, Ancker JS, Horowitz C, Kaushal R, Lin JJ. Telemedicine impact on the patient-provider relationship in primary care during the COVID-19 pandemic. *Med Care.* 2023; 61(Suppl 1): pp. S83–S88. doi: 10.1097/MLR.0000000000001808
91. Call VR, Erickson LD, Dailey NK, et al. Attitudes toward telemedicine in urban, rural, and highly rural communities. *Telemed J E Health.* 2015; 21(8): pp. 644–651. doi: 10.1089/tmj.2014.0125
92. Cimperman M, Brenčič MM, Trkman P, Stanonik MD. Older adults' perceptions of home telehealth services. *Telemed J E Health.* 2013; 19(10): pp. 786–790. doi: 10.1089/tmj.2012.0272
93. Conway N, Webster C, Smith B, Wake D. eHealth and the use of individually tailored information: a systematic review. *Health Informatics J.* 2017; 23(3): pp. 218–233. doi: 10.1177/1460458216641479
94. Nguyen MH, Bol N, King AJ. Customisation versus personalisation of digital health information: effects of mode tailoring on information processing outcomes. *Eur J Health Comm.* 2020; 1(1): pp. 30–54.
95. Fotheringham MJ, Owies D, Leslie E, Owen N. Interactive health communication in preventive medicine: internet-based strategies in teaching and research. *Am J Prev Med.* 2000; 19(2): pp. 113–120.
96. Ferguson C, Hickman LD, Turkmani S, Breen P, Gargiulo G, Inglis SC. "Wearables only work on patients that wear them": barriers and facilitators to the adoption of wearable cardiac monitoring technologies. *Cardiovasc Digit Health J.* 2021; 2(2): pp. 137–147. doi: 10.1016/j.cvdhj.2021.02.001
97. Liu P, Li X, Zhang XM. Healthcare professionals' and patients' assessments of listed mobile health apps in China: a qualitative study. *Front Public Health.* 2023; 11: p. 1220160. doi: 10.3389/fpubh.2023
98. Elbert NJ, van Os-Medendorp H, van Renselaar W, et al. Effectiveness and cost-effectiveness of ehealth interventions in somatic diseases: a systematic review of systematic reviews and meta-analyses. *J Med Internet Res.* 2014; 16(4): e110. doi: 10.2196/jmir.2790
99. Bassi G, Mancinelli E, Dell'Arciprete G, Rizzi S, Gabrielli S, Salcuni S. Efficacy of ehealth interventions for adults with diabetes: a systematic review and meta-analysis. *Int J Environ Res Public Health.* 2021; 18(17): 8982. doi: 10.3390/ijerph18178982
100. Robert C, Erdt M, Lee J, Cao Y, Naharudin NB, Theng YL. Effectiveness of ehealth nutritional interventions for middle-aged and older adults: systematic review and meta-analysis. *J Med Internet Res.* 2021; 23(5): e15649. doi: 10.2196/15649

101. Bernstein IA, Zhang YV, Govil D, et al. Comparison of ophthalmologist and large language model chatbot responses to online patient eye care questions. *JAMA Netw Open*. 2023; 6(8): e2330320. doi: 10.1001/jamanetworkopen.2023.30320
102. van Buchem MM, Boosman H, Bauer MP, Kant IMJ, Cammel SA, Steyerberg EW. The digital scribe in clinical practice: a scoping review and research agenda. *NPJ Digit Med*. 2021; 4(1): 57. doi: 10.1038/s41746-021-00432-5
103. Ayers JW, Poliak A, Dredze M, et al. Comparing physician and artificial intelligence chatbot responses to patient questions posted to a public social media forum. *JAMA Intern Med*. 2023; 183(6): pp. 589–596. doi: 10.1001/jamainternmed.2023.1838
104. Ahuja AS. The impact of artificial intelligence in medicine on the future role of the physician. *PeerJ*. 2019; 7: e7702. doi: 10.7717/peerj.7702
105. Kolata GA. Mystery in the E.R.? Ask Dr Chatbot for a diagnosis. *New York Times*. July 22, 2023.
106. Bresnick, J. Top 12 ways artificial intelligence will impact healthcare. *Health IT Analytics*. Retrieved April 30, 2018. https://healthitanalytics.com/news/top-12-ways-artificial-intelligence-will-impact-healthcare
107. Thirunavukarasu AJ, Hassan R, Mahmood S, et al. Trialling a large language model (ChatGPT) in general practice with the Applied Knowledge Test: observational study demonstrating opportunities and limitations in primary care. *JMIR Medical Education*. 2023; 9: e46599. doi: 10.2196/46599
108. Weiss DC. Judge finds out why brief cited nonexistent cases—ChatGPT did research. *ABA Journal*. May 30, 2023.
109. New report finds doctors and nurses ready to embrace generative AI to answer the pressure points facing global health systems. Elsevier website. September 7, 2023. https://www.elsevier.com/about/press-releases/new-report-finds-doctors-and-nurses-ready-to-embrace-generative-ai-to-answer
110. Dill MJ, Pankow S, Erikson C, Shipman S. Survey shows consumers open to a greater role for physician assistants and nurse practitioners. *Health Affairs*. 2013; 32(6): pp. 1135–1142.
111. Young AT, Amara D, Bhattacharya A, Wei ML. Patient and general public attitudes towards clinical artificial intelligence: a mixed methods systematic review. *Lancet Digit Health*. 2021; 3(9): pp. e599–e611. doi: 10.1016/S2589-7500(21)00132-1
112. Fritsch SJ, Blankenheim A, Wahl A, et al. Attitudes and perception of artificial intelligence in healthcare: a cross-sectional survey among patients. *Digit Health*. 2022; Aug 8; 8: p. 20552076221116772. doi: 10.1177/20552076221116772
113. McKenna J. Medscape physicians and AI report 2023: a source of help or concern? Medscape website. October 30, 2023. https://www.medscape.com/slideshow/2023-artificial-intelligence-6016743?ecd=WNL_physrep_231104_ai_etid6020523&uac=372388DZ&impID=6020523
114. Longoni C, Morewedge CK. AI can outperform doctors. So why don't patients trust it? Harvard Business Review website. October 30, 2019. https://hbr.org/2019/10/ai-can-outperform-doctors-so-why-dont-patients-trust-it
115. 60% of Americans would be uncomfortable with provider relying on AI in their own health care. Pew Research Center website. February 22, 2023. https://www.pewresearch.org/science/2023/02/22/60-of-americans-would-be-uncomfortable-with-provider-relying-on-ai-in-their-own-health-care/

116. Grunhut J, Wyatt AT, Marques O. Educating future physicians in artificial intelligence (AI): an integrative review and proposed changes. *J Med Educ Curric Dev.* 2021; 8: p. 23821205211036836. doi: 10.1177/23821205211036836
117. Regulatory considerations on artificial intelligence for health. Geneva: World Health Organization; 2023. https://iris.who.int/bitstream/handle/10665/373421/9789240078871-eng.pdf?sequence=1&isAllowed=y
118. Gupta A, Corrado G. How 3 healthcare organizations are using generative AI. Google Blog website. August 29, 2023. https://blog.google/technology/health/cloud-next-generative-ai-health/
119. Steinhubl SR, Muse ED, Topol EJ. Can mobile health technologies transform health care? *JAMA.* 2013; 310(22): pp. 2395–2396. doi: 10.1001/jama.2013.281078
120. Americans' use of mobile technology and home broadband. Pew Research Center website. January 31, 2024. https://www.pewresearch.org/internet/2024/01/31/americans-use-of-mobile-technology-and-home-broadband/
121. Emergence of application-based healthcare. AHRQ website. August 5, 2022. https://psnet.ahrq.gov/perspective/emergence-application-based-healthcare
122. Marcano Belisario JS, Huckvale K, Greenfield G, Car J, Gunn LH. Smartphone and tablet self-management apps for asthma. *Cochrane Database Syst Rev.* 2013; 2013(11): CD010013. doi: 10.1002/14651858.CD010013.pub2
123. Geuens J, Swinnen TW, Westhovens R, de Vlam K, Geurts L, Vanden Abeele V. A review of persuasive principles in mobile apps for chronic arthritis patients: opportunities for improvement. *JMIR Mhealth Uhealth.* 2016; 4(4): e118. doi: 10.2196/mhealth.6286
124. de Jongh T, Gurol-Urganci I, Vodopivec-Jamsek V, Car J, Atun R. Mobile phone messaging for facilitating self-management of long-term illnesses. *Cochrane Database Syst Rev.* 2012; 12(12): CD007459. doi: 10.1002/14651858.CD007459.pub2
125. Kim JY, Wineinger NE, Steinhubl SR. The influence of wireless self-monitoring program on the relationship between patient activation and health behaviors, medication adherence, and blood pressure levels in hypertensive patients: a substudy of a randomized controlled trial. *J Med Internet Res.* 2016; 18(6): e116. doi: 10.2196/jmir.5429
126. Chomutare T, Tatara N, Arsand E, Hartvigsen G. Designing a diabetes mobile application with social network support. *Stud Health Technol Inform.* 2013; 188: pp. 58–64.
127. Hong Y, Dahlke DV, Ory M, et al. Designing iCanFit: a mobile-enabled web application to promote physical activity for older cancer survivors. *JMIR Res Protoc.* 2013; 2(1): e12.
128. Dayer L, Heldenbrand S, Anderson P, Gubbins PO, Martin BC. Smartphone medication adherence apps: potential benefits to patients and providers. *J Am Pharm Assoc.* 2013; 53(2): pp. 172–181. doi: 10.1331/JAPhA.2013.12202
129. Pérez-Jover V, Sala-González M, Guilabert M, Mira JJ. Mobile apps for increasing treatment adherence: systematic review. *J Med Internet Res.* 2019; 21(6): e12505. doi: 10.2196/12505
130. Park HR, Kang HS, Kim SH, Singh-Carlson S. Effect of a smart pill bottle reminder intervention on medication adherence, self-efficacy, and depression in breast cancer survivors. *Cancer Nurs.* 2022; 45(6): pp. E874–E882. doi: 10.1097/NCC.0000000000001030

131. Sideri K, Cockbain J, Van Biesen W, De Hert M, Decruyenaere J, Sterckx S. Digital pills for the remote monitoring of medication intake: a stakeholder analysis and assessment of marketing approval and patent granting policies. *J Law Biosci*. 2022; 9(2): lsac029. doi: 10.1093/jlb/lsac029
132. Litvinova O, Klager E, Tzvetkov NT, et al. Digital pills with ingestible sensors: patent landscape analysis. *Pharmaceuticals (Basel)*. 2022; 15(8): 1025. doi: 10.3390/ph15081025
133. Wise J, Operario D. Use of electronic reminder devices to improve adherence to antiretroviral therapy: a systematic review. *AIDS Patient Care and STDS*. 2008; 22(6): pp. 495–504.
134. Boden C, Sit A, Weinreb RN. Accuracy of an electronic monitoring and reminder device for use with travoprost eye drops. *J Glaucoma*. 2006; 15(1): pp. 30–34.
135. Fish L, Lung CL. Adherence to asthma therapy. *Ann Allergy Asthma Immunol*. 2001; 86(6 Suppl 1): pp. 24–30.
136. Fox MC, Creinin MD, Murthy AS, Harwood B, Reid LM. Feasibility study of the use of a daily electronic mail reminder to improve oral contraceptive compliance. *Contraception*. 2003; 68(5): pp. 365–371.
137. Thakkar J, Kurup R, Laba TL, et al. Mobile telephone text messaging for medication adherence in chronic disease: a meta-analysis. *JAMA Intern Med*. 2016; 176(3): pp. 340–349. doi: 10.1001/jamainternmed
138. Beni JB. Technology and the healthcare system: implications for patient adherence. *Int J Electron Healthcare*. 2011; 6(2–4): pp. 117–137.
139. Ingersoll KS, Cohen J. The impact of medication regimen factors on adherence to chronic treatment: a review of literature. *J Behav Med*. 2008; 31(3): 213–224. doi: 10.1007/s10865-007-9147-y
140. Gollwitzer P, Schaal B. How goals and plans affect action. In: Collis JM, Messick SJ, Schiefele U, eds. *Intelligence and Personality: Bridging the Gap in Theory and Measurement*. London: Taylor & Francis Group; 2021; pp. 143–166.

Chapter 9
Individuals in the Context of Medical Systems and Public Policy

Throughout this book, we have examined individual health behaviors and considered adherence to the management of acute and chronic medical conditions. We have seen that behavior can be influenced by myriad factors including beliefs and expectations, sociocultural pressures, characteristics of treatment regimens, and the interpersonal context of healthcare. In the preceding chapters, we have offered strategies for informing, motivating, and encouraging health behavior change, and we have proposed that health professionals can be optimistic about their patients' adherence when the proper strategies are thoughtfully and carefully applied. We have also argued that success at behavior change requires frank recognition of vulnerabilities and risk factors for nonadherence, while keeping in mind the unique experience and sociocultural context of each individual. Barriers to successful behavior change and adherence are many (some of the most common, from prior chapters, are reviewed in Table 9.1), and strategies for improving adherence work best in the context of provider-patient partnerships.

In this final chapter, we broaden our lens to examine a cross-section of system-level factors that contextualize individual choices. Many of these factors were once invisible elements in the background of any healthcare experience. However, with growing rates of chronic diseases and comorbid conditions, the emergence of new pathogens, increasingly expensive treatment options, and ever more complex financial structures governing healthcare, these factors are becoming more apparent and their influence on health behavior and adherence is increasingly profound.

We note, with some dismay, that in the United States today, an individual's health and healthcare are shaped by a broad array of interests, some of which have competing goals. In this chapter, we consider some of the dynamic tensions among various "stakeholders." One example is the industry promotion of ultra-processed foods versus public health efforts to reduce

Table 9.1 Common Barriers to Adherence and Strategies for Addressing Them

Barrier	Strategy
Number of medications	Reduce polypharmacy; simplify medication schedules with combination or time-release drugs.
Regimen complexity	Simplify regimen and integrate with patient's daily schedule; link health behaviors to already existing habits (e.g., to cue action, keep medication bottle or list of exercises next to coffee maker or toothbrush).
Expected and experienced side effects	Discuss potential side effects with patients; adjust regimen to alleviate them if possible; discuss cofactors (e.g., dietary restrictions) required for effective regimen management.
Regimen rationale and outcome expectations unclear	Discuss potential outcomes with and without adherence; encourage incremental change and realistic expectations.
Financial challenges of care	Provide help with insurance claims and identifying resources for assistance; suggest low-cost alternatives (e.g., outdoor or mall-walking; generic and mail-order drugs; drugstore coupons).
Hectic schedule, no time	Suggest ways to integrate regimen with schedule; work to enhance patient commitment and motivation.
Hectic schedule, forgetting	Help patient develop habits; set reminders (including cues to action).
Lack of social support	Encourage support from family members and friends; help connect patient with support group.
Low health literacy, lack of understanding	Offer clear explanations; avoid jargon; check for understanding; build rapport; provide educational materials (interactive, if possible); provide written/visual materials to aid understanding and memory.
Low self-efficacy for health behavior	Encourage greater self-efficacy using the strategies of personal experience, vicarious experience, and verbal persuasion.
Need for positive reinforcement of regimen	Praise patient success and progress toward overall health goals; encourage family and social network reinforcement; help patient establish self-monitoring, self-evaluation, and self-reinforcement.
Limited healthcare access	Help patient identify community resources or assistance programs.
Interference of comorbidities	Work with patient to find alternative ways of carrying out desired behavior; discuss ways to coordinate all regimen requirements.

their consumption. Another involves cost-effective ways to promote population health in nonprofit and integrated healthcare systems versus costly for-profit health insurance practices that erect barriers to preventive care and chronic disease management.

In this chapter, we also examine the broader context of laws and policies that can shape health behavior and adherence, including taxes (such as on cigarettes and sugary drinks) and laws governing women's healthcare. We review public health responses to communicable disease threats, including some lessons learned from the COVID-19 pandemic. We also examine the social and psychological factors that challenge health policy in the management of current and emerging diseases.

The big picture

Health behavior change and treatment adherence are complex and multifaceted, and there is no single, simple answer to the question of how one might best form and maintain health habits. Solutions require conscious, sustained effort to manage the many internal and external forces that drive health behavior. In the big picture of their lives, individuals are influenced by systems, policies, and forces over which they have little direct control, and which may even be outside their awareness. Some of these might be supportive of their health goals, such as federal laws that protect them from harmful contaminants in their food, or local policies that promote the walkability of the neighborhoods in which they live. Others may be less helpful, however, such as messages that tempt them to eat ultra-processed snacks, and healthcare options that remain too expensive for them to afford.

Changing health behaviors and helping patients adhere to medical treatments require interventions that are wide-ranging in their implementation. Two reviews have noted that comprehensive interventions are more effective than those focusing on any single adherence barrier, and that interventions are most helpful when they target a combination of cognitive, behavioral, and affective elements of the patient's experience.[1,2] For example, a nicotine patch might indeed help a smoker to quit smoking, but an intervention will be most effective if it also includes a smoking cessation support group, a behavioral contract, and a health insurance premium discount that rewards being smoke-free. Personalized interventions that are coordinated among members of a healthcare delivery team[3-5] and tailored to the broad picture of the individual's life are most likely to achieve good results.[2]

Stakeholders in health: who owns the risk?

"Owning the risk" is a simple concept. Although a patient must ultimately deal with the daily consequences of any health challenge they face, the financial consequences are borne not only by the patient but also by other entities (like insurance providers, employers, or society). If, for example, an employer offers health insurance, the costs for care must be borne across the "risk pool" of employees; if those costs rise considerably, insurance premiums go up. When costs rise in caring for patients in publicly funded healthcare systems like Medicare, the cost increases must be borne by taxpayers and by Medicare subscribers in the form of increased premiums.

Offering optimal care is certainly a goal but so, too, is controlling costs. In the United States, the cost of healthcare surpasses $4 trillion a year and accounts for almost 20% of the Gross Domestic Product.[6] Unhealthy behaviors and patient nonadherence can, over the long term, contribute to increased costs and considerable waste of these healthcare dollars.

To understand the bigger picture of health and health behavior in the United States, we cannot ignore "stakeholders" in health, the degree to which they own the risks of healthcare costs, and whether and how those costs are shifted to other entities. In Chapter 1, for example, we looked at the costs to society of unhealthy behaviors and treatment nonadherence. Diets of ultra-processed foods, sugared beverages, and sedentary lifestyle as well as the unsafe use of alcohol and tobacco increase costs to everyone in our society, directly or indirectly. The American public collectively owns the risk of the consequences of everyone's health behaviors; they are *stakeholders* in healthcare.

Those championing the "public good" (e.g., government agencies, employers, nonprofit organizations), might press for curbs on these health risks in order (among other reasons) to control costs. There are, however, equally powerful stakeholders who have conflicting interests. These include industries that derive economic benefit from consumption of the very elements that drive up healthcare costs (e.g., tobacco, sugar, processed foods, opioid medications). The efforts of these entities (through advertising of snack foods and resistance to taxes on alcohol, for example) can work against the willpower and personal control of individuals. Even an encouraging healthcare provider and a family that is fully supportive of eating whole foods and avoiding alcohol might not stand much of a chance against these powerful forces.

Costs, health insurance, and access to care

Many of the barriers to health behavior change and adherence that we have discussed in this book are unique to individuals—rooted in their past experiences, cultural norms, and personal beliefs, attitudes, habits, and values. Some contexts of healthcare delivery can help coordinate care in order to help patients overcome their personal barriers; other contexts, however, can create and maintain barriers to effective health outcomes. Healthcare costs, health insurance challenges, and limitations in access to medical care are system-level barriers that are of major importance in understanding individuals' social-ecological contexts.

The costs of medical care have been rising significantly throughout the United States, even for those with "good" insurance.[7] A December 2023 Kaiser Family Foundation poll examined people's experiences with healthcare costs in the United States and reported that about half of adults had problems paying for their healthcare.[8] One in four said that in the past 12 months, they skipped or postponed needed care because of the cost, and one in five did not fill a prescription because they could not afford it. Even individuals with health insurance have difficulty paying for their care. About 40% said they worried about affording their health insurance premiums, and 48% said they worried about their deductible amount. Half responded that they would be unable to pay a $500 USD unexpected medical bill without incurring debt; 41% reported having debt due to medical or dental bills.

At the time of this writing, about 28 million people in the United States are without health insurance;[9] millions more are underinsured and cannot afford all the care that they need. Patients with insurance coverage are more likely to receive preventive health services, and they are particularly likely to receive preventive care if they have *both* insurance and a regular healthcare provider.[10] Insured patients also tend to adhere better to their medication regimens because they receive more consistent care and because cost is less of a barrier.[11] Patients who receive their healthcare from certain integrated delivery systems (such as the Veterans Health Administration) are less likely to cite monetary reasons for failing to take medications even when compared to those with private insurance.[11] One advantage of receiving healthcare in an integrated health system involves the relative simplicity of the financial aspects of care.

A great many insured patients in the United States face challenges in navigating the often complex and confusing landscape of employment-based for-profit insurance. Employers usually offer several plans with varying premiums, deductibles, and copayments, but trying to comprehend the options can be overwhelming. Even if they have a general understanding of how various plans might meet their needs, many individuals choose health insurance based simply on monthly premium costs, whether their doctor is currently "in-network," or their degree of trust in the insurance company involved. Few are comfortable researching options and projecting potential health challenges, including ones that might include prohibitive medication costs should a serious health problem arise. Insurance choices are important because a poor match between patients' needs and their health insurance coverage might cause them to forego preventive care or to be nonadherent to chronic disease management.

In 2001, the Institute of Medicine,[12] now called the National Academy of Medicine, offered a valuable analytic framework, still in use today, for evaluating the effectiveness of medical care and improving healthcare outcomes. The six elements of this framework are: safety, effectiveness, patient-centeredness, timeliness, efficiency, and equitability. All of these elements are challenged when individuals do not have available, affordable, and appropriate care from a usual source.[13] Patients who are able regularly to see the same team of health professionals are more likely to have their visits focused on the prevention of future health challenges instead of simply the latest emergent problems.[10,14] There are also more opportunities for patients and their providers to discuss and work toward health behavior change and adherence.[14] As we saw in Chapter 8, healthcare teams and effective technologies can help maintain the kinds of support that patients need when it will benefit them most.

When access to care that meets a patient's needs is limited, some healthcare opportunities remain underused while others, such as emergency rooms, become overused.[13,15,16] In addition to the significant expense and overcrowding of emergency departments, the use of emergency care may alleviate only the presenting symptoms; long-term planning and prevention may be ignored.[17] And, as we saw in Chapter 7, disparities in healthcare availability are well-documented. Low-income patients and those of color in the United States have significantly less access to consistent healthcare; they more often rely on emergency department care, and subsequently have poorer health outcomes.[18-20]

Integrated care systems

Health behavior change and treatment adherence, as we have emphasized throughout this book, require a multifaceted approach, provider-patient partnerships, and integrated care.[21] Uncoordinated, episodic medical care that lacks a "whole-person" orientation does not tend to foster lasting change, yet patient care is becoming increasingly fragmented[22] and many individuals feel disconnected from their healthcare providers.[23] As we saw in the analysis of the Chronic Care Model (Chapter 8), piecemeal treatment leaves patients on their own, trying to improve their health behaviors and manage their chronic conditions; typically, they don't do this very well. Healthcare team support is essential to manage the multifaceted challenges of chronic conditions. For example, moving and exercising, maintaining a healthy weight, and attending to body mechanics can help patients manage their low back pain more effectively and improve the quality of their lives; a team approach is needed to effect health behavior change and avoid expensive and questionably effective surgeries and the potential for addiction to opioid pain medications.[24]

An integrated care system of healthcare delivery ideally attempts to reduce this fragmentation, focusing on comprehensive, evidence-based treatment and incorporating principles of behavior change to improve patients' adherence. (An integrated care system can also be an Accountable Care Organization that is held accountable by funding entities like Medicaid and Medicare for providing a population with comprehensive, integrated services.) When an integrated care system offers comprehensive medical care, it is financially responsible for coordinating care that is cost-effective and avoids unnecessary treatments. Ideally, it guards against fragmentation by offering a team-based model, with complete and searchable electronic health records (EHRs), efforts at provider continuity (seeing the same health professionals), and tight coordination, consultation, and information-sharing among all professionals involved in a patient's care.

Kaiser Permanente is the largest integrated care system in the United States and an example of a health system that emphasizes disease prevention and screening to identify and treat disease conditions. This system typically offers lower costs, a coordinated experience of care, patient education, and a focus on evidence-based treatments that are shown to have value in advancing patient outcomes. In Northern California, for example, Kaiser Permanente's multifaceted hypertension management program identifies, from the

EHR, patients with high blood pressure who have poor control, have missed recommended medical visits, or have not filled their medication prescriptions in a timely way. The system reaches out to these patients, encouraging them to come in for appointments; it offers lower cost generic medications, and has clinical pharmacists available to counsel patients (and, if necessary, consult with their doctors for possible medication adjustments). Hypertension health education classes and help from chronic disease case managers are also available. Physicians are offered support for improving their communication and collaborative shared decision-making skills. With this program in place, 80% of hypertension patients experience effective disease control compared with a typical 65% in similar community settings.[25]

There are, of course, some limits to integrated care systems, and they are often unavailable outside of metropolitan areas. In systems that require primary care physician referral to specialists,[26] some patients may come to view their primary care physicians as gatekeepers rather than true partners in their care.[27] Systems also vary in the degree of integration and coordination among the health professionals on the patient care team.[28,29]

It is clear, however, that whatever the model of delivery, patients experience more positive outcomes when they are offered a greater degree of control and participation in their own healthcare.[27,30,31] Their active role allows them to better navigate the healthcare system and overcome barriers at all levels, not just the personal. The most successful healthcare organizations are those that effectively promote preventive health behaviors in addition to treating disease. They anticipate adherence challenges, and help patients overcome them.[32,33] As healthcare becomes more costly, greater emphasis must be placed on promoting primary prevention efforts through health behavior change and on enhancing patient adherence to recommended treatments. This happens best in the context of treatment that is patient-centered and involves collaborative care.

Public health and the public good

When individuals try to improve their own health behaviors and adherence, they typically focus on the direct benefits to themselves (and perhaps, by extension, their loved ones). Clinicians often take a broader view, guiding health behaviors for patients' own benefit, with an eye toward more far-reaching implications. The consequences of individuals' decisions and actions sometimes extend well beyond themselves to the well-being of their communities. One example involves childhood vaccinations, where parental decisions not to immunize their own children can have significant implications for communicable disease transmission to other, more vulnerable, children.

The reality of our health-based interconnectivity raises questions that do not have straightforward answers. What does it mean to have autonomy to make personal medical decisions? How extensive is the right of one individual to make choices that imperil others? And what role does the clinician play in this picture? Autonomy is a fundamental principle of medical ethics which relies on the central premises of choice and informed consent. But is one's degree of autonomy inextricably linked to the rights of others? As we saw in Chapter 3, in a paternalistic model, the physician disregards patient autonomy altogether and tells the patient to follow the treatment because the doctor knows best. In a patient-as-consumer model, patients might search for (and find) information of questionable accuracy or even downright misrepresentation and insist upon self-direction. There is great variability in the consequences of autonomy, and these questions encourage us to further address the complex process of making personal medical decisions, especially when they affect other people.

How others are affected depends upon many factors. As we saw above, significant overuse of medical services can drive up system wide costs. When a person is nonadherent to their hypertension and diabetes treatment and then has a stroke, or someone "at risk" of poor outcomes from flu or COVID-19 refuses vaccination and becomes seriously ill, many people suffer. Issues regarding the public good arose quite strikingly during the COVID-19 pandemic, where mitigation strategies (such as the use of masks for respiratory protection) were resisted by many people, increasing group risk.

Health education

Some of these issues are addressed in the realm of public health, specifically health education. At the most basic level, public health exists to inform and educate the public about health issues. Ideally, the first step in the

Information-Motivation-Strategy model would be sufficient to foster health behavior change (although, of course, it is not). For example, the CDC offers a program called "Step It Up! The Surgeon General's Call to Action to Promote Walking and Walkable Communities." The goal is to "increase walking by working together to increase access to safe and convenient places to walk and wheelchair roll and to create a culture that supports walking for all Americans."[34] This program offers information for multiple entities including employers, universities, healthcare institutions, media, parks and recreation, and land use entities to establish and maintain environments that support physical activity.

In the realm of food and nutrition, the U.S. government provides considerable information from nutrition science that can be easily found to help guide food choices. MyPlate[35] is a visual reminder to guide healthy choices from five food groups. The website offers many resources and ideas for building and maintaining healthy dietary patterns. Other examples include public service announcements to eliminate tobacco use, reduce the intake of alcohol, and increase vaccine uptake. These educational efforts have a modest degree of success in changing behavior. Typically, they target only the first component of the Information-Motivation-Strategy model—the information piece. We have already seen that strategies to move individuals toward action must also involve motivation and a set of effective tools that can be used to implement change.

Some health education efforts provide components in addition to information, such as posted signs that remind and motivate people to take the stairs instead of the elevator to increase their daily exercise. Some efforts actually make change possible when it might not have been, such the creation of walking trails and bike lanes; these can be very effective in changing sedentary behavior.[18,36] The effective targeting of social policies is important in order to promote good health and correct harmful habits; these policies must be built with acknowledgment of the complex associations that exist between behaviors and myriad health risk factors.[37] Sometimes, public health educational efforts fail to address the power of social network influences and do not take into account the behavioral and lifestyle patterns that dominate the daily lives of many individuals.[38] Interventions that increase the salience of information, foster individuals' motivation, and help them devise specific behavior change strategies can help foster health behavior change.[39]

Government supported programs for health behavior change

Public health policy can successfully change health behavior through direct interventions in the government-funded healthcare programs of Medicare and Medicaid. An example is the diet and exercise intervention in the 2010 Affordable Care Act signed by President Obama and targeted to roughly 86 million people with prediabetes, a condition in which individuals have blood sugar levels higher than normal, but not high enough to be considered diabetic.[40] The goal was to successfully prevent type 2 diabetes from developing by paying for certain lifestyle change programs. Trained counselors coached those at risk on developing healthier eating habits and increasing their physical activity. Participants lost, on average, 5% of their body weight and substantially reduced their risk of future diabetes. The program showed considerable financial savings by reducing the risks of health complications from diabetes; these savings more than covered the costs of the program.

Laws and public policy mandates

Public health messages, reminders, and encouragement can shift the health behaviors of some people some of the time. Despite this, however, health behavior change in response to public health efforts can be modest. Major changes are sometimes better achieved with public policies and laws. The cases of Helen and Darlene in Case Study 9.1 illustrate the effects of tax law on health behavior.

> **Case Study 9.1 Helen, Darlene, and the Price of Cigarettes and Soda**
>
> In the past, Helen—a bright, hardworking, and frugal woman—smoked at least two packs of cigarettes a day. When she moved from Virginia to New York, however, she was quite dismayed to see that cigarettes cost twice as much because of New York State's substantial tax on them. Before this blow to her budget, nothing could change Helen's smoking habits. One day, however, she decided she could no longer afford to spend so much money on cigarettes, or to give so much money to the government, and so she quit.

> Darlene is significantly overweight—obese by some standards. She loves drinking very large, sugared sodas throughout the day. She feels that they give her the energy she needs to keep going, and these sodas go well with the tasty nacho flavored chips she enjoys. Darlene was dismayed by the recent increases in the cost of sweetened drinks in her hometown, so she decided to shop at a large warehouse store only one town away, where she can buy all the soda she wants without paying the extra cost of the Sweetened Beverage Tax.

Taxes on cigarette sales have been around for a long time in the United States. In 2009, these taxes were increased considerably, and their revenue was directed to youth tobacco use prevention programs. Research demonstrates that taxes on cigarettes (and now, in some states, e-cigarettes) do reduce the amount that people smoke and prevent some young people from establishing a smoking habit. In a paper reviewing over 100 international studies, researchers found that due to the strong connections between tobacco products and both morbidity and premature death, taxes on tobacco products are highly effective in contributing to better public health.[41]

Sweetened Beverage Taxes are designed to reduce the consumption of sweetened soft drinks and sport drinks, thus decreasing the incidence of obesity and diabetes, and their associated economic costs.[42] These taxes are generally regional, and revenue is often targeted to pay for obesity prevention, nutrition education, and the health needs of individuals in the region. Of course, people can sometimes find alternative ways to continue to engage in poor health behaviors; for many, even the motivation to avoid extra costs may not be enough to abandon well-honed bad habits.

Taxes on alcohol tend to reduce its consumption. A great deal of research has addressed this issue, and there is considerable evidence that alcohol taxes help reduce the incidence of diseases that are associated with alcohol use. In one Scottish study, legislation that broadened taxation on alcohol was associated with significant reductions in alcohol-related deaths and hospitalizations. This was especially true among the economically disadvantaged, who tend to suffer the greatest harms of alcohol to their health.[43] The researchers found that cancer risk was reduced proportionally by any measures that reduced alcohol consumption (e.g., increased taxes, limits on days or times of allowed sale).[43]

Laws and public policies can also affect health behaviors through public health measures such as school vaccination mandates, educational and treatment efforts, and mandated reporting of communicable diseases. In the United States, many health-related laws and public policies vary by state. Some states are more actively protective of their populations, while others are less so, and leave many public health actions to individual choice.

Americans, on average, are more likely than people from similar countries to die prematurely (younger than age 65); there is also variability among U.S. states and regions in their laws to protect health. This variability can have significant consequences for trends in illness and death. While individual behavioral choice matters a great deal, many premature deaths could have been prevented but for decisions by local and state governments to forego public health measures. Laws mandating automobile seat-belt use, immunizations, disease mitigation strategies, healthcare support, and taxes on cigarettes and alcohol have been shown to save lives, and yet these are not in effect in some areas. Arguments that public health policies cost too much or overstep personal freedom often stand in the way of many protections that could be offered to a population.[44]

Significant health disparities also exist across the United States partly because states vary in their policies and degree of investment in longer-term population health and longevity. Examples of policies include laws regarding tobacco use and sales, expansions of Medicaid, income supports, and motor vehicle laws and enforcement.[44] The management of health safety-net funding within a state affects whether citizens can obtain needed healthcare, a factor with significant potential long-term consequences.

Data are quite clear that many public health policies can help to modify health behaviors and have demonstrably positive effects on health and survival. Two areas that have been particularly salient in the early 2020s have been women's reproductive health and vaccinations. We address each of these below, examining public health outcomes related to law and policy.

Laws and women's healthcare

As we have emphasized many times in this book, an individual's health outcomes are dependent not only on their personal choices but also on contextual factors including the availability of health promoting options and healthcare services. The legal landscape surrounding the individual can have a profound effect on the availability and reliability of healthcare.[45] Some locations, such as rural settings and impoverished inner cities, tend to have far less care available than more affluent metropolitan areas, and regional and state laws can determine healthcare options.

A recent example of this variability involves the continually evolving consequences of the *Dobbs* decision by the U.S. Supreme Court (June 24, 2022), which negated the federally protected right to abortion, overturning the landmark case of *Roe v. Wade* (1973), and returning abortion regulation to the states. Although there have been conflicting opinions about the ruling, a Kaiser Family Foundation poll of obstetricians showed that in response to this decision, there was a reported increase in maternal mortality.[46] This was a nationally representative survey of United States, office-based physicians specializing in Obstetrics and Gynecology (OB/GYN) who provided direct patient care in the majority of their work. In this study, 20% of OB/GYN physicians reported feeling personally constrained in their care of patients' miscarriages and other pregnancy-related medical emergencies; this proportion was 40% in states where abortion has been banned. Over a third of OB/GYN doctors nationally, and over half in abortion-banned states, responded that there has been a reduction in their ability to deliver the necessary standard of care to their patients. Seventy percent responded that the *Dobbs* decision worsened racial and ethnic inequities in maternal health; 64% said that pregnancy-related mortality had increased, and 55% believed that the decision reduced the ability to attract new physicians to the specialty. In states with restrictive abortion laws, highly skilled obstetricians who handle risky pregnancies have been leaving (or avoiding setting up a practice), limiting healthcare access for large parts of the population, especially in rural areas.[47] The March of Dimes has identified a large number of counties in the United States that have recently become "maternity care deserts" where there are no hospitals providing obstetric care, no birthing centers, no OB/GYN physicians, and no certified nurse midwives.[48] This shortage affects roughly 2.2 million women of childbearing age. Not only are abortion services and maternity care impacted, so are contraceptive services and the prevention, detection, and treatment of sexually transmitted diseases and some cancers. Whether for pregnant persons needing maternity care, individuals needing contraceptive services, socioeconomically disadvantaged individuals requiring basic healthcare, or individuals needing cancer screening, the availability of reliable, quality healthcare is the most necessary element required to achieve the goals of health behavior change and adherence.

Public health and the COVID-19 pandemic

As of this writing in late 2024, multiple and variable waves of pandemic activity involving SARS CoV-2 continue to draw our attention back to what are essentially behavioral issues. When levels of circulating virus are high, necessary health behaviors may again include wearing properly fitted respiratory protection, testing, and accepting vaccination boosters. From 2020 through 2022, COVID-19 vaccinations and mitigation strategies were, in some cases, managed well; they were especially successful where trusted public health officials played a central role in reaching out to, and educating, the public.[49] It is estimated, however, based on calculations of the uptake of the original COVID-19 vaccine across the United States, that as many as 200,000 people who chose to remain unvaccinated ultimately died of COVID-19.[50]

Public health officials and crafters of pandemic health policy may not have adequately anticipated the resistance that arose against medical and health policy recommendations, or the refusal of individuals to adhere to health behavior and lifestyle changes. In their May 2023 opinion piece in the *New York Times*, the Biden-Harris administration's 2020 Transition Advisory Board on Pandemic Response noted this underestimation and conceded that the influence of social context/support factors and behavioral incentives had not been adequately understood.[51]

It is important to note here that psychological and sociocultural factors have been important elements in the study of public health for at least 50 years. Indeed, the earliest models of health behavior (reviewed in Chapter 2) were developed by public health researchers. Certainly, some issues and concerns now have additional components (especially developments like social media), but the basics of behavior change are foundational in the field of public health. Given the decades-long availability of research on health behavior change and treatment adherence/nonadherence (starting in 1948), what occurred at the interface of human behavior and the SARS-CoV-2 coronavirus should probably not have been surprising. The COVID-19 pandemic reminded us that health policy is directed at human beings, who are complex in their psychology and sometimes headstrong in their resistance.

Precisely modeling and understanding the events of the COVID-19 pandemic can be difficult. So, too, is predicting what could happen if we are confronted with another pathogen for which humans have no immunity and there is no treatment. Some experts warn that more pandemics may be coming,[52,53] and that these are likely to involve airborne communicable diseases like influenza, making some of the more difficult behavioral requirements of the COVID-19 era necessary again. In order to be prepared for a future communicable disease pandemic, we must fully understand the social, psychological, and behavioral elements of the one we have recently experienced. We must also better understand human behavior in other communicable and noncommunicable diseases as well as in mental health conditions that remain widespread. The implications for population health and well-being are pervasive.

Psychological and behavioral issues are of central importance in the training of professionals in public health, population medicine, and all aspects of healthcare because the success of health directives and the management of present and future diseases require responses and policies that are sensitive to powerful psychological and sociocultural forces. Today's students will soon be the leaders in public health, medicine, and psychology; understanding the cognitive, social, and contextual factors that drive health behavior change and adherence must be essential elements of their graduate level training.

Implementation science and research on health behavior change

After more than seven decades of study, it is fair to say that a good deal is known about health behavior change and treatment adherence. Throughout the chapters of this book, we have endeavored to consolidate much of this evidence and to suggest real world applications of theory, clinical observation, and experimental research. We have argued that the application of this knowledge can improve health at many points, from acceptance and implementation of primary prevention behaviors to treatment adherence for acute and chronic disease. We have noted the applicability of much of this work to public health policy, integrated healthcare delivery, and individual daily clinical practice.

The abundance of research we have reviewed and integrated in this book has shown that although health behavior change is not easy, *it is possible.*

The broad strokes of the Information-Motivation-Strategy Model provide a template, showing us that change, at the most basic level, requires that people know what they need to do, want to do it, and are able to do it. This approach can be successfully applied if practitioners at every level of intervention are aware of its value and know how to use it. Awareness and application of knowledge do, however, require both dissemination (i.e., the spread of information, research findings, and ideas for clinical application) and implementation (i.e., integration into practice at many levels).

The field of implementation science[54] involves the development and study of dissemination and implementation, focusing on methods to be used for the adoption and integration of strategies that work at the levels of clinical practice, organization management, and population health in public policy. A related goal in this realm is the de-implementation of low-value care[55] and the successful avoidance of interventions and practices that are ineffective and may even prove counterproductive. Implementation science utilizes a wide range of methods to better understand how to apply what is known about improving individual and population health outcomes. While intervention research in health has existed for a great many decades, implementation science offers a focused and concerted effort to use that research to make changes at many levels, from the clinical to the organizational to the governmental. Implementation science utilizes many existing methodologies in medicine, public health, and behavioral science, and offers timely application of effective medical and behavioral interventions that can improve health and save lives. It demonstrates how proven interventions and evidence-based practices can be used in real world health and medical settings, and how problems that might limit their application can be avoided. Evidence-based behavioral programs, interventions, policies, and guidelines might exist but remain theoretical if they are not applied in the real-world settings of clinics and communities. Implementation science seeks to improve the speed and effectiveness of the application and impact of what is known about health behavior.

Health behavior change: now and in the future

We undertook this second and expanded edition of *Health Behavior Change and Treatment Adherence* a few years after witnessing the COVID-19 pandemic and acknowledging, yet again, what has been clear for decades: health behavior is multifaceted and changing it can be difficult. During this pandemic, hundreds of millions of people in the United States, and billions across the globe, were required to rethink what mattered to them, what they believed in, their relationships to one another, and their values and life goals—all the while in fear of a deadly disease. And now, nearly five years since COVID-19 emerged, it has taken its place in the rearview mirror for most people.

It has not been forgotten, however, by most medical, behavioral, and public health professionals who may (or may not) have been surprised that behavior change, even in the face of a deadly disease, turned out to be so difficult, and that adherence was not just "commonsense." In this book, we have seen that many aspects of human life drive health behavior and adherence, including the cognitive, emotional, social, cultural, economic, environmental, legal, and health policy contexts. We have suggested a multitude of ways that managing health behaviors can mitigate present and future threats to population health. And we have noted that, even without catastrophes like COVID-19, there are plenty of clinical health challenges with which to contend, as rates of heart disease, diabetes, obesity, and smoking-related diseases continue to rise.

In this book, we have placed particular emphasis on the need to develop, strengthen, and maintain clinician-patient relationships and partnerships, especially within the broader context of changing health systems, policies, and laws. In partnership with their healthcare teams, patients will need to be actively engaged in overcoming barriers to adherence and behavior change, navigating the healthcare system, and rising above the societal forces that threaten to derail their health efforts. For clinicians, relationship-building will be more central than ever to working with the complex and multifaceted nature of health behavior change and treatment adherence. It will also be helpful for clinicians to remember that in the pursuit of health, people will only do: *(1)* what they clearly understand and remember; *(2)* what they are motivated to do; and *(3)* what they are able to do within their unique sociocultural and environmental contexts. This is the Information-Motivation-Strategy Model, which requires us to remain aware of and understand the social-ecological framework that surrounds an individual. Health behavior is driven by beliefs, attitudes, motivations, habits, and relationships with social networks and healthcare providers. It is also influenced by financial forces, public policies and laws, and even the processed food industry. Awareness of these elements remains essential to behavior change.

Even when the individual's social-ecological framework is operating to limit and determine their choices, they can recognize that health is largely the hard-won result of their daily habits. Even after they have spent years struggling with poor health habits and nonadherence, people can strive to change and instead build and strengthen healthy behavioral patterns. They can choose to look critically at the forces that push on them, and acknowledge how strongly they can be influenced by others. They can remain mindful of health misinformation and avoid contributing to its spread. They can choose to respect science and scientific data and encourage others to do the same. Individuals can call upon their health professionals and their social support networks to help achieve and maintain their own health, and they can provide health behavior support for their family members and friends in return.

Each year, thousands of empirical studies and reviews are published that advance our knowledge of health behavior change and treatment adherence. These offer health professionals and patients the opportunity to continually learn more about how to best promote human health, whether in the realm of acute and chronic disease conditions or in the possible pandemic diseases of the future. As we bring our analysis of health behavior change and treatment adherence to a close, we encourage readers to continue learning about these issues. This book has offered a framework for understanding this vast research in medicine, public health, and the social and behavioral sciences, and can serve as a scaffolding on which thousands of research studies of the future can be organized. This book contains hundreds of published references on theory, original empirical research, and comprehensive review of what is known about how and why people change (and how and why they do not). Reading some of these primary sources can be enlightening; future issues of the journals cited here are likely to offer the latest research on these topics. The books we have recommended as suggested readings at the end of each chapter provide an additional perspective and flesh out the chapter's topics in absorbing detail. They are narratives and human stories that make the issues come alive, and they have inspired us and our students over the years. Their authors are likely to write more about these timely topics in the future, and we encourage readers to look for these works and take advantage of the expertise and perspective of these authors. We also encourage readers to pay attention to healthcare issues reported by trusted online and print news sources, and to think about how developments in healthcare might impact health administrators, educators, public health authorities, lawmakers, families and communities, clinicians, patients, and provider-patient partnerships. It is our hope that keeping an open mind and continuing to learn about the many facets of health behavior change and treatment adherence will help to improve health and healthcare now and in the future.

Summary

In Chapter 9, we broaden our perspective from previous chapters to focus on system-level factors that drive individual health behavior choices, influence adherence, and affect patients' and providers' experiences of healthcare. We examine a complex network of stakeholders in healthcare, the concept of "owning risk," and models of effective, evidence-based healthcare delivery in integrated health systems that offer comprehensive, cost-effective means to promote population health. We consider how health insurance can contribute to, or deter patients from, navigating preventive healthcare and chronic disease management. We examine the notion of public good in the face of growing numbers and rates of chronic diseases and newly emerging treatment pathogens. We examine the broader context of laws and policies that can shape health behavior and adherence (ranging from taxes on cigarettes and sugared drinks to bans on abortion). We assess public health responses to communicable disease threats, lessons learned from the COVID-19 pandemic, and the social and psychological factors that continue to challenge health policy. We examine the role of implementation science in applying research on health behavior change and treatment adherence. We assess the three factor Information-Motivation-Strategy Model in the broader contextual frameworks that drive health and healthcare choices.

Tools for instruction and self-study

Learning objectives

By the end of this chapter, readers should be able to

1. Discuss common barriers to patient adherence and approaches to address those barriers.
2. Describe various stakeholders in health and healthcare in the United States.

3. Define the concept of "owning the risk" in health and healthcare.
4. Discuss issues of healthcare cost and health insurance in relationship to patient behavior and access to care.
5. Explain the role of integrated systems in healthcare delivery.
6. Identify examples of how individual health behaviors can benefit the public good.
7. Discuss how laws related to women's healthcare, taxes related to health behavior, and public policy mandates can affect individual health behaviors and healthcare availability.
8. Explain how psychological, behavioral, and sociocultural factors were at the interface of public health efforts during the COVID-19 pandemic.
9. Discuss how implementation science is relevant in health and medical settings.
10. Describe the three components of the Information-Motivation-Strategy Model as related to health behavior change and patient adherence.

Review questions

1. List at least four common barriers to adherence and provide one specific strategy for addressing each.
2. Explain a "multifaceted intervention" and give an example.
3. Describe the concept of "owning the risk." Give three examples of stakeholders in the United States and describe their relationship to owning risk in health and healthcare.
4. Give two examples of how healthcare costs can affect patient behavior and access to care.
5. Explain how integrated systems in healthcare delivery can affect treatment adherence.
6. According to the Institute of Medicine, now the National Academy of Medicine, what are the six elements of care that are essential for improving healthcare outcomes?
7. Explain public good, and the role of public health and health education.
8. Provide an example of an individual health decision that can impact the health of a broader community.

9. Describe the role of laws, taxes, and public policy mandates in health behaviors and healthcare availability.
10. Describe some public health lessons from the COVID-19 pandemic.
11. Explain the concept of implementation science.

Prompts for discussion and further study

1. Individual freedoms may sometimes compete with the greater good. How can these contradictions be managed? What factors must be considered?
2. In the United States, large disparities exist between individuals in their access to quality (and sometimes any) healthcare. What are some of the implications of the fact that the United States is the only developed country in which healthcare is not available to all?
3. What are some lessons about health behavior and adherence that we have learned from the COVID-19 pandemic? Do you think our society will be ready if another such pandemic occurs? Why or why not?

Suggested reading

1. Dorsey GM, Caron RM, eds. *Health and Freedom in the Balance: Exploring the Tensions Among Public Health, Individual Liberty, and Governmental Authority.* Nova Science Pub Inc; 2017.
2. Welch G. *Less Medicine, More Health: 7 Assumptions That Drive Too Much Medical Care.* Beacon Press; 2015.
3. Gawande A. *The Checklist Manifesto: How to Get Things Right.* Metropolitan Books; 2009.
4. Gawande A. *Better: A Surgeon's Notes on Performance.* Metropolitan Books; 2007.

References

1. Roter DL, Hall JA, Merisca R, Nordstrom B, Cretin D, Svarstad B. Effectiveness of interventions to improve patient compliance: a meta-analysis. *Med Care.* 1998; 36(8): pp. 1138–1161.

2. van Eijken M, Tsang S, Wensing M, de Smet PA, Grol RP. Interventions to improve medication compliance in older patients living in the community: a systematic review of the literature. *Drugs Aging*. 2003; 20(3): pp. 229–240.
3. DeBusk RF, Miller NH, Superko HR, et al. A case-management system for coronary risk factor modification after acute myocardial infarction. *Ann Intern Med*. 1994; 120(9): pp. 721–729.
4. Miller NH, Hill M, Kottke T, Ockene IS. The multilevel compliance challenge: recommendations for a call to action. A statement for health care professionals. *Circulation*. 1997; 95(4): pp. 1085–1090.
5. Peters AL, Davidson MB, Ossorio RC. Management of patients with diabetes by nurses with support of subspecialists. *HMO Pract*. 1995; 9(1): pp. 8–13.
6. Amadeo K. The rising cost of health care by year and its causes. The Balance. Oct. 21, 2022. https://www.thebalancemoney.com/causes-of-rising-healthcare-costs-4064878
7. Rosenthal E. How the high cost of medical care is affecting Americans. *New York Times*. December 18, 2014.
8. Lopes L, Montero A, Presiado M, Hamel L. Americans' challenges with health care costs. Kaiser Family Foundation website. Dec 21, 2023. https://www.kff.org/health-costs/issue-brief/americans-challenges-with-health-care-costs/
9. Cohen RA, Cha AE. Health insurance coverage: early release of estimates form the National Health Interview Survey, 2022. Centers for Disease Control and Prevention, National Center for Health Statistics. Released May 2023. https://www.cdc.gov/nchs/data/nhis/earlyrelease/insur202305_1.pdf
10. DeVoe JE, Fryer GE, Phillips R, Green L. Receipt of preventive care among adults: insurance status and usual source of care. *Am J Public Health*. 2003; 93(5): pp. 786–791.
11. Piette JD, Wagner TH, Potter MB, Schillinger D. Health insurance status, cost-related medication underuse, and outcomes among diabetes patients in three systems of care. *Med Care*. 2004; 42(2): pp. 102–109.
12. Institute of Medicine. *Crossing the Quality Chasm: A New Health System for the Twenty-first Century*. Washington, DC: National Academies Press; 2001.
13. Berry LL, Seiders K, Wilder SS. Innovations in access to care: a patient-centered approach. *Ann Intern Med*. 2003; 139(7): pp. 568–574.
14. Ettner SL. The relationship between continuity of care and the health behaviors of patients: does having a usual physician make a difference? *Med Care*. 1999; 37(6): pp. 547–555.
15. McGinnis JM. Investing in health: the role of disease prevention. In: Blank RH, Bonnicksen AL, eds. *Emerging Issues in Biomedical Policy: An Annual Review*. Vol. 1. New York: Columbia University Press, 1992; pp. 13–26.
16. Sickles EA. Mammography screening and the self-referred woman. *Radiology*. 1988; 166(1 Pt 1): pp. 271–273.
17. Smedley BD, Stith AY, Nelson AR. *Unequal Treatment: Confronting Racial and Ethnic Disparities in Health Care*. Washington, DC: National Academies Press; 2002.
18. Adler NE, Newman K. Socioeconomic disparities in health: pathways and policies. *Health Aff (Millwood)*. 2002; 21(2): pp. 60–76.
19. Adler NE, Ostrove JM. Socioeconomic status and health: what we know and what we don't. *Ann N Y Acad Sci*. 1999; 896: pp. 3–15.

20. Keppel KG. Ten largest racial and ethnic health disparities in the United States based on Healthy People 2010 objectives. *Am J Epidemiol.* 2007; 166(1): pp. 97–103. doi: 10.1093/aje/kwm044
21. Safran DG. Defining the future of primary care: what can we learn from patients? *Ann Intern Med.* 2003; 138(3): pp. 248–255.
22. Kern LM, Ringel JB, Rajan M, et al. Ambulatory care fragmentation and total health care costs. *Med Care.* 2024; Apr 1; 62(4): pp. 277–284. doi: 10.1097/MLR.0000000000001982
23. Zulman DM, Haverfield MC, Shaw JG, et al. Practices to foster physician presence and connection with patients in the clinical encounter. *JAMA.* 2020; 323(1): pp. 70–81. doi:10.1001/jama.2019.19003
24. Deyo RA. *Watch Your Back.* Ithaca, NY: ILR Press, Cornell University; 2014.
25. Kleinsinger F. The unmet challenge of medication nonadherence. *Perm J.* 2018; 22: pp. 18–33. doi: 10.7812/TPP/18-033
26. Retchin SM, Brown B. Management of colorectal cancer in Medicare health maintenance organizations. *J Gen Intern Med.* 1990; 5(2): pp. 110–114.
27. Forrest CB, Shi L, von Schrader S, Ng J. Managed care, primary care, and the patient-practitioner relationship. *J Gen Intern Med.* 2002; 17(4): pp. 270–277.
28. Clement DG, Retchin SM, Brown RS, Stegall MH. Access and outcomes of elderly patients enrolled in managed care. *JAMA.* 1994; 271(19): pp. 1487–1492.
29. Roulidis ZC, Schulman KA. Physician communication in managed care organizations: opinions of primary care physicians. *J Fam Pract.* 1994; 39(5): pp. 446–451.
30. Greenfield S, Kaplan S, Ware JE, Jr. Expanding patient involvement in care. Effects on patient outcomes. *Ann Intern Med.* 1985; 102(4): pp. 520–528.
31. Guadagnoli E, Ward P. Patient participation in decision-making. *Soc Sci Med.* 1998; 47(3): pp. 329–339.
32. Yach D, Hawkes C, Gould CL, Hofman KJ. The global burden of chronic diseases: overcoming impediments to prevention and control. *JAMA.* 2004; 291(21): pp. 2616–2622.
33. Cowen EL. The wooing of primary prevention. *Am J Community Psychol.* 1980; 8(3): pp. 258–284.
34. Brown DR, Carlson SA, Kumar GS, Fulton JE. Research highlights from the Status report for Step It Up! The Surgeon General's Call to Action to Promote Walking and Walkable Communities. *J Sport Health Sci.* 2018; 7(1): pp. 5–6. doi: 10.1016/j.jshs.2017.10.003
35. Tagtow A, Raghavan R. Assessing the reach of MyPlate using National Health and Nutrition Examination Survey data. *J Acad Nutr Diet.* 2017; 117(2): pp. 181–183. doi: 10.1016/j.jand.2016.11.015
36. Sallis JF, Bauman A, Pratt M. Environmental and policy interventions to promote physical activity. *Am J Prev Med.* 1998; 15(4): pp. 379–397.
37. Friedman HS. Healthy life-style across the life-span: The heck with the Surgeon General. In: Suls J, Wallston K, eds. *Social Psychological Foundations of Health and Illness.* Blackwell Publishing; 2003; pp. 3–21.
38. Hornik RC, ed. *Public Health Communication. Evidence for Behavior Change.* Lawrence Erlbaum; 2002.
39. Napoli PM. Consumer use of medical information from electronic and paper media: a literature review. In: Rice RE, Katz JE, eds. *The Internet and Health Communication.* Sage; 2000; pp. 79–89.

40. Pear R. Medicare proposal takes aim at diabetes. *New York Times*. March 23, 2016.
41. Bader P, Boisclair D, Ferrence R. Effects of tobacco taxation and pricing on smoking behavior in high-risk populations: a knowledge synthesis. *Int J Environ Res Public Health*. 2011; 8(11): pp. 4118–4139. doi: 10.3390/ijerph8114118
42. Andreyeva T, Marple K, Marinello S, Moore TE, Powell LM. Outcomes following taxation of sugar-sweetened beverages: a systematic review and meta-analysis. *JAMA Netw Open*. 2022; 5(6): e2215276. doi: 10.1001/jamanetworkopen.2022.15276
43. Wyper GMA, Mackay DF, Fraser C, et al. Evaluating the impact of alcohol minimum unit pricing on deaths and hospitalisations in Scotland: a controlled interrupted time series study. *Lancet*. 2023; 401(10385): pp. 1361–1370. doi: 10.1016/S0140-6736(23)00497-X
44. Couillard BK, Foote CL, Gandhi K, Meara E, Skinner J. Rising geographic disparities in US mortality. *J Econ Perspect*. 2021; 35(4): pp. 123–146. doi: 10.1257/jep.35.4.123
45. Phelan JC, Link BG, Tehranifar P. Social conditions as fundamental causes of health inequalities: theory, evidence, and policy implications. *J Health Soc Behav*. 2010; 51 Suppl: pp. S28–40. doi: 10.1177/0022146510383498
46. Frederiksen B, Ranji U, Gomez I, Salganicoff A. A national survey of OB/GYNs' experiences after Dobbs. Kaiser Family Foundation website. June 21, 2023. https://www.kff.org/womens-health-policy/report/a-national-survey-of-obgyns-experiences-after-dobbs/
47. Stolberg SG. As abortion laws drive obstetricians from red states, maternity care suffers. *New York Times*. September 7, 2023.
48. Brigance C, Lucas R, Jones E, et al. Nowhere to go: maternity care deserts across the U.S. (2022 report). March of Dimes website. Retrieved March 22, 2024. https://www.marchofdimes.org/maternity-care-deserts-report
49. Karlamangla S. How Marin County changed its reputation on vaccines. *New York Times*. October 11, 2022.
50. Hotez PJ. *The Deadly Rise of Anti-Science: A Scientist's Warning*. Johns Hopkins University Press; 2023.
51. Emanuel EJ, Borio L, Bright R, Osterholm MT, Jim J, Michaels D. We worked on the U.S. pandemic response. Here are 13 takeaways for the next health emergency. *New York Times*. May 11, 2023.
52. Garrett L. *The Coming Plague: Newly Emerging Diseases in a World Out of Balance*. Penguin; 1995.
53. Osterholm M, Olshaker M. *The Big One: How to Prepare for World-Altering Pandemics to Come*. Little, Brown Spark; February 4, 2025.
54. Nilsen P. Making sense of implementation theories, models and frameworks. *Implement Sci*. 2015; 10:53. doi: 10.1186/s13012-015-0242-0
55. Nilsen P, Ingvarsson S, Hasson H, von Thiele Schwarz U, Augustsson H. Theories, models, and frameworks for de-implementation of low-value care: a scoping review of the literature. *Implement Res Pract*. 2020; 1:2633489520953762. doi: 10.1177/2633489520953762

Index

For the benefit of digital users, indexed terms that span two pages (e.g., 52–53) may, on occasion, appear on only one of those pages.

abortion, 303–304
Acceptance and Commitment Therapy (ACT), 234
Accountable Care Organizations, 296
Accreditation Council for Graduate Medical Education, 72
actor-observer asymmetry, 85–87
adherence. *See also* nonadherence
   agreeableness and, 185
   automated reminder technologies and, 275
   barriers to, 25, 26t, 290, 294–295, 291t
   benefits of, 24
   chronic stress and, 229–231
   conscientiousness and, 185
   costs as potential obstacle to, 26t, 291t, 294
   empathy and, 86b
   family conflict and, 208
   health insurance and, 294–295
   health literacy and, 97–98
   implementation science research and, 305–306
   integrated care systems and, 296–297
   intentions and, 2–3
   medication *versus* lifestyle regimens and, 23
   mobile health technologies and, 273–278
   models of, 39–58
   perceived severity of disease and, 42–43
   Social Determinants of Health approach and, 56–57
   social-ecological perspective on, 26–28
   telemedicine and, 265
   trauma and, 229–231b
   trust in provider-patient relationship and, 22, 220, 227, 228
adverse effects of medical treatment (AEMTs), 228
Affordable Care Act (2010), 251–252, 254, 300
African Americans, 223–224b, 225–227
agreeableness, 184t, 185
Ajzen, Icek, 40
alcohol abuse
   correlation with other risk behaviors and, 12–14
   financial costs of healthcare treatment for, 293
   health risks associated with, 13, 38
   managing ups and downs regarding, 195t
   pervasiveness of, 1–2
   provider-patient communication and, 14
   public health campaigns against, 299
   religious prohibitions against, 213–214
   self-efficacy and, 150
   taxes as means of reducing, 293, 301, 302
American Heart Association, 20–21, 259–260
amygdaloid complex, 101
a posteriori probabilities, 112
a priori probabilities, 111–112
artificial intelligence (AI)
   chatbots and, 268, 271
   digital transcription and, 268–269
   empathic communication and, 269–270b
   large language models (LLMs) and, 268, 271–273
   limitations of, 260–261, 268
   medical diagnosis and, 260–261, 268, 271–273
   medical education and, 272–273
   online psychological support and, 172
   patient care and, 268–273
   patients' and providers' perceptions of, 272–273
   patients' consulting of, 248, 260
   warnings regarding, 273
Association of American Medical Colleges, 72
attitudes
   behavioral change and, 39–40
   beliefs and, 40, 43
   definition of, 39–40
   emotions and, 43
   in Theory of Planned Behavior, 45, 46f
   in Theory of Reasoned Action, 43–44, 44f
automated health care systems, 261–262

back-channeling, 83–84
back pain, 196, 228, 296
Bandura, Albert, 150
Bayesian methods, 110–113
Becker, M.H., 41
behavioral contracts, 143–144, 177–178, 197, 292
behavior change. *See also* habits; health behaviors
  accessibility and, 190, 291*t*
  attitudes and, 39–40
  barriers to, 40–42, 42*f*, 51, 189–197, 290, 291*t*, 294
  beliefs and, 39–40, 43
  discomfort and, 187
  financial costs and, 190, 291*t*
  gradual nature of, 157, 170
  mobile health tools and, 275–278*b*
  subjective norms and, 43–44
behaviorism, 172–173
beliefs
  attitudes and, 40, 43
  behavioral change and, 39–40, 43
  cognitive filtering and, 104
  definition of, 39–40
  information processing and, 102*t*, 104
  religious beliefs and, 213–214
  in Theory of Reasoned Action, 43
BetterHelp, 267
body mass index (BMI), 9–11
brain plasticity, 101

Cacioppo, J.T., 106–107
cancer
  loss-framed messaging and, 146
  nonadherence to treatments for, 23
  patient involvement in decision-making regarding, 122–123
  physical activity as means of reducing risk of, 17
  premature deaths from, 7
  radon gas and, 51
  screenings for, 20–21, 145, 146, 262
  tobacco use and, 12–13
  treatments for, 13–14
Cassell, Eric, 66
caveat emptor, 69
Chat GPT, 268–269, 271
Chronic Care Model (CCM), 252–253, 296
chronic illness
  acute illness compared to, 37
  chronic stress and, 232–233
  consequences of, 38*b*
  definition of, 37
  depression as comorbidity of, 37, 232–233
  empathy and, 233–234
  group medical visits and, 255–256
  irrational health-related behaviors and, 38–39
  medical teams' role in managing, 249–250
  mobile health technologies and, 274
  prevalence of, 170
  prevention strategies and, 38
  telemedicine and, 265
  tobacco use as risk factor in, 38*b*
chunking, 108
Church of Jesus Christ of Latter-day Saints, 213–214
Cialdini, Robert, 186–187
classical conditioning, 49, 174, 205
climate change, 229
closed-ended questions, 75–76*b*, 88–89
Cognitive Behavior Therapy (CBT), 172, 196–197, 234
cognitive dissonance, 54–55, 103–104, 159*b*
cognitive filters, 104–105
Collaborative Care Model (CoCM), 253–254
conditioning
  classical, 49, 174, 205
  operant, 49, 174–175, 205, 275–276
condom use, 44
conscientiousness, 185, 193–194, 184*t*
consciousness raising, 46–49
constructive thinking, 149, 164
contingency contracts and plans, 177–178, 197–198
COVID-19
  airborne transmission of, 16, 217
  deaths of unvaccinated individuals from, 304
  Health Belief Model and, 42
  lack of information and conflicting information during early pandemic stages and, 109–110, 217, 219–220, 228
  primary prevention actions and, 15*b*, 15–16, 298, 304
  psychological and sociocultural dimensions of responses to, 304–305
  social media and, 138*b*, 217–218*b*
  social norms regarding mitigation measures and, 213
  societal implications of risks from, 25
  Sturgis Motorcycle Rally (2020) and, 140*b*

telemedicine and online interactions during pandemic of, 263–265
vaccinations against, 15–16, 39, 138b, 139–140, 218b, 298, 304
culture
bias and, 234
definition of, 211
medical care informed by, 234–235

decision-making. *See also* risk assessment
aids for, 262–263
Bayesian methods and, 110–113
decision trees and, 110, 122–123b, 124f
marketing and, 109
medical decision analysis and, 110–113
participatory tools for, 122–125
patient involvement in, 121–127, 252–253, 262–263
depression
Chronic Care Model and, 252–253
chronic illness and, 37, 232–233
health professionals' inquiries to patients regarding, 233, 254
nonadherence and, 231
social media use and, 220
diabetes
as chronic illness, 37
cognitive dissonance and, 54b, 54–55
financial costs associated with treating, 24
follow-up care and, 251
group medical visits and, 256b
health behavior change and, 171b, 176b, 181b
health complications associated with, 24–25, 38
medication for, 171b, 176b
obesity and, 11
peer support and, 274
perceived behavioral control and, 215
physical exercise and, 18–19
processed foods and, 10
screenings for, 20–21
sleep patterns and, 147–148
treatment of, 8–9
DiClemente, C.C., 47, 49
diet
breaking bad habits regarding, 176b, 179, 182b
cultural norms regarding, 104–105
family influence on, 206, 209b
financial costs influencing, 190
goal setting and, 147

healthiest options for, 10
health status and, 2–3, 7
managing ups and downs regarding, 194, 195t
mobile health technologies and, 274, 276b
practitioners' recommendations regarding, 137
primary prevention and, 8–10
processed foods and, 9–10
public health education campaigns and, 299
reinforcement schedules and, 176b
religious beliefs and, 213–214
teachable moments and, 144
Dietz, William H., 57
disease screenings, 20–21, 145, 146, 230, 262
Dobbs v. Jackson Women's Health Organization, 303–304
Duhigg, Charles, 162

eHealth technologies. *See* technologies in healthcare
Elaboration Likelihood Model (ELM), 106–107
Electronic Medical Records (EMRs), 248, 264, 267, 296
empathy
actor-observer asymmetry and, 85–87
adherence to treatment and, 86b
artificial intelligence and, 269–270b
assessment tools for, 84–85
chronic illness and, 233–234
defining qualities of, 83
pain experienced by patients and, 226
paralinguistic cues and, 83–84
in provider-patient relationship, 14, 64b, 71–72, 83–85, 154b, 226
touch and, 83
training in, 84–85
voice tone and, 84
extraversion, 184t
Eye Movement Desensitization and Reprocessing (EMDR), 234

Facial Action Coding System, 82–83
"fail-safe N," 120
Festinger, Leon, 214
First 5 Program (California), 205–206
Fishbein, Martin, 40
flashbulb memory, 101
Freidson, Eliot, 66
frequentism, 111

gain-framed messages, 145–146
gender
  disease risk and, 121
  information processing and recall and, 105
  women's health care and, 302–304
Geronimus, Arline, 229–230
goals
  constructive thinking and, 149, 164
  cost-benefit perceptions and, 151–152
  desires of others and, 148, 151–152
  expectations of success and, 148
  framing of, 152–156
  intrinsic rewards and, 152
  optimism and, 149
  pursuit of, 148
  reasoned decision-making and, 147
  self-efficacy and, 148, 150, 151*t*, 152–153
  setting of, 146–152
  social comparisons and, 146–147
  social support and, 206–211*b*
  subgoals and, 153–154*b*
  targeting and, 153–156, 158–159
  unrealistic, 153
group medical visits, 255–256*b*

habits
  addictive behaviors and, 180
  behavioral contracts and, 143–144, 177–178, 197, 292
  belief and, 189–190
  breaking of bad habits and, 176*b*, 179–182*b*
  choosing right environments and, 186–187
  classical conditioning, 174
  cognitive behavior modification and, 172, 196–197
  contingency plans and, 177–178, 197–198
  definition of, 172–173, 197
  early life experiences' effects on, 205
  encoding process in, 173–174
  feedback and, 178–179
  forming of, 173–177
  intrinsic motivation and, 178–179
  involuntary forms of, 172–174
  long-term impact of, 170
  mindfulness and balancing of, 152–156
  mobile health technologies and, 275–278
  neural processing and, 173–174
  "not doing" and, 181*b*, 181–182
  nudges and, 186–187, 188*t*
  operant conditioning and, 174–175, 275–276
  personality and, 183–186
  reinforcement schedules and, 175–176*b*
  repetition and, 180
  rewards for behaviors and, 174–180
  self-efficacy and, 189–190
  self-knowledge and, 183
  self-monitoring and, 190–192
  small behavior changes and, 182–183, 187
hazard ratios, 116–117
Health Behavior Internalization Model, 192–194
health behaviors
  agreeableness and, 185
  chronic stress and, 229–231
  conformity and, 213–214
  conscientiousness and, 185, 193–194
  cultural distrust of medicine and, 139–140, 227–228
  family influences on, 205–206, 209*b*, 207*t*
  feedback and, 216–217
  government-supported programs to help change, 300
  gradual nature of change in, 157–158, 170
  implementation science research and, 305–306
  integrated care systems and, 296–297
  managing ups and downs and, 194–196, 195*t*
  mental health challenges and, 229
  mobile health technologies and, 273–278
  models of, 39–58
  multilevel determinants approach to, 55*b*, 55–57
  neuroticism and, 185
  pets and, 193
  poverty and, 229–230
  proactive coping and, 194–196
  reasons for failures to change, 25, 26*t*
  social-ecological perspective on, 28–29
  social media and, 217–220
  social norms and social comparisons' influences on, 213–217
  social support and, 26*t*, 206–211*b*
  telemedicine and, 265
  trauma and, 229–231*b*
Health Belief Model
  cues to action and, 40–41, 42*f*, 42
  demographic characteristics and, 40–41, 42*f*
  intentions and, 41
  origins of, 40
  perceived barriers to health behavior change and, 40–42, 42*f*

perceived benefits of health behavior change and, 40, 42f, 42
perceived self-efficacy and, 41, 42f, 42, 50
perceived severity of a disease and, 40–41, 42f, 42–43
perceived susceptibility to a disease and, 40, 42f, 42
health care costs in the United States, 7, 13, 196, 293, 294
Health Insurance Portability and Accountability Act (HIPAA), 273
health literacy
  adherence and, 97–98
  cultural influences on, 211
  definition of, 97–98
  information processing and recall and, 102t, 127
  the internet and, 26t
  notations in medical records regarding, 98
  pervasive low levels of, 97–98
  provider-patient communication and, 78, 97–99
  providers' overestimation of patients' levels of, 98
  teach-back method and, 98–99
  universal precautions for, 98
heart disease
  diabetes as risk factor for, 24
  nonadherence and, 21, 25
  obesity as risk factor for, 11
  pervasiveness of, 307
  physical activity and, 17, 19
hippocampus, 103
Hippocrates, 68
HIV (human immunodeficiency virus), 7, 23, 24, 261–262, 275
Hotez, Peter, 218b
HPV (human papillomavirus), 52, 139–140, 221–222

implementation science research, 305–306
influenza, 15, 137–138, 222, 298, 305
Information-Motivation-Strategy Model, 52–54, 53f, 99, 104–105, 298–299, 305–307
information processing and recall
  age and, 100–101, 105
  beliefs and, 102t, 104
  brain plasticity and, 101
  chronic stress and, 103
  chunking and, 108
  cognitive filtering and, 104–105
  cultural context and, 104–105
  digital aids and, 248, 258
  duration of medical visits and, 106
  emotion and, 101–103, 102t, 127
  encoding of information and, 99–100
  focusing of attention and, 100, 105–106
  gender and, 105
  health literacy levels and, 102t, 127
  long-term memory and, 100–101, 105–106
  long-term potentiation and, 101
  memory aids and, 99, 105, 107–108, 102t
  mnemonics and, 102t, 108
  primacy effects and, 102t, 108
  public health messaging and, 99
  recency effects and, 102t, 108
  retrieval of information and, 99–100
  self-enhancement bias and, 103–104
  short-term memory and, 100–101
  sleep deprivation and, 105–106
  storage of information and, 99–101
  strategies for improving, 99, 102, 106–107, 102t
  tailoring of information and, 106–107, 102t
  working memory and, 100–101, 105
integrated care systems, 296–297
the internet
  decision aids and, 262–263
  health literacy and, 26t
  misinformation on, 259–260
  patients' consulting of, 121, 219, 248, 258–259
  quality of information available on, 112–113

Kahneman, Daniel, 186–187
Kaiser Permanente, 296–297

LGBTQIA individuals, 229–230
life expectancies, racial and socioeconomic disparities in, 223–224
Loma Linda (California), 213–214
long-term potentiation (LTP), 101
Lorber, Judith, 66
loss-framed messages, 145–146

maternal health, 303–304
Medicaid, 300, 302
medical teams
  automated healthcare systems and, 261–262
  biopsychosocial approach to healthcare and, 251
  care for the whole person and, 251–255
  chronic disease management and, 249–250

medical teams (*Continued*)
  communications among, 248–250
  complexity of contemporary healthcare and, 249
  division of tasks and, 249
  follow-up care and, 251
  ideal size of, 249–250
  integrated care systems and, 296–297
  as means of overcoming resource and time constraints, 248–249
  mental health professionals and, 254–255
  nurse practitioners and, 249–250
  planning and agenda-setting for medical visits by, 250–251
  team goals and, 249
Medicare, 293, 300
memory. *See* information processing and recall
meta-analysis, 119–120
mHealth (mobile health technologies), 258, 273–278*b*
Miller, William, 158–159
mnemonics, 102*t*, 108
motivation
  definition of, 156
  expectations of likely benefits and, 158
  intrinsic motivation and, 178–179
  motivational communication and, 158–162
  readiness to change and, 154*b*, 170
  self-efficacy and, 154*b*
Multilevel Determinants Model, 55*b*, 55–57
MyPlate website, 299

neonatal mortality, 114
neuroticism, 184–185, 184*t*
nonadherence. *See also* adherence
  actor-observer asymmetry and, 85–86*b*
  depression and, 231
  financial costs of, 24–25
  human costs of, 25
  intentional nonadherence and, 22, 227–228
  internet searches for medical information and, 259
  nonfulfillment and, 21
  non-persistence and, 21
  prevalence of, 22–24
  provider-patient communication and, 21–24, 26*t*, 64*b*, 64, 66–67, 79, 127
  public health consequences of, 298
  unintentional nonadherence and, 21–22
Noom, 267
nudges, 186–187, 188*t*

obesity
  bariatric surgery and, 12
  body mass index and, 9–11
  chronic disease and health risks associated with, 9–10, 12
  cultural values regarding, 9
  dietary change therapy and, 11
  drug treatments and, 9, 12
  pediatric obesity and, 11
  pervasiveness of, 1–2, 8, 307
  physical activity and, 11, 16–17
  physiological factors and, 180
openness to experience, 184*t*
operant conditioning, 49, 174–175, 205, 275–276
opioids, 226, 228, 293, 296
Osler, William, 72

paternalism, 65–66, 68–69
Patient-Centered Medical Home (PCMH)
  Affordable Care Act and, 254
  care for the whole person and, 254
  group visits and, 255
  medical teams and, 254
  official designations for, 254
  patient satisfaction assessments and, 254
  psychological comorbidities and, 79
Patient Self-Determination Act, 69
Pavlov, Ivan, 174
perceived behavioral control, 45, 46*f*, 207–208, 215–216
persuasion
  advertising and, 137
  conversion compared to, 138
  definition of, 137–138
  desire for consistency and, 143–144, 141*t*
  expectations and, 138*b*, 141*t*, 146
  expertise and, 69, 141*t*, 142, 142*t*
  fear induction and, 141*t*, 144
  liking for the messenger and, 142–143, 141*t*
  media articles and, 147–148
  message framing and, 145–146, 141*t*
  perceptions of scarcity and, 141*t*, 143
  physical activity and, 137–138
  reciprocity and, 141*t*, 143
  resistance to, 137–140
  self-efficacy and, 150, 151*t*
  subliminal messages and, 140–141
  teachable moments and, 144–145, 141*t*
  vaccinations and, 137–138*b*
physical activity
  breaking bad habits and, 182*b*

INDEX 321

factors influencing levels of, 18–19
goal setting and, 147
health benefits associated with, 16–17, 19*b*
managing ups and downs regarding, 195*t*
mobile health technologies and, 274, 276*b*
motivation and, 154*b*
obesity prevention and, 11, 16–17
perceived behavioral control and, 215
pervasive failure to meet guidelines regarding, 8, 17–18
practitioners' recommendations and persuasion messaging regarding, 137–138
provider-patient communication and, 19*b*, 19
public health campaigns promoting, 298–299
reinforcement schedules and, 175–176*b*
self-efficacy and, 150
social comparisons and, 215–216
soreness and discomfort as obstacles to, 190
pneumonia vaccines, 222
Precaution Adoption Process Model
barriers to behavioral change and, 51
individuals' changes over time and, 51–52
origins of, 51
radon exposure example and, 51
stages of behavioral change and, 51, 52*f*, 52
testing of, 52
Primary Care Behavioral Health model (PCBH), 253–254
primary prevention, 7–20
proactive coping, 194–196
Prochaska, James, 47, 49, 157
Profile of Nonverbal Sensitivity (PONS), 82–83
prostate-specific antigen (PSA) screening, 262
provider-patient communication. *See also* provider-patient relationship
age of patient and, 72
computers in exam rooms and, 74, 267
distress indicators and, 82
empathy and, 14, 64*b*, 71–72, 83–85, 154*b*, 226
health literacy and, 78, 97–99
information exchange and, 78
internet misinformation and, 260
nonadherence and, 21–24, 26*t*, 64*b*, 64, 66–67, 79, 127
nonverbal communication and, 81–83
open-ended questions and, 75–77*b*
pain sensitivity indicators and, 82–83
patient memory and, 97

patients' narrativizations and, 78–81*b*
pharmaceutical advertising and, 260
physical environment of medical appointments and, 73–74
privacy and, 73
refraining from interruption and, 77–78
"rolling with resistance" and, 154*b*
socioeconomic status of patient and, 72
somaticizers and, 79–80*b*
Transtheoretical Model of health behavior change and, 49
trust and, 71–87, 142–143
verbal communication and, 74–81
provider-patient relationship
appropriate contexts for different roles and, 70*t*, 77
consumerism and, 69
differential diagnosis and, 75
expertise and, 69
the internet's impact on, 219
mutuality and, 70–71
paternalism and, 65–66, 68–69
patient involvement in decision-making and, 121–127, 252–253, 262–263
patients' preferences and, 67*b*, 68
premature closure and, 75
rapport and, 66–67
social contract model and, 65–66
telemedicine and, 265–267*b*
trust and, 64, 66, 71, 218–219
public health
autonomy and, 298, 302
health education and, 298–299
informational ambiguity and, 219–220
nonadherence and, 298
optimistic bias and, 219–220
psychological and sociocultural dimensions of, 304–305
public policy mandates and laws promoting, 218–219, 300–305
"sin taxes" and, 300*b*, 301
social media and, 218–219
social network influences and, 299
vaccinations and, 297–299

quality-adjusted life years (QALYs), 125–127

racism and disparities in medical care, 225–227, 229
Respiratory Syncytial Virus (RSV), 15
risk assessment. *See also* decision-making
base rates and, 117, 117*t*

risk assessment (*Continued*)
  cardiovascular disease example and, 119–120
  conflicting information and, 118–119
  cumulative *versus* interactive effects and, 120–121
  hazard ratios and, 116–118
  meta-analysis and, 119–120
  neonatal mortality example and, 114
  odds ratios and, 113–114, 118
  risk ratios and, 114–116, 117*t*, 117–118
  tobacco use examples and, 113–114
Roe v. Wade, 303–304
Rollnick, Stephen, 158–159

Salles, Arghavan, 227
secondary prevention, 7–8, 20–21
self-efficacy
  enactive attainments and, 151*t*
  feedback and, 216
  improvement and, 216
  persuasion and, 150, 151*t*
  physiological arousal and, 150, 151*t*
  strategies for increasing, 150, 151*t*
  vicarious experiences and, 150, 151*t*
self-enhancement bias, 103–104
Seventh-day Adventists, 213–214
sex, 1–2, 12, 14–15, 44, 221–222
Skinner, B.F., 172–173
smoking. *See* tobacco use
Social Cognitive Model
  classical and operant conditioning in, 49, 205
  cultural influences and, 211–212
  environmental factors and, 49, 50*f*, 50–51, 205
  family social influences and, 205–206, 207*t*, 209*b*
  personal expectancies and, 49–50, 50*f*, 205
  self-efficacy and, 50
  self-regulation and, 50
  social expectations and, 205, 213–220
  social support and, 206–211*b*
social media
  COVID-19 pandemic and, 138*b*, 217–218*b*
  depression and emotional distress associated with use of, 220
  as "lay referral network," 217
  misinformation and, 217, 220
somaticizers, 79–80*b*
statistical significance measures, 119
Sturgis Motorcycle Rally (2020), 140*b*

taxes
  on alcohol, 293, 301, 302
  on sweetened beverages, 300*b*, 301
  on tobacco, 300*b*, 301–302
teams. *See* medical teams
technologies in healthcare. *See also* artificial intelligence (AI)
  automated health care systems and, 261–262
  automated reminder technologies and, 275
  decision aids and, 258, 262–263
  digital divide as obstacle to, 257
  Electronic Medical Records (EMRs) and, 248, 264, 267, 296
  medical communication technologies and, 264–268
  medication packaging technology and, 263–264
  mental health and, 267
  mobile health technologies and, 258, 273–278*b*
  telemedicine and, 258, 264–268*b*
  virtual support groups and, 263
tertiary prevention, 7–8, 21
Thayer, Julian, 223–224
Theory of Cognitive Dissonance, 54*b*, 54–55, 103–104
Theory of Planned Behavior
  attitudes and, 45, 46*f*
  intentions and, 45–46, 46*f*
  origins of, 45
  perceived behavioral control, 45, 46*f*
  subjective norms and, 45–46, 46*f*
Theory of Reasoned Action
  attitudes and, 43–44, 44*f*
  beliefs and, 43
  condom use example and, 44
  intentions and, 44*f*, 44
  origins of, 43
  subjective norms and, 43–44, 44*f*
tobacco use
  cancer and other health risks associated with, 2–3, 7, 8, 12–13, 38*b*, 38, 43–44, 113, 301
  cessation support groups and, 292
  cognitive dissonance and, 54*b*, 54–55
  correlation with other risk behaviors and, 12
  cost-benefit analysis regarding, 151
  financial costs of healthcare treatment for, 293
  managing ups and downs and, 195*t*
  perceived behavioral control and, 45

pervasiveness of, 1–2, 307
provider-patient communication and, 14
public health campaigns against, 299
religious prohibitions against, 213–214
risk assessment regarding, 113–114
self-efficacy and, 150
social-ecological perspective on, 26–27
social support of efforts to quit, 208
subjective norms and, 43–44
taxes as means of reducing, 300*b*, 301–302
teachable moments and, 144–145
Transtheoretical Model of health behavior change and, 47–49.
Transtheoretical Model
action and, 47–48, 48*f*, 154*b*
addictive behaviors and, 48–49
choosing among options and, 46–47
consciousness raising and, 46–49
contemplation and, 47–48, 48*f*, 48–49, 154*b*
contingency control and, 46–47
maintenance and, 47–48, 48*f*, 48–49, 154*b*
motivational communication and, 158
origins of, 46–47
patients' involvement in decision-making and, 122
precontemplation and, 47–48, 48*f*, 48–49, 154*b*
preparation and, 47–48, 48*f*, 154*b*
provider-patient communication and, 49
stages of behavioral change and, 47
treatment adherence. *See* adherence
trust in provider-patient relationship
adherence and, 22, 220, 227–228
adverse effects of medical treatment and, 228

cooperative intent and, 71
definition of trust and, 71
provider-patient communication and, 71–87, 142–143
Tuskegee Syphilis Study, 139–140, 227
Tversky, Amos, 186–187
Type I and Type II errors, 119

vaccinations
avoidance of, 1–2, 15, 39, 220–221, 298
beliefs and, 40
childhood diseases and, 139–140, 221–222, 297–298
COVID-19 and, 15–16, 39, 138*b*, 139–140, 218*b*, 298, 304
health benefits of, 2–3
healthcare professionals' beliefs regarding, 220–223
HPV (human papillomavirus) and, 221–222
influenza and, 222
innovations in, 1
pneumococcal pneumonia vaccine and, 222
practitioners' recommendations and persuasion messaging regarding, 137–138*b*
provider-patient communication and, 121–122
public health consequences of, 297–299
school mandates regarding, 302
TDAP (tetanus-diphtheria-pertussis) and, 222

Wagner, Edward, 252
women's healthcare, 302–304